PERSPECTIVES IN PEDIATRIC CARDIOLOGY

Series Editor
Robert H. Anderson, M.D.

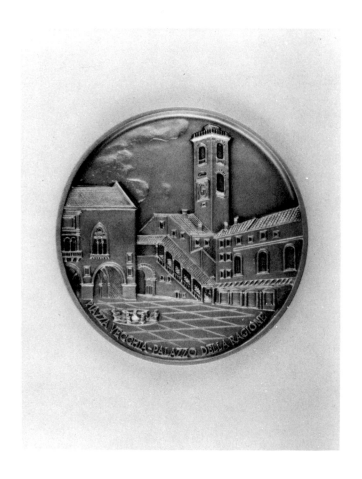

PERSPECTIVES IN PEDIATRIC CARDIOLOGY

Volume 2

Pediatric Cardiac Surgery

Part 3

Editors

Giancarlo Crupi, M.D.
Cardiac Surgeon
Department of Cardiac Surgery
Ospedali Riuniti
Bergamo, Italy

Lucio Parenzan, M.D.
Surgeon-in-Chief
Ospedali Riuniti
Bergamo, Italy

Robert H. Anderson, B. Sc., M.D., F.R.C. Path.
Joseph Levy Professor of
Paediatric Cardiac Morphology
National Heart and Lung Institute
University of London
London, United Kingdom

**Futura Publishing
Company, Inc.**
Mount Kisco, NY
1990

Contributors

Mohamed Rashid Al Fagih
Armed Forces Hospital
Riyadh, Saudi Arabia

Lindsey D. Allan
Guy's Hospital
London, U.K.

Joseph J. Amato
The Children's Hospital of Newark
Newark, New Jersey, U.S.A.

John Anderson
New England Medical Center
Boston, Massachusetts, U.S.A.

Robert H. Anderson
National Heart & Lung Institute
London, U.K.

Manuel J. Antunes
University of Witwatersrand
Johannesburg, South Africa

Ken-Ichi Asano
University of Tokyo, Tokyo, Japan

Metin Avkiran
The Rayne Institute,
St. Thomas' Hospital
London, U.K.

Peter Bardos
Klinikum Aachen
Aachen, West Germany

Albrecht Beitzke
Children's Hospital–Hospital of Graz
Graz, Austria

Mark V. Braimbridge
The Rayne Institute,
St. Thomas' Hospital
London, U.K.

J. M. Brito Perez
Hospital Ramon Y Cajal
Madrid, Spain

Gerald D. Buckberg
U.C.L.A. Medical Center, School of
Medicine
Los Angeles, California, U.S.A.

Joachim H. Bursch
University of Göttingen
Göttingen, West Germany

Louise A. Calder
Green Lane Hospital
Auckland, New Zealand

Mario Carminati
Ospedali Riuniti
Bergamo, Italy

Alain Carpentier
Hospital Broussais
Paris Cedex, France

Sylvain Chauvaud
Hopital Broussais
Paris Cedex, France

Ing-Sh Chiu
National Taiwan University Hospital
Taipei, Taiwan

Kyung J. Chung
University of California
San Diego, California, U.S.A.

Antonio Corno
Ospedale "Bambin Gesù"
Roma, Italy

Giancarlo Crupi
Ospedali Riuniti
Bergamo, Italy

Carmine A. Curcio
GaRankuwan Hospital
Medical University of Southern Africa
GaRankuwan, South Africa

Charles A. Dietl
Hospital Guemes
Buenos Aires, Argentina

Kenneth E. Fellows
Children's Memorial Hospital
Boston, Massachusetts, U.S.A.

Vincenzo Gallucci
University of Padova
Padova, Italy

William J. Greeley
The Duke Heart Center
Durham, North Carolina, U.S.A.

Andreas I. Haàn
Hungarian Institute of Cardiology
Budapest, Hungary

Yorikazu Harada
The Heart Institute of Japan
Tokyo Women's Medical College
Tokyo, Japan

Istvàn Làszlò Hartyanszky
University Medical School
Hungarian Institute of Cardiology
Budapest, Hungary

Paul H. Heintzen
Christian Albrechts Universitat
Kiel, West Germany

Roland Hofstetter
Faculty of Medicine–RWTH
Aachen, West Germany

Stanley John
Christian Medical College & Hospital
Vellore, India

Jean Kachaner
Hopital Necker-Enfants Malades
Paris Cedex, France

Harald Korb
University of Göttingen
Göttingen, West Germany

Munetaka Kumate
Kurume University
Fukuoka, Japan

Hillel Laks
University of California
Los Angeles, California, U.S.A.

Jerome Le Bidois
Hopital Necker-Enfants Malades
Paris Cedex, France

Leon Levinsky
Beilison Medical Center
Sackler School of Medicine
Tel Aviv, Israel

James E. Lock
Children's Memorial Hospital
Boston, Massachusetts, U.S.A.

Torsten Malm
University Hospital
Uppsala, Sweden

Alessandro Mazzucco
University of Padova
Padova, Italy

Milton A. Meier
State University of Rio de Janeiro
Rio de Janeiro, Brazil

James L. Monro
Wessex Regional Centre for Cardiothoracic
Surgery
Southampton, U.K.

Carlos A. Moraes
Federal University of Pernambuco
Recife, Brazil

Jaume Mulet
Hospital Clinico Y Provincial
Hospital San Juan De Dios
Barcelona, Spain

Charles E. Mullins
Texas Children's Hospital
Houston, Texas, U.S.A.

Francesco Musumeci
Harefield Hospital
Harefield, U.K.

Yasuaki Naito
Wakayama Medical College
Osaka, Japan

Jorg Ostermeyer
University of Düsseldorf
Düsseldorf, West Germany

Alessandro Pellegrini
Ospedale Niguarda
Milano, Italy

Fernando M. Picchio
University of Bologna
Bologna, Italy

Roberto Piva
Hospital "Lancisi"
Ancona, Italy

C. J. Preusse
University of Düsseldorf
Düsseldorf, West Germany

Manuel Quero Jimenez
Hospital Ramon Y Cajal
Madrid, Spain

Raul Ivo Rossi Filho
Institute of Cardiology
Porto Alegre, Brazil

Jean E. Rubay
Cliniques Universitaire Saint-Luc
Bruxelles, Belgium

David J. Sahn
University of California
San Diego, California, U.S.A.

Timo Savunen
University of Turku
Turku, Finland

Peter Schupbach
University of Bern
Bern, Switzerland

Rui Sequeira de Almeida
Hospital Evangelico de Curitiba
Curitiba, Brazil

Francesco Siclari
Hannover Medical School
Hannover, West Germany

Umberto Squarcia
University di Parma
Parma, Italy

Gaetano Thiene
University of Padova
Padova, Italy

Janice Anne Till
Brompton Hospital
London, U.K.

Atanas Todorov
National Center of Cardiovascular Disease
Medical Academy
Sofia, Bulgaria

Michael J. Tynan
Guy's Hospital
London, U.K.

Ross M. Ungerleider
Duke University Medical Center
Durham, North Carolina, U.S.A.

Richard Van Praagh
Children's Hospital
Harvard Medical School
Boston, Massachusetts, U.S.A.

Choompol Vongprateep
Children's Hospital
Bangkok, Thailand

Fumio Yamamoto
National Cardiovascular Center
Suita, Japan

Yong-Soo Yun
Children's Hospital–
Seoul National University
Seoul, Korea

Collaborators

A. Agnetti
Parma, Italy

Y. Al Faraidi
Riyadh, Saudi Arabia

A. Al Kasab
Riyadh, Saudi Arabia

A. Alonso
Madrid, Spain

U. Althaus
Bern, Switzerland

F. Andou
Fukuoka, Japan

S. Aoyagi
Fukuoka, Japan

S. Aranki
Harefield, U.K.

N. Arnaudov
Sofia, Bulgaria

A. Ashmeg
Riyadh, Saudi Arabia

P. Austoni
Milano, Italy

L. Bacchi Reggiani
Bologna, Italy

N. Banner
Harefield, U.K.

C. Barriuso
Barcelona, Spain

S. L. Bassi
Curitiba, Brazil

H. Becker
Los Angeles, California, U.S.A.

J. Ben-Ari
Tel Aviv, Israel

L. Bendig
Budapest, Hungary

M. Berant
Tel Aviv, Israel

J. Bertoletti
Porto Alegre, Brazil

A. Billingsley
Los Angeles, California, U.S.A.

W. Bircks
Düsseldorf, West Germany

S. Biscaglia
Bologna, Italy

A. Borowski
Göttingen, West Germany

H. G. Borst
Hannover, West Germany

U. Bortolotti
Padova, Italy

S. Bowald
Uppsala, Sweden

P. R. Brofman
Curitiba, Brazil

E. Buffolo
Rio de Janeiro, Brazil

J. Bushong
Newark, New Jersey, U.S.A.

A. Bylock
Uppsala, Sweden

N. Carano
Parma, Italy

I. S. Casagrande
Rio de Janeiro, Brazil

I. Castro
Porto Alegre, Brazil

I. Cavalcanti
Recife, Brazil

C. Cavalli
Parma, Italy

M. E. Cazzaniga
Buenos Aires, Argentina

K. A. Chacko
Boston, Massachusetts, U.S.A.

C. H. Chalant
Bruxelles, Belgium

S.-F. Chao
Taipei, Taiwan

S. L. Checa
Madrid, Spain

T. Colombo
Milano, Italy

J. V. Cotroneo
Newark, New Jersey, U.S.A.

S. L. Cronjé
Pretoria, South Africa

G. Crupi
Bergamo, Italy

L. Daliento
Padova, Italy

N. S. Daudt
Porto Alegre, Brazil

J. C. de Andrade
Rio de Janeiro, Brazil

E. R. De Vivie
Göttingen, West Germany

P. Diaz
Madrid, Spain

J. I. Diez
Madrid, Spain

F. Donatelli
Milano, Italy

D. Drinkwater
Los Angeles, California, U.S.A.

G. Faggian
Padova, Italy

R. G. Favaloro
Buenos Aires, Argentina

A. Fehér
Budapest, Hungary

C. Firpo
Porto Alegre, Brazil

G. Fita
Barcelona, Spain

T. Fujita
Suita, Japan

K. Fujiwara
Osaka, Japan

S. Fukuchi
Tokyo, Japan

R. J. Galdieri
Newark, New Jersey, U.S.A.

M. M. Gebhard
Göttingen, West Germany

B. George
Los Angeles, California, U.S.A.

P. Gersbach
Bern, Switzerland

M. Goenen
Bruxelles, Belgium

C. Gomar
Barcelona, Spain

R. Gomez
Madrid, Spain

S. Guarnera
Paris, France

J. C. Haertel
Porto Alegre, Brazil

A. Haverich
Hannover, West Germany

D. J. Hearse
London, U.K.

E. Heldmann
Newark, New Jersey, U.S.A.

G. Herrmann
Hannover, West Germany

S. Higashiue
Osaka, Japan

A. Hoeft
Göttingen, West Germany

C. Y. Hong
Seoul, Korea

D. Horstkotte
Düsseldorf, West Germany

C. Hung
Taipei, Taiwan

Y. Imai
Tokyo, Japan

M. Inberg
Turku, Finland

K. Ishihara
Tokyo, Japan

F. Isobe
Suita, Japan

P. Jaumin
Bruxelles, Belgium

P. L. Julia
Los Angeles, California, U.S.A.

K. Kadar
Budapest, Hungary

H. C. Kallfelz
Hannover, West Germany

T. Kamiya
Suita, Japan

M. Kawada
Tokyo, Japan

Y. Kestens-Servaye
Bruxelles, Belgium

A. Khaghani
Harefield, U.K.

H. Kishimoto
Suita, Japan

J. A. Kisslo
Durham, North Carolina, U.S.A.

E. Kleinhans
Aachen, West Germany

K. Kocherscheidt
Düsseldorf, West Germany

E. F. Kofsky
Los Angeles, California, U.S.A.

E. Koncz
Budapest, Hungary

H. Kurosawa
Tokyo, Japan

K. Kosuga
Fukuoka, Japan

A. Krian
Düsseldorf, West Germany

S. Lambreva
Sofia, Bulgaria

J. Lammer
Graz, Austria

S. Lasarov
Sofia, Bulgaria

M. Lengyel
Budapest, Hungary

J. P. Leon
Madrid, Spain

C. Lepeniotis
Newark, New Jersey, U.S.A.

M. J. Levy
Tel Aviv, Israel

F. Loogen
Düsseldorf, West Germany

D. R. Loures
Curitiba, Brazil

F. Lucchese
Porto Alegre, Brazil

H.-C. Lue
Taipei, Taiwan

M. J. Maitre Azcarate
Madrid, Spain

A. Matta
Bruxelles, Belgium

N. Medeiros
Porto Alegre, Brazil

J. T. Mendonca
Rio de Janeiro, Brazil

B. J. Messmer
Aachen, West Germany

S. Mihaileanu
Paris, France

A. Milano
Padova, Italy

C. Mortera
Barcelona, Spain

I. Nesralla
Porto Alegre, Brazil

J. W. Neto
Rio de Janeiro, Brazil

J. Y. Neveux
Paris, France

K. Nishigaki
Suita, Japan

B. O'Connor
Boston, Massachusetts, U.S.A.

K. Ohara
Suita, Japan

K. Ohishi
Fukuoka, Japan

A. Ohryoji
Fukuoka, Japan

M. Okuno
Suita, Japan

Y. Ono
Suita, Japan

V. Oprea
Budapest, Hungary

I. Palik
Budapest, Hungary

A. Pangrazi
Ancona, Italy

J. Pearl
Los Angeles, California, U.S.A.

E. Pedroni
Paris, France

J. Philips
Durham, North Carolina, U.S.A.

J. F. Piechaud
Paris, France

V. Pilosof
Sofia, Bulgaria

J. C. Prates
Porto Alegre, Brazil

E. Quani
Milano, Italy

R. Radley-Smith
Harefield, U.K.

C. Rapezzi
Bologna, Italy

J. G. Reves
Durham, North Carolina, U.S.A.

E. J. Ribeiro
Curitiba, Brazil

M. L. Rigby
London, U.K.

E. Riva
Milano, Italy

J. V. Rodrigues
Recife, Brazil

E. Rosenkranz
Los Angeles, California, U.S.A.

E. Rowland
London, U.K.

M. Rubino
Padova, Italy

P. Sakornpant
Bangkok, Thailand

M. Salazar
Madrid, Spain

C. A. Salles
Rio de Janeiro, Brazil

P. A. Sanchez
Madrid, Spain

J. R. Sant'Anna
Port Alegre, Brazil

C. L. Santos
Recife, Brazil

W. Sawyer
Riyadh, Saudi Arabia

A. Schachner
Tel Aviv, Israel

T. Schonfeld
Tel Aviv, Israel

H. D. Schulte
Düsseldorf, West Germany

D. Sidi
Paris, France

I. A. Simpson
San Diego, California, U.S.A.

N. Slavkov
Sofia, Bulgaria

T. Sluysmans
Bruxelles, Belgium

L. R. Smith
Durham, North Carolina, U.S.A.

F. E. Stark
Newark, New Jersey, U.S.A.

D. S. Steed
Los Angeles, California, U.S.A.

J. I. Stein
Graz, Austria

G. Stellin
Padova, Italy

F. Stoker
Bern, Switzerland

K. P. Suh
Seoul, Korea

C. Suppan
Graz, Austria

A. Suzuki
Suita, Japan

E. Tiso
Padova, Italy

A. R. Torres
Buenos Aires, Argentina

G. Touati
Paris, France

A. Tschirkov
Sofia, Bulgaria

M. Turri
Padova, Italy

S. Utapisarnsuradi
Bangkok, Thailand

D. Velitschkova
Sofia, Bulgaria

D. Vellibre
Madrid, Spain

T. Verebely
Budapest, Hungary

F. Villagra
Madrid, Spain

E. Vitali
Milano, Italy

M. Vitanova
Sofia, Bulgaria

A. Vliers
Bruxelles, Belgium

G. Von Bernuth
Aachen, West Germany

P. Vouhe
Paris, France

J. K. Wang
Taipei, Taiwan

I. W. Weber
Bern, Switzerland

J. Winter
Düsseldorf, West Germany

A. Wu
Los Angeles, California, U.S.A.

M. H. Wu
Taipei, Taiwan

M. Yacoub
London, U.K.

T. Yagihara
Suita, Japan

E. Yamamoto
Fukuoka, Japan

Y. Yano
London, U.K.

L. Zavota
Parma, Italy

P. Zielinsky
Porto Alegre, Brazil

G. Ziemer
Hannover, West Germany

Preface and Acknowledgments

The three parts of this volume, the second in our series offering perspectives in the diagnosis and treatment of cardiological disease of the young, gather together the written manifestations of the topics discussed at the First World Congress of Pediatric Cardiac Surgery, held in Bergamo, Italy, over the period June 19 through 23, 1988. The meeting itself was carefully designed so that all important and growing areas of pediatric cardiac surgery and their related cardiological disciplines would be covered in detail by recognized experts. We were delighted that virtually all those invited as experts accepted their role and, furthermore, took considerable care to prepare their work in the form of manuscripts, following our chosen format. This process, in itself, ensured that the books which emerged would not represent mere transcriptions of the proceedings of the symposium. But, although the invited experts ensured detailed coverage of the crucial areas, we were immensely gratified by all the other workers in the field who came in their multitudes to Bergamo, offering papers for presentation which stood shoulder to shoulder with the contributions of our chosen panelists. These investigators also prepared manuscripts following our instructions. Taken together, therefore, the body of material represents a true panorama of all that is important in the world of diagnosis and treatment of heart disease in the young. We, as editors, have tried to arrange this material in uniform fashion, so that the books, as much as is possible, read with a reasonable degree of continuity. Inevitably, some of the manuscripts required more work than others, since English is not the native tongue of many of our contributors. We hope that our efforts to provide uniformity have not been too draconian, and that all still recognize their original drafts! In several instances, topics proved controversial. We have not tried to shirk such controversy, rather we have chosen to highlight potential disagreements by the use of editorial notes. These will indicate the appropriate points at which editorial license has been taken. The number of contributors to our three-part volume is considerable. Had we listed all as "authors", the resulting catalogue would have been almost as long as the overall book! We have compromised, therefore, by listing the first authors as "contributors". The various co-workers are grouped as "collaborators". We hope all thus cited will appreciate the reasons for such economy.

We were satisfied beyond our wildest expectations at the success of the First World Congress and for this we are grateful to all our medical colleagues of the Department of Cardiac Surgery of Ospedali Riuniti, Bergamo, for their continuous help and support. We are equally excited with the contents of these books. They could not have been prepared and edited so swiftly and successfully without the considerable care and secretarial efforts of Mrs. Hilda Oprandi. She worked far beyond the call of duty in transcribing and modifying the manuscripts. We are indebted also to the editorial staff of Futura, who continued our initial efforts with their customary efficiency.

Giancarlo Crupi
Lucio Parenzan
Robert H. Anderson

Contents

Section II Imaging in Congenital Heart Disease

Section III Valve Disease in Children

Section VI   Cardiopulmonary Bypass and Myocardial Protection

Section VII   Miscellaneous

Interventional Cardiology

Introduction

Michael Tynan

When Dr. William Rashkind introduced effective therapeutic catheterization with balloon atrial septostomy,[1] he exposed a whole generation of pediatric cardiologists for what they are—surgeons manqué. At that time, we did not call it "interventional catheterization"—but we all did it! Balloon septostomy, however, was not the first attempt to use cardiac catheterization for the purpose of treatment. In 1953, Rubio-Alvarez[2,3] and his colleagues in Mexico attempted valvoplasty using a catheter and a guide wire assembly that prefigured the Park septostomy blade[4] in an attempt to "saw" through stenosed valves. It is difficult, when reading their publications, to be certain that this approach was successful. In any event, it did not catch on. Although further attempts at relief of stenotic lesions were reported,[5] it was not until techniques pioneered in atheromatous disease[6] were applied to congenital heart disease, following considerable experimental work,[7–12] that consistent success has been achieved. Thus, in 1982, Kan and her colleagues[13] reported relief of valvar pulmonary stenosis. This technique is now accepted as the treatment of first choice in most centers. Its success is illustrated in the chapter of Yun and his colleagues from Korea (Chapter 1.4), who have treated 72 such patients, with good results, in only 2 years. The momentum of balloon angioplasty in treatment of congenital heart dis-

eases has now increased markedly, with its use spreading both geographically and in the number of pathologies treated. This is illustrated in the chapters by Hofstetter and colleagues (Chapter 1.7), Picchio and colleagues (Chapter 1.3) and Beitzke and colleagues (Chapter 1.6). Congenital valvar aortic stenosis has also proved to be amenable to this treatment[14] and, even if it is only a palliative procedure, what else is surgical valvotomy in children? Postoperative restenosis of aortic coarctation has been successfully treated[15] but, contrary to our original belief, aneurysms can be caused. We have certainly observed this complication in our unit. The use of balloon angioplasty in the primary treatment of aortic coarctation remains controversial. The technique is effective but aneurysmal formation is again a problem[16] and its frequency of occurrence is unknown. It does not appear to be related to technical aspects, such as size of the balloon, but is probably an inherent anatomical risk of the technique. An anatomical study[17] has suggested that aneurysms could ensue in up to one-third of patients undergoing dilatation. Furthermore, one histological study suggested that cystic medial necrosis of the aorta is common in coarctation[18] thus conferring an additional risk for aneurysmal formation.

More experimental applications of balloon angioplasty include its use in the palliation of the tetralogy of Fallot[19] and in the treatment of subvalvar aortic stenosis.[20] As yet, both applications need further evaluation but, in our unit, we now routinely use the technique for palliation of tetralogy with acceptable results.

The list of lesions in which balloon angioplasty has been used, therefore, continues to grow. As discussed, it is problematical in some conditions, such as aortic coarctation. Success appears to depend on careful selection of suitable cases. This is particularly evident in the setting of peripheral pulmonary stenosis where discrete single stenoses, particularly of short tubular pattern, or stenoses occurring after surgery appear to respond well, but multiple stenotic lesions do not. Perhaps, in this latter situation, the combination of angioplasty and implantation of stents may prove beneficial. Improved selection of cases may render balloon angioplasty more acceptable in treatment of aortic coarctation by reducing the risk of aneurysmal formation. Here, the improved characterization of the tissues made possible by resonance imaging may hold the key.

Other applications of balloon angioplasty include dilatation of stenosed venous channels after atrial redirection operations for complete transposition; dilatation of stenosed Blalock (or other) shunts; and treatment of pulmonary arterial stenoses resulting from insertion of such shunts or prosthetic conduits, as reported in the chapters of Hofstetter and Squarcia and their colleagues (Chapters 1.7 and 1.8). In these applications, angioplasty is used as an adjunct to surgery. No doubt the list will grow. An overall view of the uses of balloon angioplasty is provided in the chapter by Kachaner and his colleagues (Chapter 1.2). But an indication of the widespread acceptance of these techniques is the range of lesions dealt with in the report of Beitzke and his associates (Chapter 1.6), modestly qualified as being from a "small unit." In their chapter (Chapter 1.5), Piva and Pangrazi illustrate

the applicability of balloon angioplasty even in the very young.

The other major area of therapeutic catheterization is the use of embolization for the closure of congenital and acquired shunts. The equipment used includes detachable latex balloons, implantable coils, gelfoam fragments, and special devices such as the Rashkind occluder for closure of the arterial duct. Tissue adhesives have also been employed, but they are now rarely used, although they still have their adherents. Embolization with coils is useful in occluding arteriovenous malformations in the lung and in the coronary circulation;[21] and for closure of major systemic-to-pulmonary collateral arteries and unwanted shunts. Formulas for deciding on the appropriate size of coil have been suggested. It is reasonable to start with one that is approximately the same size as the vessel to be occluded. In some instances, nonetheless, flow continues through the center of the coil. In these cases, several coils may be needed, and these may have to be of different sizes. Complete occlusion is then effected by a "nest" of coils. Care must be taken not to use coils so small that they embolize from their chosen site, particularly into the systemic circulation. Detachable balloons are particularly useful in vessels of large calibre where coils may not cause cessation of flow. The balloon may be inflated with silicone polymer or with dilute contrast medium. The former has the advantage that deflation cannot occur, but the disadvantage that, once the silicone has been introduced, the position of the balloon cannot be modified and the balloon cannot be deflated. Thus, errors of positioning cannot be corrected while embolization remains a major risk. Inflation with contrast medium has the advantage that, at any point up to the moment of detachment, the balloons can be deflated and withdrawn or repositioned. Spontaneous deflation, however, may occur with the later risk of embolization. When embolization occurs into the pulmonary circulation, there appear to be no detectable adverse effects. When it occurs to the systemic circulation, in contrast, there are obvious dangers. When approaching any embolization procedure, therefore, it is as well to have both coils and detachable balloons available, since they can be used together with advantage. The detachable balloon obstructs flow while the coils promote thrombosis. Complete occlusion without risk of balloon embolization can then be achieved.

The application of these methods of embolization to patients with congenital heart disease is somewhat limited, and the indications for their use are relatively rare. The introduction of devices specifically designed for closure of common congenital defects is in the process of altering this picture. For some years, a method for closing the arterial duct has been available.[22] Pioneered by Porstman and collegues in Berlin, its disadvantage was the size of the catheter needed for introduction, which has been so large as to preclude its use in children. In Chapter 1.9, Kumate and colleagues describe a modification of this technique which allows its use in children down to 4 years of age. This development has occurred over the same period during which Rashkind perfected his double umbrella device for ductal occlusion. Mullins presents this latter technique from an incomparable experience (Chapter 1.10). The Rashkind method, as modified by Mullins,[23] now enjoys a worldwide popularity. But the efforts of the Japanese, along with the development of an alternative device by Soviet doctors[24] show that there is more than one way to skin a cat. The Rashkind device has also been used to close ventricular septal defects, systemic-to-pulmonary arterial shunts and postoperative interatrial defects. We ourselves have successfully closed a postinfarction ventricular septal defect with it. Such unorthodox use of the Rashkind duct occluder, and developments towards a device designed specifically for occlusion of septal defects, are discussed by Lock in Chapter 1.11.

Already there has been a revolution in the treatment of structural congenital cardiac malformations. Now, therapeutic catheterization accounts for half the work in our laboratory for cardiac catheterization in children and amounts to 30%. of the total "surgical" work performed in our unit. Several advantages accrue, including shorter hospital stays. Most patients spend only 1 or 2 nights in hospital and, in some instances, the procedures are performed as day cases. There is less pressure on intensive care beds and on scarce nursing resources. The morbidity is lower and both patients and their parents prefer the nonsurgical approach. The indications are that this type of work will increase, with consequent lower morbidity for the patients and financial savings. The continued development in this area is the best tribute we can make to the man who as teacher, and for many of as a friend, got us started in this direction and who made us keep going: William Rashkind.

References

1. Rashkind WJ, Miller WW. Creation of an atrial septal defect without thoracotomy. J Am Med Assoc 1966;196:991–2.
2. Rubio-Alvarez V, Limon Lason R, Soni J. Valvotomias intraccardiacas por medio de un catheter. Arch Inst Cardiol Mexico 1953;23:183–92.
3. Rubio-Alvarez V, Limon Lason R. Comisurotomia tricuspidea por medio de un catheter modificado. Arch Inst Cardiol Mexico 1955;25:57–69.
4. Park SC, Neches WH, Zuberbuhler JR, et. al. Clinical use of blade atrial septostomy. Circulation 1975;58:600–6.
5. Semb BKH, Tijonneland S, Stake G, et al. "Balloon valvulotomy" of congenital pulmonary valve stenosis with tricuspid valve insufficiency. 1979;2:239–41.
6. Gruntzig A, Hopff H. Perkutane Rekanalisation chronischer arterieller Verschlusse mit einem neuen Dilatationskatheter: Modification der Dotter-Technic. Deutsch Med Wschr 1974;99:2502–5.
7. Lock JE, Neimi BA, Enzig S, et al. Transvenous angioplasty of experimental branch pulmonary artery stenosis in newborn lambs. Circulation 1981;64:886–93.

8. Castaneda-Zuniga WR, Lock JE, Vlodaver Z, et al. Transluminal dilatation of coarctation at the abdominal aorta: An experimental study in dogs. Radiology 1982;143:693–7.

9. Lock JE, Neimi BA, Burke B, et al. Transcutaneous angioplasty of experimental aortic coarctation. Circulation 1982,66:1280–6.

10. Sus T, Sniderman KW, Rettek-Sos B, et al. Percutaneous transluminal dilation of coarctation of the thoracic aorta post-mortem. Lancet 1979;9:970–71.

11. Luck JE, Castenada-Zuniga WR, Bass JL, et al. Balloon dilatation of excised aortic coarctation. Radiology 1982;143:698–91.

12. Kan JS, Anderson JH, White RI Jr. Experimental basis for balloon valvoplasty of congenital pulmonary valvar stenosis, Proc Sect Cardiol Am Acad Ped, New York, October 1982, pp. 101A.

13. Kan JS, White RI Jr, Mitchell SE, et al. Percutaneous balloon pulmonary valvoplasty: A new method for treating congenital pulmonary valve stenosis. N Engl J Med 1982; 307:540–2.

14. Lababidi Z, Wu J, Walls JT. Percutaneous balloon aortic valvuloplasty: Results in 23 patients. Am J Cardiol 1984;53: 194–7.

15. Lorber A, Ettedgui JA, Baker EJ, et al. Balloon aortoplasty for recoarctation following the subclavian flap operation. Int J Cardiol 1986;10:57–63.

16. Wren C, Peart I, Bain H, et al. Balloon dilatation of unoperated coarctation: Immediate results and one year follow up. Br Heart J 1987;58:369–76.

17. Pellegrino A, Deverall PB, Anderson RH, et al. Aortic coarctation in the first three months of life. An anatomopathological study with respect to treatment. J Thorac Cardiovasc Surg 1985;89:121–7.

18. Isner JM, Donaldson RF, Fulton D, et al. Cystic medial necrosis in coarctation of the aorta: A potential factor contributing to adverse consequences after percutaneous balloon angioplasty of coarctation sites. Circulation 1987;75:689–95.

19. Qureshi SA, Kirk CR, Lamb RK, et al. Balloon dilatation of the pulmonary valve in the first year of life in patients with tetralogy of Fallot: A preliminary study. Br Heart J 1988;60:332–5.

20. Suarez de Lezo J, Pan M, Sancho M, et al. Percutaneous transluminal balloon dilatation for discrete subaortic stenosis. Am J Cardiol 1986;88:619–21.

21. Reidy JF, Jones ODH, Tynan ML, et al. Embolization procedures in congenital heart disease. Br Heart J 1985;54:184–92.

22. Porstmann W, Wierny L, Warnke H. Closure of persistent ductus arteriosus without thoracotomy. Thoraxchirurgie 1967;15:199–201.

23. Rashkind WJ, Mullins CE, Hellenbrand WE, et al. Nonsurgical closure of patent ductus arteriosus: Clinical application of the Rashkind PDA Occluder System, Circulation 1987; 75:583–92A.

24. Савельев СВ: Отдаленные результаты лечения больных открытым артериальным протоком методом эндоваскулярнои окклюэии. Кардиологэя, 1988, 28:77–80.

Percutaneous Balloon Dilatation of Right-Sided Cardiovascular Lesions

J. Kachaner, J. F. Piechaud, J. Le Bidois, S. Guarnera, and E. Pedroni

Introduction

Congenital or acquired right-sided lesions of the heart were the first to be successfully submitted to percutaneous techniques for balloon dilatation.[1] A few years later, these methods have become routine in many obstructive conditions, such as typical pulmonary valvar stenosis. Balloon procedures have been attempted in a great number of other lesions with varying results and still remain somewhat experimental.[2] In this article, we will summarize the state of this art in pediatric patients.

Pulmonary Valvar Stenosis

Pulmonary valvar stenosis can be considered typical when it appears as an isolated lesion due to fusion of thin leaflets along their commissures. The orifice is no more than a tiny hole at the distal end of a dome-shaped valve. Balloon pulmonary valvoplasty, using oversized balloons, is easy to achieve and is both safe and effective in relieving the obstruction, even if it leaves a degree of infundibular stenosis which is usu-

ally moderate and transient.[3,4] Balloon dilatation is thus recognized as the treatment of choice in these patients, removing the need for surgery. We recommend valvotomy in every case with a transvalvar pressure gradient greater than 40 mmHg.

Some cases, nonetheless, remain more difficult to manage and may still require surgical help. These are, first, the so-called dysplastic forms of pulmonary valvar stenosis. In these, the leaflets are thick and myxoid. In addition, the ventriculo-arterial junction as well as the pulmonary trunk can have small dimensions. The condition is often familial and may be part of a syndrome such as Noonan's syndrome, leopard syndrome, or Watson's syndrome. Balloon valvoplasty is difficult to perform in these patients, early and late results are poor, and surgery is usually needed when the transvalvar pressure gradient remains high.

The same is true for all cases with hypoplastic ventriculo-pulmonary junctions bearing either a normal or a dysplastic valve. Ballooning these valves may improve some patients, but the procedure is palliative. Again, therefore, surgery is very often required. On the same standpoint, patients with tetralogy of Fallot may present very early in life because they have severe hypoplasia of the right ventricular outflow tract, the ventriculo-arterial junctions, and the entire pulmonary arterial tree. Balloon dilatation of the valvar component of this stenosis may be helpful—as the Brock operation was—in increasing pulmonary blood flow, improving oxygen saturation, and delaying the need for any urgent surgical procedure.[5]

Pulmonary valvar stenosis presenting in the first few days of life is usually called critical pulmonary stenosis and deserves special attention. The anatomic features resemble those described in patients with pulmonary atresia and intact ventricular septum. They include some degree of right ventricular underdevelopment and a particularly small orifice within the dome of the valve. The pathophysiology is also unfavorable. Even after relief of the obstruction, the poor compliance of the right ventricle does not always allow a significant increase in pulmonary blood flow. A right-to-left transatrial shunt may thus persist, and the need for an aortopulmonary shunt may not be eliminated. Furthermore, technical problems often arise in these patients, mainly because of the small dimensions of the vessels and the cardiac structures to be traversed by the devices. Balloon valvoplasty is more difficult to perform and is associated with more complications and with a lower success rate than in older children.[4]

A recent French cooperative study includes 45 neonates aged from 1 to 17 days with a mean ($\pm$SD) of 5.4 days ($\pm$3.1) with severe pulmonary stenosis as assessed by right ventricular pressures ranging from 80 to 180 mmHg, mean 106 mmHg ($\pm$22). The ventriculo-pulmonary junction was 7–9 mm in diameter. Balloon valvoplasty was attempted in all patients, but the pulmonary valve could not be traversed in 14 (31%). Six major complications (20%) occurred in the 31 cases that were effectively dilated, including myocardial infarction in two, hemopericardium with tamponade in three, and

rupture of the ventriculo-arterial junction in one. Four patients died, while 14 had a bad or fair result requiring another valvoplasty or subsequent surgery. Only 13 (42%) had a good long-term result.

Better results have been reported recently.[2] Our personal experience has also improved so that, up to May 1988, we tried to dilate 22 neonates with critical pulmonic stenosis, with only five failures (23%), one major complication (5%), and 14 early successes in the 17 effective dilatations. We feel, therefore, that percutaneous balloon valvoplasty should be recommended as the first intervention in all neonates with critical pulmonic stenosis.

Obstructive Lesions of the Branch Pulmonary Arteries

Arterial lesions of the pulmonary trunk and branches, either short stenoses or extensive areas of hypoplasia, are difficult to treat surgically, so that balloon dilatation is now commonly attempted using balloons with diameters which are two to four times the diameter of the stenotic segment.[6] The aim is to tear the internal layers of the vessel[7] and to enlarge its diameter by at least 50%.[2] The anomalies may be either congenital (appearing as part of a complex syndrome and then often being associated with dysplastic pulmonary valves) or, more commonly, acquired after an operation (shunts, repair of tetralogy of Fallot with or without pulmonary atresia, Fontan procedure, banding of the pulmonary trunk, arterial switch operation for complete transposition).

The procedure is not absolutely safe. A mortality rate of 1.7%[2] and varying complications have been reported, including rupture of the arteries,[7] pulmonary arterial thrombosis, hemoptysis, and formation of aneurysms.[2,6] It is often difficult to assess the results since multiple stenoses are common, needing multiple procedures. On the whole, the success rate is about 50%[2] and better results have been obtained in the younger patients (less than 3 years). Balloon angioplasty, therefore, may provide significant improvements in some patients with stenoses of branch pulmonary arteries in whom conventional surgery is usually unsuccessful.

Other Right-Sided Obstructive Lesions

Balloon dilatation may also be a successful means of relieving the venous obstruction which can follow an atrial redirection operation for complete transposition. Large balloons should be used, and the best cases are those where the obstruction is intracardiac at the site of the suture of the baffle to the atrial septum.[8]

Bioprosthetic valves inserted in either the tricuspid or the pulmonary position or in conduits between the right ventricle and the pulmonary arteries (see also article 1.7) are known to calcify and to become obstructive in the pediatric age group. These lesions are amenable to balloon dilatation, and successes have been reported.[9] Even if the obstruction is not entirely relieved, partial success may be beneficial to the patient in delaying a subsequent difficult reoperation.

References

1. Kan JS, White RI, Mitchell SE, Gardner TJ. Percutaneous valvuloplasty: A new method for treating congenital pulmonary valve stenosis. N Engl J Med 1982;307:540–2.
2. Perry SB, Kean JF, Lock JE. Interventional catheterization in pediatric congenital and acquired heart disease. Am J Cardiol 1988;61:109–17.
3. Ben Shachar G, Cohen MF, Sivakoff MC, et al. Development of infundibular obstruction after percutaneous pulmonary balloon valvuloplasty. J Am Coll Cardiol 1985;5:574–6.
4. Piechaud JF, Voshtani H, Kachaner J, et al. Problèmes posés par la valvuloplastie pulmonaire percutanée chez l'enfant. Arch Mal Coeur 1987;80:413–9.
5. Wright JGC, Arnold R, Bini RM, et al. Percutaneous balloon dilatation of right ventricular outflow tract and pulmonary valve in patients with tetralogy of Fallot. Br Heart J 1986;55:516(abstr).
6. Ring JC, Bass JL, Marvin W, et al. Management of congenital stenosis of a branch pulmonary artery with balloon dilation angioplasty. Report of 52 procedures. J Thorac Cardiovasc Surg 1985;90:35–44.
7. Edwards BS, Lucas, RV, Lock JE, Edwards JE. Morphologic changes in the pulmonary arteries after percutaneous balloon angioplasty for pulmonary arterial stenosis. Circulation 1985;71:195–201.
8. Lock JE, Bass JL, Castaneda-Zuniga W, et al. Dilatation angioplasty of congenital or operative narrowings of venous channels. Circulation 1984;70:457–64.
9. Lloyd TR, Marvin WJ Jr, Mahoney LT, Lauer RM. Balloon dilatation valvuloplasty of bioprosthetic valves in extracardiac conduits. Am Heart J 1987;114:268–74.

Italian Multi-Institutional Study on Balloon Dilatation in Congenital Heart Disease

F. M. Picchio, C. Rapezzi, L. Bacchi Reggiani, and S. Biscaglia

Introduction

In this article, we present the preliminary results of a retrospective multicentric study of balloon dilatations. Twelve Italian centers participated to produce a total number of 448 consecutive procedures performed between January 1, 1984, and May 30, 1988 (Table 1). We have reviewed the first 401 procedures comprising 301 pulmonary valvoplasties, 36 aortic valvoplasties, and 64 angioplasties for aortic coarctation. Particular attention has been addressed during analysis to the technical aspects, the immediate and intermediate-term results, the incidence of complications, and the incremental risk factors for complications and failure of the procedure.

Balloon Valvoplasty for Pulmonary Valvar Stenosis

Three hundred and one procedures were performed in 283 patients aged 9 days

This study was supported by the Italian Group for Hemodynamic Studies (GISE) and the Italian Society of Pediatric Cardiology.

to 68 years (mean 6.7 ± 9.6 years). A single balloon catheter was used in 258 cases, a dual balloon procedure in 30, while a triple balloon procedure was employed in three cases. Dilatation using double balloons was performed in 11 cases. The ratio of the diameter of the balloon to that of the ventriculo-arterial junction averaged 1.2 ± 0.2. A mean of 3.6 ± 1.2 inflations were performed (range 1-7).

The peak systolic gradient decreased from 71 ± 30 to 29 ± 19 mmHg ($p < 0.000001$) with a mean reduction of 61%. A linear correlation was found between the predilatation gradient and the pressure gradient drop ($r = 0.63$, $p < 0.001$). An excellent result (residual gradient < 30 mmHg) was achieved in 204 procedures (68%). A significant (30 to 79 mmHg) residual gradient was measured in 57 (19%), while no change in predilatation gradient was obtained in 35 cases (12%). Five procedures (2%) were attempted but not completed because of technical problems. In 27 procedures (7%), reactive infundibular stenosis was documented. In seven neonates with critical pulmonary stenosis, the peak systolic gradient decreased from 100 ± 13 to

Table 1

Types and Numbers of Procedures for Each Participating Center

Center	Pulmonary valvoplasty	Aortic valvoplasty	Aortic coarctation angioplasty	Postop coarctation angioplasty	Total
Ancona	33	7	36	3	79
Bergamo	73	20	1	3	97
Bologna	19	—	—	—	19
Firenze	6	—	—	—	6
Genova	24	3	3	—	30
Milano	32	4	15	2	53
Napoli	36	5	—	4	45
Padova	5	—	—	—	5
Parma	18	—	—	—	18
Roma	73	—	—	—	73
Torino	6	—	—	—	6
Vicenza	15	—	—	2	17
Total	340	39	55	14	448

46 ± 9 mmHg ($p < 0.0005$). Where we compared different subgroups in terms of the hemodynamic results, only a dysplastic valve and age less than 1 month proved to be incremental risk factors for an unsatisfactory result. It was noted, however, that the predilatation gradient was higher in the group with significant residual gradients (80 ± 37 vs. 68 ± 26 mmHg, $p < 0.05$).

The right ventricular end-diastolic pressure (measured in 84 cases before and after the valvoplasty) decreased from 9.4 ± 3.7 to 7.3 ± 1 ($p < 0.0005$). Since it is reasonable to assume that cardiac output did not decrease (cardiac output was not measured but systolic arterial pressure did not change), this observation could be explained by an improvement of right ventricular diastolic function.

Five major complications (2%) were reported. There were two deaths: one, in a neonate, was unexplained; the other in an infant, was due to perforation of the infundibulum. Cerebral embolism occurred in two cases, and there was one episode of transient cerebral ischemia, all in infants.

A follow-up period with a mean of 10.6 ± 8.8 months was available in 156 patients. The final gradient (measured by cardiac catheterization or, in most cases, by continuous wave Doppler) was similar to the postprocedure gradient (28 ± 19 vs. 30 ± 19 mmHg, NS). In detail, the further reduction of the gradient seen in 12% was counterbalanced by an increase in the gradient in 13%, the latter being particularly frequent when the postdilatation gradient was greater than 45 mmHg. A second balloon valvoplasty was performed in 17 patients and a third procedure in one.

Balloon Valvoplasty for Aortic Valvar Stenosis

Thirty-six procedures were performed in 34 patients, who were aged from 4 days to 19 years (mean 6.9 ± 5.2 years). The age was less than 1 month in six cases. Seven patients had associated cardiac defects and five had previously undergone aortic valvotomy.

A single balloon catheter was employed in 27 procedures, a two-step procedure in six, and double balloons were used in two. The ratio of the diameters of the balloon to the ventriculo-aortic junction was $0.91 \pm$

0.16 (range 0.40–1.25) for the first balloon and 0.80 ± 0.30 (0.32–1.25) when a second one had to be used. A mean of 3.6 ± 1.4 inflations were performed (range 2–7).

The peak systolic gradient decreased from 80 ± 31 to 32 ± 23 mmHg (p < 0.0005) with a mean reduction of 60%. The aortic valvar area increased significantly (from 0.44 ± 0.13 to 1.69 ± 0.24 cm^2/m, p < 0.00005). No correlation was found between the predilatation gradient and the drop in the pressure gradient. An excellent or good result (residual gradient less than 30 mmHg) was achieved in 22 cases (61%). A significant (30 to 69 mmHg) residual gradient was measured in eight cases (22.2%). The procedure was ineffective in five occasions (16.5%) and was attempted but not completed in one patient.

The left ventricular end-diastolic pressure (measured in 29 cases before and after the dilatation) decreased from 15.3 ± 5.8 to 13.2 ± 4.9 mmHg, p < 0.001). Since it is reasonable to assume that cardiac output did not decrease (cardiac output was not measured, but systolic arterial pressure slightly increased from 91 ± 14 to 97 ± 20 mmHg, p < 0.05), these data might be explained by an improvement of left ventricular diastolic function.

In respect to the cases with either no or minimal improvement, the subgroup with a good result was characterized by a lower age (69 ± 57 vs. 104 ± 64 months, p < 0.05) and a greater ratio of balloon size to ventriculo-aortic junction (0.95 ± 0.14 vs. 0.84 ± 0.17, p < 0.05).

Nine major complications (25%) were reported, including two deaths, two cases of femoral arterial thrombosis, and three cases of severe aortic incompetence. The age was significantly lower in these patients (4.4 ± 5 vs. 7.7 ± 5.1 years, p < 0.05).

At a mean period of follow-up of 6.4 ± 4 months, the peak systolic gradient (measured in 18 patients by cardiac catheterization or continuous wave Doppler) and aortic valvar area (measured in nine) did not change significantly.

Balloon Angioplasty for Aortic Coarctation

Fifty-two procedures were performed for dilatation of native aortic coarctations in 43 patients aged from 9 days to 28 years with a mean of 3.1 ± 5.7 years. The age was less than 1 month in 20 and between 1 month and 1 year in 15 patients. Associated anomalies were present in 36 patients.

A single balloon was employed in 43 cases and two successive balloons in nine. The ratio of the diameter of the balloon to the coarcted segment averaged 3.1 ± 1 (range 1.5–6.4) for the first balloon and 3.3 ± 0.5 (range 2.5–4.2) when a second balloon was employed. A mean of 4.6 ± 1.4 inflations was performed (range 2–8).

The peak systolic gradient decreased from 46 ± 22 to 11 ± 13 mmHg (p < 0.00001), while the coarctation diameter increased from 2.3 ± 1.1 to 6.3 ± 3 mm (p < 0.00001). The result of the procedure was considered excellent or good (resulting in a postdilatation gradient less than 35% of the basal) in 35 cases (68%) and only satisfactory (a postdilatation gradient between 25% and 50% of the basal) in six (11%). The result was unsatisfactory (a postdilatation gradient greater than 50% of the basal) in six cases (11%). In five patients (10%), the procedure was attempted but not completed. No statistically significant difference was found in the clinical, angiographic, and technical characteristics between successful and unsuccessful procedures.

The ratio between pulmonary and systemic cardiac output (measured before and after the procedure in 20 patients with associated septal defects) decreased from 3.1 ± 1.5 to 2.4 ± 0.9 (p < 0.005).

Seven major complications (13.5%) were reported: two deaths (one related to iliac arterial laceration); four cases of femoral or iliac artery occlusion; and one case of injury to the brachial plexus. No development of aortic aneurysms was reported. The incidence of complications was 20%

among the newborns and only 6% among the children older than 1 year. A mean period of follow-up of 8.6 ± 10 months was available in 25 patients with a good immediate result. In 16 (64%), the peak systolic gradient increased significantly, and the procedure was repeated in nine.

A small group of 12 angioplasties performed for postoperation residual coarctation was also available for analysis. The mean age of these patients was 5.2 ± 6.2 years. A single balloon was employed in each case. The ratio of the diameter of the balloon to the stenotic area ranged from 1 to 3.3 (mean 2.1 ± 0.9), and the mean number of inflations was 3.6 ± 2. The peak systolic gradient decreased from 48 ± 17 to 13 ± 15 mmHg (p < 0.00005), while the di-

ameters of the coarcted segment increased from 5.6 ± 4.2 to 8.7 ± 4.1 mm (p < 0.00001). The procedure was attempted in two patients but not completed. The result was good in the other cases. No complication was reported. In the four patients in whom follow-up was available (31 ± 12 months), the gradient was unchanged.

Discussion

The preliminary results of this large multicenter study confirm the clinical utility of interventional procedures for the treatment of congenital heart disease with ventricular outflow obstruction. As previously reported,[1-3] pulmonary balloon valvoplasty

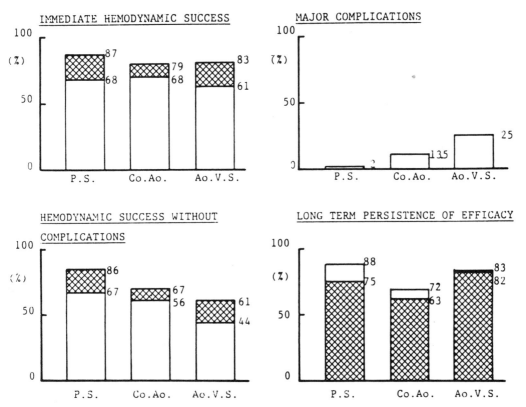

Figure 1. Hemodynamic results and complications of the three interventional procedures. The numbers are expressed as percentages. The white columns include only the cases with good or excellent results. The shaded columns include also the cases with a mild improvement. P.S., balloon valvoplasty for pulmonary stenosis; Co.Ao., balloon angioplasty for native aortic coarctation; Ao.V.S., balloon valvoplasty for aortic stenosis.

appears to be an effective and long-lasting procedure with relatively low risk (Fig. 1). An immediate hemodynamic success occurs in 87% of the cases. The diastolic function of the right ventricle also improves. Major complications are seen in only 2% of cases (mortality 0.7%). An effective procedure without major complications can, therefore, be expected in 85% of the cases (Fig. 1). The best hemodynamic results are obtained in patients without dysplastic valves who are older than 1 year. After an intermediate-term period of follow-up, the efficacy of the procedure persists in up to 75% of the cases. The procedure is clinically effective in neonates with critical pulmonary stenosis, but a relatively high residual gradient has to be expected, and a repeat valvoplasty or a surgical intervention must be considered in the follow-up.

The experience concerning balloon valvoplasty for aortic stenosis is not as good, although the procedure is now well established.[2,4,5] Our data show acceptable results in 83% of the cases, especially if balloons equal to the diameter of the ventriculo-aortic junction are employed. The diastolic function of the left ventricle also improves. The procedure remains efficacious during an intermediate-term period of follow-up in up to 83% of patients. The incidence of major complications, however, is high (25%), and mortality is 5.5%. Only in 61% of the cases can an acceptable result without major complications be expected. This percentage drops to 44% if only good or excellent results are considered (Fig. 1).

As could be predicted from the literature,[6-8] balloon angioplasty for native aortic coarctation provides excellent results in two-thirds of cases, but the rate of complications is relatively high (13.5%) and mortality is 3.8%. A good result free of complications, therefore, is expected in only 56%

of the procedures (Fig. 1). Complications are particularly frequent in the neonate. The procedure must be considered palliative. Indeed, a strong tendency for recoarctation at follow-up has already been documented.[6-8] In contrast, good or excellent results with no complications are to be anticipated in 83% of cases with recoarctation occurring after surgical interventions.

At present, balloon aortic valvoplasty and coarctation angioplasty remain investigational procedures that should be limited to a selected number of centers. The available data are still insufficient to be compared with advantages and disadvantages of traditional surgical treatments.

References

1. Lababidi Z, Wu JR. Percutaneous balloon pulmonary valvuloplasty. Br Heart J 1985;53:520–4.
2. Walls JT, Lababidi Z, Curtis JJ, Silver D. Assessment of percutaneous balloon pulmonary and aortic valvuloplasty. J Thorac Cardiovasc Surg 1984;88:352–6.
3. Mullins CE, Ludomirsky A, O'Laughlin MP, et al. Balloon valvuloplasty for pulmonic valve stenosis. Two-year folow-up: Hemodynamic and Doppler evaluation. Catheterization Cardiovasc Diagn 1988;14:76–81.
4. Lababidi Z, Wu JR, Walls JT. Percutaneous balloon aortic valvuloplasty: Results in 23 patients. Am J Cardiol 1984;53:194–7.
5. Helgason H, Keane JF, Fellows KE, et al. Balloon dilatation of the aortic valve: Studies in normal lambs and in children with aortic stenosis. J Am Coll Cardiol 1987;9:816–22.
6. Lababidi Z, Daskalopoulos DA, Stoeckle H Jr. Transluminal balloon coarctation angioplasty: Experience with 27 patients. Am J Cardiol 1984;54:1288–91.
7. Saul JP, Keane JF, Fellows KE, Lock JE. Balloon dilatation angioplasty of postoperative aortic obstructions. Am J Cardiol 1987;59:943–8.
8. Cooper RS, Ritter SB, Rothe WB, et al. Angioplasty for coarctation of the aorta: Long-term results. Circulation 1987;75:600–4.

Percutaneous Balloon Angioplasty in Children with Pulmonary Valvar Stenosis

Y. S. Yun, C. Y. Hong, and K. P. Suh

Introduction

Percutaneous transluminal angioplasty was first introduced in 1964 by Dotter and Judkins.[1] Application of the technique, however, was limited by the size of the telescoping catheter. Since development of the balloon-tipped flexible catheter by Gruntzig and associates,[2] the technique of angioplasty has been widely used for relief of coronary, renal, and peripheral vascular stenoses.[3,4] Relief of pulmonary valvar stenosis by balloon dilatation during cardiac catheterization was first reported in 1982.[5] Subsequently, the results of this procedure have been reported in large series of patients with a wide range of age.[6,7] Some have been concerned with residual stenosis, but it is well recognized that there is spontaneous regression of residual systolic pressure gradients across the right ventricular outflow tract after surgical pulmonary valvotomy.[8] In this article, we describe our experience with 72 consecutive cases of congenital pulmonary valvar stenosis seen in children who underwent percutaneous balloon valvoplasty.

Patients and Methods

From September 1985 through December 1987, 72 consecutive patients (45 males and 27 females) thought to have moderate or severe pulmonary stenosis (diagnosed by auscultation, electrocardiography, and Doppler and cross-sectional echocardiography) underwent cardiac catheterization, cineangiography, and percutaneous transluminal valvoplasty. The ages ranged from 8 months to 15 years with a median age of 6.3 years. Initially we measured the diameter of the pulmonary ventriculo-arterial junction during the systolic phase by cross-sectional echocardiography and estimated transpulmonary pressure gradients by means of continuous wave Doppler studies. Thereafter, under light anesthesia, right heart catheterization was performed, the transpulmonary pressure gradient was measured, and right ventriculography achieved via an NIH sidehole catheter. Valvoplasty was then attempted following the technique described by Kan et al.[5] and Lababidi and Wu.[6] The diameters of the balloons were chosen, in most cases, to be about 20–40% greater than that of the pulmonary ventriculo-arterial junction. The entire procedure was monitored by means of fluoroscopy. After the valvoplasty, both measurements of the transpulmonary pressure gradient and right ventriculography were repeated. Follow-up by means of electrocardiography, radiography, and echocardiography were conducted at intervals of one, three and six months after the procedures.

Results

Initial valvoplasty was successful in 70 patients (97%). Two patients were resistant to dilatation and proved to have dysplastic valves during a subsequent surgical valvotomy. The transpulmonary systolic pressure gradients ranged from 15 mmHg to 250 mmHg (mean ± SD: 79 ± 47 mmHg) before dilatation, and from 4 to 140 mmHg (mean ± SD: 37 ± 21 mmHg) immediately after the

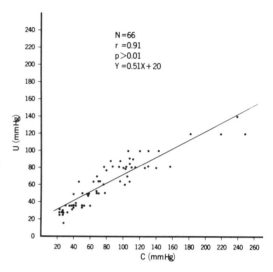

Figure 2. Correlation between the systolic pressure gradients measured at catheterization and predicted by Doppler echocardiography in 66 patients with pulmonary stenosis.

procedure (Fig. 1). There were seven patients who had residual transpulmonary systolic pressure gradients of 60 mmHg or more after the initial valvoplasty. Repeat cardiac catheterization has been performed in four of them 1 year after the initial procedure and a further decrease in the pressure gradients has been observed in two of them. Two patients with high residual gradients underwent successful repeat dilatation with a double balloon. In 21 patients, we initially used a single balloon of 20 mm diameter and failed to achieve effective dilatation. Our second attempt in these patients with a double balloon was successful. The stenotic valve orifice was too small in three patients to permit a balloon catheter of appropriate size to pass into the pulmonary trunk. In these cases, the stenotic valve was dilated successfully by means of a gradual increase in the size of the catheter employed. Good correlation ($r = 0.91$) was found between the gradients measured at catheterization and those predicted by Doppler in 66 patients (Fig. 2).

Immediately after the procedure, the murmur had been reduced to grade I in 44 patients and grade II in 23 patients. A sys-

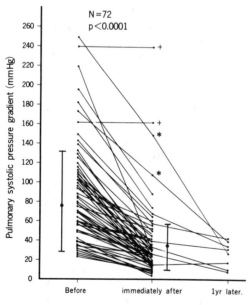

Figure 1. Pulmonary systolic pressure gradients before, immediately after, and one year after balloon dilatation of the pulmonary valve. $^{+}$ Surgical valvotomy due to dysplastic valve. * Repeat balloon dilatation 1 year later.

tolic thrill had been palpable in 50 patients before dilatation and became impalpable in 36 cases after the dilatation. A systolic click had been audible in 16 patients and disappeared in 12 after the procedure. The height of the R wave in V1 was seen to decrease rapidly during the first month after dilatation and then gradually with time. Complications were mild. Transient bradycardias and systemic hypotension occurred in all cases during inflation of the balloon, but they resolved after the balloon was deflated. A mild degree of pulmonary regurgitation (Grade I–II) was noted by Doppler echocardiography in 31 patients (44%) after the procedure. This complication had also been noted by Griffith and colleagues[8] in 70% of children after surgical valvotomy and proved not to be serious. Thus far, we have found no evidence of restenosis, and the results have been gratifying during the period of follow-up.

References

1. Dotter CT, Judkins MP. Transluminal treatment of arteriosclerotic obstruction. Description of a new technique and a preliminary report of its application. Circulation 1964; 30:654–700.
2. Gruntzig AR, Senning A, Siegenthaler WE. Nonoperative dilatation of coronary artery stenosis: Percutaneous transluminary coronary angioplasty. N Engl J Med 1979;301:61–8.
3. Tegneyer CJ, Dyer R, Teats CD, et al. Percutaneous dilatation of the renal arteries. Technique and results. Radiology 1980;135:589–99.
4. Spence RK, Freiman DB, Gatenby R, et al. Longterm results of tranluminal angioplasty of the iliac and femoral arteries. Arch Surg 1981;116:1377–86.
5. Kan JS, White RI Jr, Mitchell S, et al. Percutaneous balloon valvuloplasty: A new method for treating congenital pulmonary valve stenosis. N Engl J Med 1982;307:540–2.
6. Lababidi Z, Wu J-R: Percutaneous balloon pulmonary valvuloplasty. Am J Cardiol 1983; 52:560–62.
7. Rocchini AP, Kveselis DA, Crowley D, et al. Percutaneous balloon valvuloplasty for treatment of congenital pulmonary valvular stenosis in children. J Am Coll Cardiol 1984; 3:1005–12.
8. Griffith BP, Hardesty RL, Siewers RD, et al. Pulmonary valvulotomy alone for pulmonary stenosis; Results in children with and without muscular infundibular hypertrophy. J Thorac Cardiovasc Surg 1982;83:577–83.

Balloon Angioplasty in Very Young Patients

R. Piva and A. Pangrazi

Introduction

The use of balloon angioplasty in the dilatation of congenital heart malformations is, by now, widespread, yet experience in very young infants is still limited. We present our experience in this chapter.

Patients Studied

From February 1984 to December 1987, we attempted at least one balloon angioplasty in each of 32 critically ill infants younger than 3 months of age. A left ventricular outflow tract obstruction was present in 23, valvar in 2, and at the aortic isthmus in 21. Nine had right ventricular obstruction, which was at valvar level. The associated malformations are shown in Table 1.

Results

Two neonates, 13 and 6 days old, respectively, underwent balloon aortic valvoplasty. The procedure failed in the first because of failure to cross the valve with the balloon. A very temporary success was achieved in the other. A second procedure was necessary three days later, and this produced a satisfactory outcome such that the patient was stable when seen at latest follow-up at the age of 18 months. The initial systolic pressure gradient of 40 mmHg was completely abolished in this patient. Dilatation of aortic coarctation was performed in 21 babies whose mean age was 20 days. Of these, 14 were in the first month of life: four were up to 10 days old, six were 11 to 20 days old, and four were 21–30 days old. The procedure failed in two because of technical difficulties.

Among the 19 immediate successes, judged in terms of a residual pressure gradient less than 10 mmHg, obvious morphological change, and immediate clinical improvement, one death occurred within 24 hours. This was related to iatrogenic damage of the right common iliac artery, this being the portal for catheterization. A blood transfusion was needed at the end of the procedure in three patients, and absence of the femoral pulse on the side of the arterial puncture was irreversible in four more. Table 2 shows the clinical evolution of the patients. Another death occurred in the period immediately after the dilatation and was unrelated to the procedure. This occurred in a baby 47 days old who was in critically

Table 1

Associated Pathology

	PAPVC	ASD	VSD	AVSD	DORV	TGA	TF	SAS	HCM	PAD
AVS(2)	—	—	—	—	—	—	—	1	—	2
IS(21)	1	4	9	1	2	1	—	—	—	15
PVS(9)	—	OF9	—	—	—	—	2	—	1	8

AVS = aortic valve stenosis; IS = isthmic stenosis; PVS = pulmonary valve stenosis; PAPVC = partial anomalous pulmonary venous connection; ASD = atrial septal defect; VSD = ventricular septal defect; AVSD = atrioventricular septal defect; DORV = double-outlet right ventricle; TGA = complete transposition; TF = tetralogy of Fallot; SAS = subaortic stenosis, HCM = hypertrophic cardiomyopathy; PAD = patent arterial duct; OF = oval foramen.

poor clinical condition prior to the dilatation. Three patients underwent surgical treatment for the associated malformations within two months of the procedure, and nine other patients presented with recoarctation. Of these, two underwent surgery and seven underwent a second balloon dilatation, which has proven successful in six after a mean period of follow-up of 10 months. The remaining five immediate successes were all stable at a mean period of 20 months follow-up. Interestingly, of five patients who had a ventricular septal defect as the solitary associated cardiac malformation, spontaneous closure was observed in two and attenuation of the intracardiac shunt occurred in one. Thus, dilatation results in stable clinical improvement at a mid-term period of follow-up in 11 of the 17 surviving patients.

Balloon pulmonary valvoplasties were performed in nine infants at a mean age of 24 days. Success was presumed when the ventricular pressures final ratio was equal to or less than 1, there was substantial clinical improvement, and it proved possible to discontinue prostaglandins. On this basis, two procedures were considered failures. In a neonate, one failure was technical, while in the other patient, 2.5 months old, the dilatation was ineffective. A grossly dysplastic

Table 2

Follow-Up of Balloon Dilatation of Isthmal Coarctation

(21 patients)

Outcome	Short-term*		Mid-term
Failure (2)	2 Surgery		
Immediate success (19)	2 early deaths	related (1) / unrelated (1)	
	3 early surgery	1 complete transposition / 2 ventricular sepal defect	
	9 recoarctaction	re-dilatation (7) / surgery (2)	stable (6) → stable (10m) / surgery (1)
	5 stable		→ stable (20m)

* Within 2 months; ( ) n° of patients.

pulmonary valve and hypertrophic cardiomiopathy were present in this baby, and he died within 24 hours of the procedure because of an arrthythmic event. No iatrogenic injury was noted at autopsy. In two other patients, 1 and 3 days old respectively, the valvoplasty produced an apparent hemodynamic improvement, but their clinical condition was unstable and both underwent surgery within one week. Another patient 2-day-old with Fallot's tetralogy underwent emergency surgery because of an infundibular perforation produced during the procedure. The valvoplasty was effective in four patients, whose clinical evolution is summarized as follows: In two, the first dilatation (at the ages of 1 day and 2 months, respectively) was only temporarily successful. A second procedure was needed (at the age of 2.5 and 3 months, respectively) to achieve mild and stable residual pressure gradient (20 and 30 mmHg at the age of 30 and 36 months, respectively. One patient underwent successful dilatation at 17 days of age. This was more than one year ago, and he is now awaiting surgical repair of associated tetralogy of Fallot. The fourth neonate was submitted to a left subclavian to pulmonary arterial anastomosis and intraoperative balloon valvoplasty at the age of 1 day. When he was 13 days old, the shunt had closed and the valve was still severely stenotic. A second dilatation was performed. A severe restenosis was detected 16 months later and a third dilatation accomplished. The residual pressure gradient was 20 mmHg one year later.

Conclusions

From our limited experience, it seems that balloon angioplasty in very young patients is associated with greater technical difficulties and greater risk of anatomical damage. Nevertheless, it achieves useful neonatal palliation in life-threatening obstructive lesions of both the right and left ventricles, thus opening the door for more radical treatments later in infancy.

Experience of a Small Unit with Balloon Valvoplasty and Angioplasty in Treatment of Congenital Heart Malformations

A. Beitzke, J. I. Stein, J. Lammer, and C. Suppan

Introduction

Balloon valvoplasty and angioplasty have become the treatment of choice for treatment of certain cardiac malformations, such as valvar pulmonary stenosis or postoperative aortic coarctation.[1,2] In other lesions, such as valvar aortic stenosis or native aortic coarctation, the long-term results are less well established.[3,4] With these facts in mind, we report here our experience in a small unit with balloon valvoplasty and angioplasty with various cardiac lesions from January 1986 through June 1988.

Patients and Methods

Forty dilatations were performed in 37 patients, who were aged 8 months to 16 years and who weighed 8–52 kg. The clinical diagnoses, as determined clinically, were pulmonary stenosis in 19, aortic stenosis in nine, aortic coarctation in five, and obstruction of the superior caval vein in four pa-

tients. The indications for valvoplasty and/or angioplasty were systolic gradients of more than 50 mmHg in pulmonary and aortic stenosis, gradients over 30 mmHg in aortic coarctation, and gradients over 3 mmHg together with clinical signs of inflow obstruction for obstruction of the superior caval vein. The gradients prior to dilatation were known from previous catheterizations or from continuous wave Doppler studies. All dilatations were performed under general anesthesia. Angiograms were taken before and after the procedure, and the diameters of the balloons were selected according to the particular lesion. In pulmonary stenosis, a diameter was chosen that was 20% greater than the diameter of the ventriculo-arterial junction. In aortic stenosis, the diameter of the balloon was chosen to equal three times the diameter of the narrowest segment. Obstruction of the superior caval vein was always dilated with balloons of increasing size, which, however, never exceeded the diameter of the prestenotic segment of the vein. If the diameter of a valve was too large for a single balloon (in other words, over 20 mm), we used either a large trefoil catheter or two balloon catheters.[5] When using two balloons, we added another 20% to the calculated diameter for a single balloon, the sum being divided by two to give the diameter of each balloon. Balloon catheters were introduced, positioned, and the procedures performed as has been described previously.[1,3,6,7] A transseptal approach was used in patients with aortic stenosis so as to place an additional catheter within the left ventricle. We never attempted to pass a catheter over a freshly dilated segment of a vessel without the use of a guide wire.

Results

The age of the patients with pulmonary stenosis ranged from 11 months to 15 years, and they weighed 8.5–46 kg. Four had previously undergone surgery, two for repair of Fallot's tetralogy and two for pulmonary atresia with intact ventricular septum. A trifoil catheter was used in three patients, and a double balloon technique in one (Fig. 1a). One patient with a dysplastic valve under-

went a second dilatation which, however, was not successful. Overall, gradients of 63.0 ± 13.2 mmHg were reduced to 20.2 ± 14.6 mmHg (p < 0.0005). Systolic pressures within the right ventricle fell from 76.8 ± 22.6 mmHg to 41.3 ± 14.5 mmHg. There were no complications.

The patients with aortic stenosis ranged in age from 5 to 16 years and weighed from 18 to 52 kg. One patient had previously undergone a surgical valvotomy. Our first attempt at dilatation of aortic stenosis was completely ineffective. Thereafter, in all the patients, a mean gradient of 63.9 ± 11.4 mmHg was reduced to 31.1 ± 15.4 mmHg (p < 0.0005). A trifoil catheter was used in three patients and a double balloon technique in four (Fig. 1b). Arterial injuries occurring as a consequence of catheterization in three patients needed surgical revision, while moderate aortic incompetence developed in one patient.

Of the five patients with aortic coarctation treated by balloon angioplasty, four had developed recoarctation after a primary surgical repair in the neonatal period (two had undergone subclavian flap operations

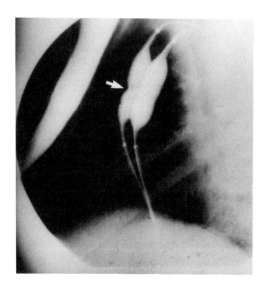 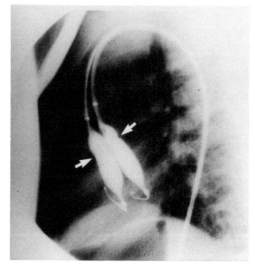

Figure 1. A lateral view of the use of a double balloon technique for dilatation of valvar pulmonary (a) and aortic (b) stenosis.

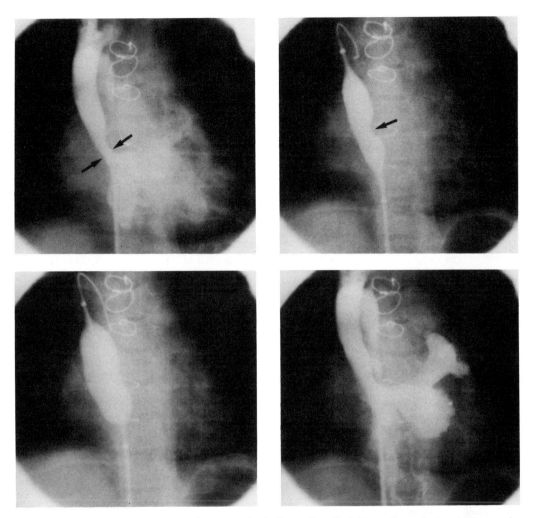

Figure 2. This sequence shows the use of a balloon for dilatation of an obstructed superior caval vein. The predilatation angiogram revealing the stenosis (arrows) as seen in the frontal projection is shown in (a). Dilatation with increasing size of the balloon and a typical waist (arrows) is seen in (b) and (c), while (d) is a postdilatation angiogram showing a good result.

while end-to-end anastomoses had been performed in the other). The remaining patient had native coarctation of the aorta. Balloon angioplasty was done one to seven years after the operative procedures and at the age of 11 months in the patient with native coarctation. Gradients of 40–60 mmHg were completely abolished in all cases. Arterial injuries occurred in two patients, and they were treated by surgical intervention and thrombolysis, respectively.

Obstruction of the superior caval vein was treated six times in four patients who had previously undergone a Senning[2] or Mustard[2] repair for complete transposition (Fig. 2a–d). The time interval between operation and dilatation was 3 months to 9 years. Gradients of 10–5 mmHg were initially reduced to 0–4 mmHg. One to two years later, however, two patients again developed signs of inflow obstruction and underwent redilatation. Gradients of 6 and 5 mmHg were reduced on this second occasion to 2 and 0 mmHg, respectively. Single balloons only were used in this group. There were no complications.

Discussion

Standards for balloon dilatation of various congenital and acquired malformations have now been established[1-8] so as to avoid damage to outflow tracts, valves, and vessel walls. A double balloon technique has been used in some lesions.[5,8] The technique has been shown to be easy to perform and without risk when used for pulmonary stenosis and gives excellent results.[1,5,7] Some rare patients with dysplastic pulmonic valves, however, respond poorly.[1] It can safely be stated that balloon valvoplasty has now replaced surgery for the treatment of valvar pulmonary stenosis.

For many patients with aortic stenosis seen in infancy and childhood, surgical valvotomy is no more than a palliative solution because of the dysplastic nature of the valves or the small size of the ventriculo-arterial junction. In these circumstances, it seems justifiable to attempt balloon valvoplasty, bearing in mind that complications of the catheterization, such as perforations, aortic incompetence, or arterial injuries, are frequent, especially in smaller children.[3,6,9] We produced three arterial complications in our nine patients along with one instance of aortic incompetence. Together with two arterial injuries in the group of patients with aortic coarctation, we produced a 33% incidence of arterial lesions when employing an arterial approach for balloon catheterization (five of 15). We have now decided to attempt balloon valvotomy for aortic stenosis only in older children with pressure gradients greater than 70 mmHg. Perhaps the double balloon technique using two smaller balloons might be a useful means of reducing arterial trauma, since arterial injuries in our hands occurred only with the use of larger single catheters. Postoperative

aortic coarctation presents little risk for balloon angioplasty since scar tissue forms around the previous site of operation. The reported results are excellent,[2] as is our own experience. Good results have also been reported for native coarctation, but late formation of aneurysms has occurred in some patients.[4,7,10] If native aortic coarctation is dilated (as in one of our cases), careful long-term observations of the configuration of the aortic arch, either by cross-sectional echocardiography or magnetic resonance imaging, is mandatory.

Small numbers of patients have undergone balloon dilatation for postoperative obstruction of the superior caval vein.[8] The initial results reported generally have been good, as endorsed by our experience, but restenoses are known to occur. Despite this, further dilatations even at repeated intervals, may be more effective than surgical reoperations.

References

1. Tynan M, Baker EJ, Rohmer J, et al. Percutaneous balloon pulmonary valvuloplasty. Br Heart J 1985;53:520–4.
2. Lock JE, Bass JL, Amplatz K, et al. Balloon dilatation angioplasty of aortic coarctations in infants and children. Circulation 1983;68:109–16.
3. Lababidi Z, Wu JR, Walls JT. Percutaneous balloon aortic valvuloplasty: Results in 23 patients. Am J Cardiol 1984;53:194–7.
4. Morrow WR, Vick III GW, Nihill MR, et al. Balloon dilation of unoperated coarctation of the aorta: Short- and intermediate-term results. J Am Coll Cardiol 1988;1:133–8.
5. Khan MAA, Al Yousef S, Mullins CE. Percutaneous transluminal balloon pulmonary valvuloplasty for the relief of pulmonary valve stenosis with special reference to double-balloon technique. Am Heart J 1986;112:158–66.
6. Choy M, Beekman RH, Rocchini AP, et al. Percutaneous balloon valvuloplasty for valvar aortic stenosis in infants and children. Am J Cardiol 1987;59:1010–3.
7. Syamasundar Rao P. Transcatheter treatment of pulmonary stenosis and coarctation of the aorta: experience with percutaneous balloon dilatation. Br Heart J 1986;56:250–8.

8. Lock JE, Bass JL, Castaneda-Zuniga W, et al. Dilatation angioplasty of congenital or operative narrowings of venous channels. Circulation 1984;70:457–64.

9. Fellows KE, Radtke W, Keane JF, Lock JE. Acute complications of catheter therapy for congenital heart disease. Am J Cardiol 1987;60:679–83.

10. Wren C, Peart I, Bain H, Hunter S. Balloon dilatation of unoperated aortic coarctation: Immediate results and one year follow-up. Br Heart J 1987;58:369–73.

Balloon Dilatation of Valved Conduits Inserted Between Right Ventricle and Pulmonary Trunk in Children

R. Hofstetter, E. Kleinhans, B. J. Messmer,
and G. von Bernuth

Introduction

Conduits bearing a bioprosthetic valve are used frequently in order to create continuity between the right ventricle and pulmonary trunk. Unfortunately, these conduits tend rapidly to become stenotic, especially in children. In an attempt to delay reoperation, we performed balloon dilatation of such valves in five children. This article describes our experience in these five patients with a follow-up between 6 and 22 months.

Patients and Methods

Four patients initially had a common arterial trunk, while one had pulmonary atresia with ventricular septal defect. The age at operation varied between 10 months and 8 years. In all, a conduit had been implanted between the right ventricle and the pulmonary arteries containing a Shiley valve in three patients and a Hancock and Tascon valve in one patient each. This was already the second conduit implanted in two pa-

tients three and five and a half years after the first operation, respectively, because of valvar stenosis. The overall data are listed in Table 1.

All children had a right ventricular thrust on physical examination along with a loud systolic murmur suggestive of insufficiency of the valve within the conduit. The chest x-ray showed calcification of the valve in three cases.

Catheterization was performed two to four years after operation. It revealed right ventricular hypertension at systemic levels with a right ventricular to systemic peak systolic pressure ratio of 0.68 or more due to conduit stenosis in all patients. Two patients had an additional stenosis at the origin of the right pulmonary artery. After measurements of pressure and angiocardiography, a balloon dilatation catheter was introduced percutaneously into the right femoral vein during the same procedure and advanced into the pulmonary trunk. The balloon was selected according to the size of the conduit. A trefoil balloon was used in one patient. After ascertaining that the catheter was positioned correctly, dilatation was performed

Table 1
Balloon Catheters used in 6 Dilatations of Stenotic Bioprosthetic Valves

Patient	Diagnosis	Age at operation (years)	Conduit valve (size)	Interval Op.-Dil. (years)	Balloon diameter (mm)
1	Common trunk	$4\frac{1}{12}$	18 Shiley	$4\frac{3}{12}$	15; 18
2	PA + VSD	$8\frac{1}{12}$[a]	20 Shiley	3	18
3	Common trunk	$\frac{10}{12}$	14 Shiley	$4\frac{1}{12}$	15
4	Common trunk	$1\frac{6}{12}$	16 Hancock	$4\frac{1}{12}$	19[Trf]; 6[b]; 8[b]
	Common trunk	$1\frac{6}{12}$	16 Hancock	$2\frac{7}{12}$	15
5	Common trunk	$7\frac{8}{12}$[a]	25 Tascon	$2\frac{1}{12}$	19; 15[b]; 19[b]

[a] Replacement of a stenotic conduit valve.
[b] Dilatation of the right pulmonary artery. Trf, Trefoil-catheter; PA + VSD, pulmonary atresia with ventricular septal defect.

one to three times while monitoring the systemic arterial pressure. The stenosis at the origin of the right pulmonary artery was also dilated using two catheters of increasing size in both cases. After dilatation, measurements of pressure and right ventricular angiography were repeated. During the period of follow-up, the right ventricular to pulmonary arterial pressure gradient was assessed by continuous-wave Doppler.

Results

The high ventricular to systemic pressure ratio was reduced significantly by dilatation of the stenotic valve within the conduit in three patients (Fig. 1). In one patient with additional stenosis of the right pulmonary artery, the pressure ratio could be reduced significantly only after redilatation seven months later. In the second patient with additional stenosis of the right pulmonary artery, the pressure ratio could not be reduced. The pressure gradient at the valve, however, was lowered significantly. Early postoperative pressure gradients between the right ventricle and the pulmonary arteries were available in four patients and the predilatation gradients in all five patients. In four of these, the gradient was higher than 50 mmHg. A gradient of only 25

mmHg was found in the fifth patient, who had a significant additional stenosis at the origin of the right pulmonary artery. The peak systolic right ventricular to systemic pressure ratio in this patient was 0.68.

Dilatation of the valve within the conduit resulted in a decrease of the right ventricular to pulmonary arterial systolic pressure gradient in all patients (Fig. 2). The patient with the smallest regression (from 59 to 42 mmHg), who had undergone dilatation with a trefoil balloon catheter, developed significant restenosis within seven months. Redilatation at that time resulted in a drop of the gradient to 33 mmHg. Within an interval of five months, however, the gradient had once more reached 56 mmHg as measured by continuous-wave Doppler echocardiography. In two other patients, postdilatation right ventricular to pulmonary arterial gradients of 25 and 33 mmHg had risen to 40 and 50 mmHg within 14 and 16 months, respectively. Thereafter, they remained stable up to 18–22 months after dilatation. The gradient in one patient dropped from 65 mmHg before to 37 mmHg immediately after dilatation and, thereafter, up to an interval of 19 months, remained at roughly 30 mmHg. The patient undergoing dilatation most recently is one of the two with additional stenosis in the right pulmonary artery. His gradient, of only 25

Balloondilatation
of Bioprosthetic Valves

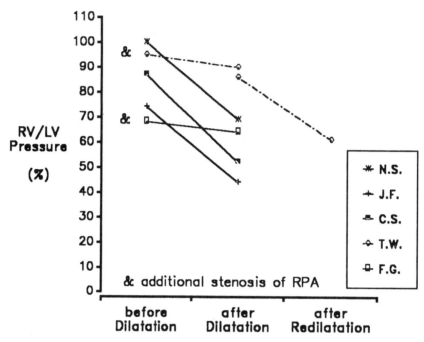

Figure 1. The ratios between right and left ventricular peak systolic pressures before and after balloon dilatation in five patients (one patient was redilated).

mmHg before dilatation, fell to 15 mmHg afterwards and remains so six months later.

Insufficiency of the valves within the conduits did not increase significantly after valvoplasty in any patient, as demonstrated by physical examination, pulmonary angiography and Doppler sonography. It should be noted that the maximal systolic pressure gradients were measured during the period of follow-up by means of continuous-wave Doppler sonography in the unsedated child. The values obtained tend to be higher than the peak-to-peak gradients obtained invasively under deep sedation. As discussed already, a stenosis at the origin of the right pulmonary artery was also dilated in two children. Predilatation right ventricular angiography in these patients had shown hypoperfusion of the right pulmonary artery.

This nearly normalized after dilatation, as demonstrated by the change in the right pulmonary arterial pressure tracing. Repeat angiography and pulmonary perfusion scintigraphy showed nearly identical perfusion with the right and left pulmonary arteries.

Complications

The balloon ruptured during the first three dilatations, possibly because of laceration by calcifications within the conduit. The rupture was longitudinal in two cases, and the catheter could easily be removed. In the third case, however, the rupture was circular, and the balloon-bearing tip of the catheter could only be withdrawn into the

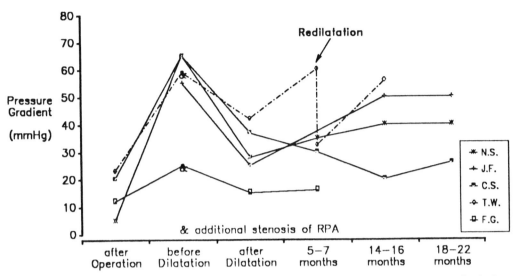

Figure 2. The pressure gradients between the right ventricle and the pulmonary arteries before and immediately after balloon dilatation occurring between 6 and 22 months after valvoplasty in five patients.

femoral vein, from where it had to be removed by surgical dissection.

The ensuing dilatations were performed using stiffer guidewires in order to minimize kinking of the filled balloon by right ventricular contractions. We used a trefoil catheter in one patient, presuming that rupture of all three balloons would be unlikely and that incomplete obstruction of the conduit by the inflated balloon might reduce stress on the right ventricle during dilatation.[1] At the present time, however, it is impossible to decide whether use of a trefoil catheter has any advantage over the conventional catheters when used in this situation.

Discussion

Conduits containing bioprosthetic valves, when implanted during childhood, tend to become stenotic within relatively short intervals thus necessitating early reo-

perations.[2] As an alternative, we (along with two other groups,[3,4]) performed balloon dilatation of the stenosed valves in five children, producing a satisfactory decrease in the gradient of right ventricular to pulmonary arterial pressures in each. The conduit was dilated twice within seven months in one patient. In this, and in another patient, additional stenosis at the origin of the right pulmonary artery was also dilated. The results suggest that dilatation of stenosed valves may delay replacement of stenosed valved conduits for a limited period which, for a growing child, is certainly an advantage.

It should be noted, nonetheless, that dilatation of a valve within a calcified conduit carries a higher risk of rupture of the balloon than does dilatation of a native pulmonary valve. The balloon ruptured during dilatation in all our first three patients. In one of these cases, the rupture was circular, and the catheter could only be removed by surgical dissection of the femoral vein. This particular problem was also encountered by Lloyd and his coworkers.[4] In their series of six dilatations, two ruptures occurred and one of these was circular. In this latter case, the catheter could only be removed by dissection of the iliac vein.

References

1. Jonas RA, Freed MD, Mayer JE, Castaneda AR. Long-term follow-up of patients with synthetic right heart conduits. Circulation 1985;72 (suppl II):77–83.

2. Meier B, Friedli B, Oberhansll I. Trefoil balloon for aortic valvuloplasty. Br Heart J 1986; 56:292–3.

3. Waldman JD, Schoen FJ, Kirkpatrick SE, et al. Balloon dilatation of porcine bioprosthetic valves in the pulmonary position. Circulation 1987;76:109–14.

4. Lloyd TR, Marvin WJ, Mahoney LT, Lauer RM. Balloon dilatation valvuloplasty of bioprosthetic valves in extracardiac conduits. Am Heart J 1987;114:268–74.

Percutaneous Balloon Angioplasty in Postoperative Patients with Pulmonary Arterial Stenosis Following the Fontan Procedure

U. Squarcia, A. Agnetti, L. Zavota, N. Carano, and C. Cavalli

Introduction

The Fontan procedure represents a good surgical alternative for a large number of congenital heart malformations. The operative mortality is low, but the long-term fate of the patients depends upon many factors.[1-4] One of the most important is a completely unobstructed flow of blood from the caval veins and the right atrium into the pulmonary circuit. Obstruction of either a conduit or a direct anastomosis between right atrium and pulmonary arteries and/or the development of peripheral pulmonary stenoses (generally at the site of a previous systemic-to-pulmonary shunt) are among the most relevant complications of the Fontan operation. Pressure gradients in the pulmonary circuit are not well tolerated, and even mild gradients at rest may increase significantly with exercise[5] and cause severe congestive heart failure. The experience described in this chapter concerns two patients with previous systemic-to-pulmonary shunts who had a Fontan procedure and, subsequently, developed severe congestive heart failure over the period of a few months after the surgery.

Methods and Results

The first patient is 15 years old, with double-inlet ventricle and pulmonary atresia in the setting of a right-sided heart, and had had a Potts operation at the age of 22 months and a Fontan procedure at the age of 15 years. The second patient, a 10-year-old girl with tricuspid atresia and pulmonary stenosis, underwent a Waterston shunt at the age of 1 year and a Fontan operation seven years later.

In the first case, the hemodynamic and angiographic study revealed almost complete exclusion of the left pulmonary arteries due to a dual peripheral arterial stenosis. In the second case, a solitary segment of stenosis was seen at the origin of the left pulmonary artery. The gradients between the right atrium and peripheral pulmonary arteries were 16 and 14 mmHg, respectively.

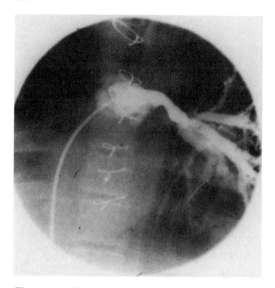
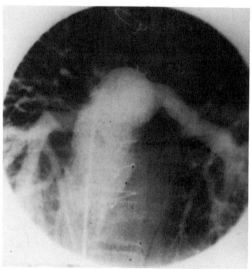

Figure 1. First patient: Selective injection of contrast medium in the left pulmonary artery shows the dual peripheral stenoses (left). Injection after the dilatation shows that the stenoses have disappeared (right).

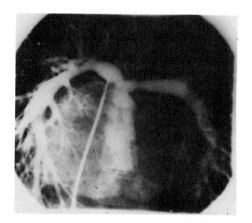
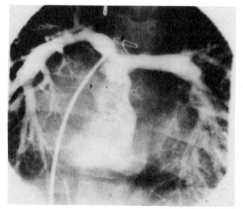

Figure 2. Second patient: The stenosis at the origin of the left pulmonary artery (left), is almost completely obliterated after the dilatation (right).

Table 1
Patient Data

	Predilatation				Postdilatation			
N	PA diameter (mm)	RA–PA gradient (mmHg)	RA pressure (mmHg)	C.I. (L/min/m²)	PA diameter (mm)	RA–PA gradient (mmHg)	RA pressure (mmHg)	C.I. (L/min/m²)
1	5.8 4.4	16	38/16	2.0	12.4 11.7	2	32/14	3.3
2	3.6	14	25/12	2.0	9.5	2	20/12	2.2

PA: pulmonary arteries; RA: right atrium; CI: cardiac index.

The diameters of the stenotic segments were measured from the angiograms, and a balloon catheter about four to five times the diameter of the stenotic area was used for dilatation. The pressures of inflation ranged from four to six atmospheres and the time of dilation ranged from 12 to 20 seconds of maximum inflation. The procedure was repeated six to seven times for each area of stenosis. Both gradients dropped to 2 mmHg after dilatation and angiography showed enlargement of the previous stenotic segments by more than 100% (Figs. 1 and 2). A significant clinical improvement was noted a few hours after the procedures. The pre- and postdilatation data are shown in Table 1.

Discussion

The Fontan operation has changed significantly the natural course of many complex malformations, but the absence of the right ventricle predicates a chronic instability in the hemodynamic status of those treated in this way. The best results are seen when all the criteria for operability are met, so that the pressures in the systemic venous circuit and in the right atrium will not increase above 15 mm of mercury. In this situation, therefore, even minimal subsequent hemodynamic changes may have a marked detrimental effect on the immediate or midterm postoperative course. Peripheral pulmonary stenosis, often occurring at the site of a previous systemic-to-pulmonary arterial shunt, can represent an important factor in further elevation of the systemic venous pressure and can cause severe congestive heart failure, as observed in both our patients.

In the face of an unfavorable postoperative course after a Fontan procedure, a peripheral pulmonary stenosis must be listed among the likely causes and cardiac catheterization is mandatory. If identified,

surgical correction of a pulmonary arterial stenosis is a major procedure which carries a considerable risk. Furthermore, the results are uncertain, depending largely upon the site of the obstruction.

Our experience, although limited, proves that percutaneous balloon dilatation has to be considered the natural choice of treatment in patients developing pulmonary arterial stenosis after the Fontan procedure. Recent experience[6-8] suggests that the best results are obtained when catheters with balloons of large diameter (four to five times the diameter of the stenosis) are used for dilatation. Furthermore, inflation should be maintained as long as possible, and the balloon should be positioned so that the stenotic area is at its middle, where the force of dilatation is maximal.

References

1. De Vivie ER, Ruppzath G. Long-term results after Fontan procedure and its modifications. J Thorac Cardiovasc Surg 1986;91:690-7.
2. Juaneda E, Haworth SG. Pulmonary vascular structure in patients dying after Fontan procedure. Br Heart J 1984;52:575-80.
3. Matsuda H, Kawashima Y, Kishimoto H, et al. Problems in the modified Fontan operation for univentricular heart of the right ventricular type. Circulation 1987;76(suppl III):45-52.
4. Warnes CA, Somerville J. Tricuspid atresia in adolescents and adults: Current state and late complications. Br Heart J 1986;56:535-43.
5. Shachar GB, Fuhrman BP, Wang Y, et al. Rest and exercise hemodynamics after the Fontan procedure. Circulation 1982;65:1043-8.
6. D'Orsogna L, Sandor GG, Cutham JAG et al. Successful balloon angioplasty of peripheral pulmonary stenosis in Williams syndrome. Am Heart J 1987;114:647-8.
7. Locke JE, Castaneda-Zuniga WR, Fuhzman BP, et al. Balloon dilatation angioplasty of hypoplastic and stenotic pulmonary arteries. Circulation 1983;67:962-7.
8. Rocchini AP, Kveselis D, MacDonald D, et al. Use of balloon angioplasty to tract peripheral pulmonary stenosis. Am J Cardiol 1984; 54:1069-73.

Transcatheter Closure of Persistent Arterial Duct without Thoracotomy (Porstmann's Procedure) in Children

M. Kumate, K. Ohishi, E. Yamamoto, A. Ohryoji, F. Andou,
S. Aoyagi, and K. Kosuga

Introduction

The technique of transcatheter closure of the arterial duct was invented by Porstmann and his colleagues in 1968[1] and was introduced in Japan by Takamiya[2] in 1973. We have now performed the procedure in 179 patients since December 1974, failing in only 10 cases (5.6%), to give a rate of success of 94.4%. Most of our failures occurred during the early stages when the technique could be considered experimental. More recently, we have used a new set of more stringent criteria to select patients for closure and the rate of success has become 100%. In this chapter, we will describe the findings in the 95 of the 179 patients who were children under 16 years of age.

Method

Porstmann's procedure is, in essence, the technique of using a catheter to insert a plug made of Ivalon sponge into the persis-tent arterial duct, thus producing its closure (Fig. 1). Patients undergo spinal anesthesia and the catheter is introduced via a small incision (approximately 4–5 cm) on the right side of the inguinal line. Then, having passed the catheter through the femoral and inferior caval veins into the right atrium, it is maneuvered through the right ventricle and the persistent duct (Fig. 1A) into the descending aorta. Further threading then permits the tip of the catheter to be removed from the femoral artery, thus producing a transductal loop.[3] A 0.4-mm-diameter piano guide wire is then inserted into the loop and the Ivalon plug attached to the guide wire, using an applicator to protect the femoral artery during its insertion. The plug is then fed along the guide wire into the open duct, advancing it by means of a second "pushing" catheter (Fig. 1B). Having pushed the plug into the duct by means of the pushing catheter from the arterial side, it is anchored in the duct by pulling the entire loop towards the venous side (Fig. 1C). Radiopaque contrast medium is injected at this point to confirm the fixation of the plug within the duct. If

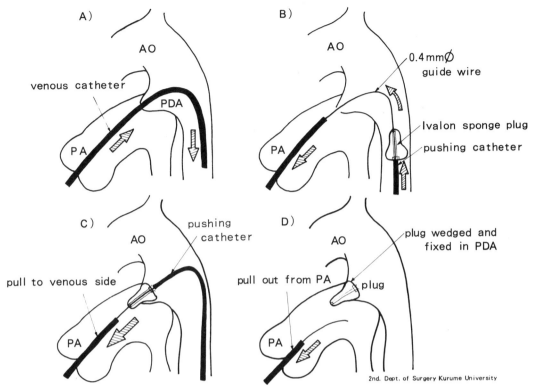

Figure 1. Diagram showing the technique of insertion of the Ivalon plug. AO, aorta; PA, pulmonary trunk; PDA, arterial duct.

insertion is judged satisfactory, the guide wire is withdrawn towards the venous side, leaving the plug firmly inserted and closing the duct (Fig. 1D). The pushing catheter is then removed, and the femoral artery is closed with an over-and-over running suture. The loop is removed from the venous side, and the groin opening is closed, thus completing the operation.

Purpose

Porstmann's procedure has the advantages that the duct is closed without leaving any surgical scar on the chest and with minimal operative influences on the patient.[1,2] Since persistent patency of the ductus is quite frequent among females, the procedure is also aesthetically advantageous. Another advantage is that it is safe in the aged and can be used in cases of recanalization of a previously closed duct. Its disadvantages are that it cannot be used until the patients grow to a certain body size and that it is not suitable for closure of either the oversized duct or those already complicated by pulmonary hypertension.[4,5] This latter point is important in determining the applicability of the technique for children. Initially, the criteria we used to judge suitability were weight over 20 kg, age over 4 years, a shunt ratio below 60% and the pulmonary to systemic pressure ratio below 60%. Now, so as to establish more stringent criteria, we have examined statistically the results in our 95 patients under the age of 16.

Clinical Material

Of the 95 ducts closed in patients between the ages of 4 and 16, 89 cases (93.7%) were successful and six (6.3%) were unsuccessful. We compared the features of those undergoing successful closure under the age of 16 with, respectively, the patients suffering unsuccessful closure under 16, those closed successfully above the age of 16 (80 cases), and a group of patients undergoing surgical closure; the operations were performed over the same period as the cases treated by transcatheter closure.

Results

The results of our analysis are shown in Table 1. The significant differences in weight and height found in those closed successfully over the age of 16 are obviously due to the difference in age of the patients. We also found that the cardiothoracic ratio and the diameters of the duct were significantly greater in the older age patients. It follows from this that the larger the body, the greater are the indications for this procedure. These findings also indicate that the diameter of the duct does not decrease with increasing age. The pulmonary to systemic pressure ratio is smaller in the older than in the younger group of patients. This is probably because blood pressure increases as one gets older and is sometimes accompanied by systemic hypertension. All of the differences noted with the group of patients having surgical closure were significant. For cases such as these, with a large persistent arterial duct, small bodies, and high values in all the featured parameters, therefore, surgical closure must still be recommended. When compared with the patients having an unsuccessful attempted closure, the "failed" patients showed significantly higher diameters for the persistent duct, greater systolic to pulmonary arterial pressures, and increased pulmonary to systemic pressure ra-

tios. The same result was found when we conducted similar statistical analysis for the entire 179 cases having the Porstmann procedure. Our overall analysis of the correlations between the various parameters permitted us to construct the formula shown at the bottom of Table 1. Weight is correlated with the size of the femoral artery. The larger the size, the more easily this procedure can be performed. In contrast, if the systolic pulmonary arterial pressure is high and the duct is large, then difficulties must be anticipated. When considered in terms of this formula, the successful cases all showed indicated values under 10, whereas most of the cases attempted without success, and most of those undergoing surgical closure, showed values between 10 and 300. The formula, therefore, has proved to be a reliable index for determining the suitability of the procedure. In brief, if the calculated value is less than 10, the procedure can be expected to prove successful.

Discussion

In collaboration with our department of pediatrics, it is now our policy to perform surgical closure of the duct at an early stage for all those who are under 1 year of age exhibiting congestive heart failure. When the shunt can be controlled medically, however, we wait for the patients to reach a size at which Porstmann's procedure becomes feasible. During this period, the patients are carefully monitored and, if the congestive heart failure is aggravated, if the systolic pulmonary arterial pressure begins to increase, or if there is evidence of infective endocarditis, we immediately perform surgical closure. When used in this way, the procedure has been shown to be both safe and advantageous, with minimal operative influences on the patients. In the 89 children undergoing a successful procedure, the heart murmur along with the symptoms disappeared as soon as the plug was inserted into the persistent duct. The average length

Table 1

Parameters Measured in Various Groups and Formula Devised to Determine Suitability of the Technique

	Porstmann's procedure successful < 16 yr n = 89	Porstmann's procedure failed < 16 yr n = 6		Surgical division < 16 yr n = 83		Porstmann's procedure successful ≥ 16 yr n = 80	
Age (years)	9.40 ± 3.04	11.16 ± 6.79	N.S.	2.63 ± 2.53	$p < 0.01$	19.09 ± 13.43	$p < 0.01$
Weight (kg)	29.16 ± 16.65	28.50 ± 9.11	N.S.	10.49 ± 5.58	$p < 0.01$	50.04 ± 8.31	$p < 0.01$
Height (cm)	129.97 ± 15.62	131.16 ± 13.37	N.S.	83.93 ± 20.09	$p < 0.01$	155.03 ± 7.97	$p < 0.01$
CTR (%)	48.50 ± 5.18	54.66 ± 5.50	$p < 0.05$	58.79 ± 5.08	$p < 0.01$	51.52 ± 6.39	$p < 0.01$
Systolic PAP (mmHg)	32.39 ± 10.04	57.16 ± 28.90	$p < 0.01$	62.55 ± 26.29	$p < 0.01$	30.62 ± 9.91	N.S.
Shunt ratio (%)	41.35 ± 16.76	48.35 ± 27.49	N.S.	58.88 ± 14.86	$p < 0.01$	44.89 ± 15.54	N.S.
Qp/Qs	2.01 ± 1.22	2.55 ± 1.09	N.S.	2.98 ± 1.49	$p < 0.01$	2.04 ± 0.83	N.S.
Rp/Rs (%)	14.60 ± 7.00	23.33 ± 17.10	$p < 0.05$	23.90 ± 14.90	$p < 0.01$	13.70 ± 6.70	N.S.
Pp/Ps (%)	26.60 ± 8.60	46.30 ± 25.5	$p < 0.01$	55.30 ± 22.80	$p < 0.01$	24.80 ± 8.60	$p < 0.05$
PDA diameter (mm)	3.69 ± 0.92	7.50 ± 3.39	$p < 0.01$	6.91 ± 2.70	$p < 0.01$	4.66 ± 1.87	$p < 0.01$
PDAD (mm) × Pp/Ps (%) / Weight (kg)	3.367 ± 2.436	12.181 ± 3.677	$p < 0.01$	45.431 ± 39.072	$p < 0.01$	2.397 ± 1.658	$p < 0.01$

of hospitalization is about 10 days. To date, there have been no instances of recanalization or surgical complications and, on follow-up, the patients are growing at the expected rates. Mortality is zero and postprocedural results are all excellent. It is a great pleasure for us to describe our experience with such satisfactory results.

References

1. Porstmann W, Wierny L, Warnke H. Der Verschluss des ductus arteriosus persistent ohne thoracotomie 2. Fortschr Roentgenstr 1968; 109:133–48.
2. Takamiya M. Ductus closure without thoracotomy. Jpn J Thorac Surg 1973;26:749–53.
3. Shimizu Y, Suehiro S, Ohashi H, et al. Closure of PDA of window type by a Porstmann method and a technical improvement of catheter manipulation: A case report. Jpn J Thorac Surg (in press) (Japanese).
4. Porstmann W, Hieronymi K, Wierny L, et al. Nonsurgical closure of oversized patient ductus arteriosus with pulmonary hypertension: Report of a case. Circulation 1974;50:376–81.
5. Naito Y, Okamoto S, Kamo Y, et al. Closure of patent ductus arteriosus of window type with artificial plug without thoracotomy: A case report Shinzo (Heart) 1974;6:1614–8 (Japanese).

Use of Rashkind Umbrella Device for Closure of Arterial Duct

C. E. Mullins

Introduction

The nonsurgical occlusion of the patent arterial duct, some atrial septal defects, and many abnormal systemic to pulmonary and systemic arterial to venous communications can be accomplished in the cardiac catheterization laboratory. All of these procedures are still considered investigational. Devices designed for the closure of atrial septal defects have been available for almost 14 years. Each device to date, however, has had significant problems with delivery, and none has gained wide clinical usage. The first of these, developed by King et al. in 1975,[1] required a very large (greater than 20 French) catheter for delivery and was very rigid in its implanted configuration. A different device, developed by Rashkind, utilizes a slightly smaller catheter for delivery but attaches to the septum by means of tiny fishhooks.[2] These hooks, unfortunately, had a tendency to catch on other structures within the left atrium, so that six of the first nine attempted implants proved unsuccessful. Because of this problem, and with the development of what appears to be a far superior and safer device for closure of atrial septal defects, the hooked device and the elective trials of its use have virtually been abandoned.

The most successful and most promising of all the techniques for nonsurgical occlusion of congenital malformations, therefore, has been that used for closure of the arterial duct. Porstmann et al. first described a technique for this procedure in 1968.[3] Although this technique is still in use in several centers (Kumate et al. Chapter 1.9), it required a very large and very complex system for its delivery, involving a combined approach through arterial and venous pathways. As a consequence, this system never gained wide clinical usage or acceptance. Rashkind independently developed a smaller device and reported the successful closure of a duct in a 3.5-kg infant in 1975. Rashkind's device was modified and became the subject of a collaborative clinical investigational trial in 1981. The use of this device, including its modifications and the results of its use at Texas Children's Hospital, the primary center, are detailed in this chapter.

Patients and Methods

As of May 1988, 147 patients have undergone attempted closure of an arterial duct at Texas Children's Hospital. All patients over 8 kg (as well as several smaller patients) who presented with patency of the duct were accepted for attempted occlusion. Their age ranged between 4 months and 76 years and their weights from 3.7 to 100 kg. The duct varied in diameter from 1.5 to 9.0 mm and occurred in all varieties of shape, length, and configuration. No patients were excluded from an attempt at transcatheter occlusion because of ductal size or configuration. The present device used for occlusion, a modification of the original device designed by Rashkind, is a double umbrella, each one activated by springs. The struts of the umbrellas are stainless steel, and the fabric is composed of polyurethane foam. The two umbrellas fold away from each other in opposing directions for delivery. The opened device is secured in the duct by the opposing spring mechanisms as the umbrellas open.

A transvenous approach is used routinely in all patients at Texas Children's Hospital. After the size and anatomy of the duct are established, a long 8 French Mullins' transseptal sheath is advanced through the right heart from the femoral vein and is threaded through the duct into the descending aorta. It is advanced over either an 8 French catheter or a dilator. Once the tip of the sheath is in the descending aorta, the catheter or dilator is removed. The sheath is allowed to bleed back and is then attached to the system used for flushing.

The occluding device is then attached to the delivery wire, collapsed and then loaded into the distal metal pod of the catheter used for delivery, using a specially designed device for the mechanism of loading. The delivery catheter is introduced into the previously positioned long sheath and advanced until the pod containing the collapsed device reaches the area of the right atrium. The catheter is fixed in this position while the delivery wire within the catheter is advanced. This maneuver advances the still-collapsed device into the sheath, which now serves as an extension of the delivery catheter. The tip of the sheath should, at this time, be in the descending aorta just at the aortic end of the duct. The delivery wire is carefully advanced further until the legs of the distal umbrella are seen to spring open (perpendicular to the sheath) as they extend out of the sheath. The entire system (sheath, catheter, delivery wire, and attached device) are then withdrawn carefully as a single unit until the open legs are seen to bend or flex in the duct. The delivery wire is then fixed in this position while the sheath is carefully withdraw several centimeters. This allows all of the legs of the proximal umbrella to open on the pulmonary side of the duct and fixes the device in the duct. The extent of fixation is tested by a gentle to-and-from motion of the delivery wire. When the operator is confident that the device is secure, the release mechanism is activated. The delivery wire and sheath are then carefully withdrawn. An aortogram is performed in the descending aorta adjacent to the duct to confirm the site of the device and occlusion of the duct.

Results

Occlusion has been attempted in 147 patients at Texas Children's since 1981. Initially there were difficulties with the devices themselves, in the techniques of delivery, and with embolization of the devices. These problems resulted in changes in the design of both the device and its delivery technique. In the last 112 patients, there have been no embolizations. Delivery has been 96% successful and has resulted in 83% total occlusion of the duct. After 6–12 months, the majority of the ducts not completely closed are not dectable by auscultation, being seen only by means of high-quality color flow echo/Doppler examination or angiographic studies. There are already proposals for further changes in technique and design that should totally eliminate these tiny residual leaks. Failure of the technique in six patients left residual shunts that were larger and that could be detected at auscultation. A second device has been used in those patients after intervals of 6–18 months with successful occlusion of the residual defect.

Discussion

Even with the early embolizations, there were no complications ensuing from either the device or its delivery that resulted in any permanent sequelae or prolongation of hospitalization. In the early experience, those patients suffering embolization of the device underwent surgical removal of the device along with a standard surgical repair of the still patent duct. In the more recent cases, the errant devices have been removed using a long sheath retrieval system and the duct has been occluded with a second device.

There are currently 12 centers utilizing the device designed for closure of the duct, collaborating so as to produce a carefully controlled study. The positive experience from this study should result in approval of the Rashkind device by the United States Federal Drug Administration by the fall of 1988. As more operators in more centers become trained and gain experience, it should become accepted as the standard treatment of a patent arterial duct in patients weighing more than 8–10 kg.

References

1. King TD, Thompson SL, Steiner C, Mills NL. Secundum atrial septal defect: nonoperative closure during cardiac catheterization. J Am Med Assoc 1976;235:2506–9.
2. Rashkind WJ. Transcatheter treatment of congenital heart disease. Circulation 1983;67:711–16.
3. Porstmann W, Wierny L, Warnke H: Der Verschluss des ductus arteriosus persisters ohne thoracotomie 2. Fortschr Roentgenstr 1968; 109:133–48.

Transcatheter Closure of Congenital Cardiac Defects

J. E. Lock

Introduction

Between May 1984 and March 1988, we attempted transcatheter closure in 195 patients with various congenital cardiac defects. Coil embolization of vessels or shunts was attempted in 104, while umbrella closure of various lesions was tried in the other 91. Over the last four years, we have modified our methodology for coil embolization using slightly oversized coils in all vessels; preshaped or balloon tipped catheters have been employed so that their tips can be secured distally in each vessel whenever possible; the coils have been soaked in topical thrombin whenever the vessel, prior to delivery, was receiving high flow; the distal part of the coil has been delivered into a very short vessel with subsequent nestling of a coil into the aortic end of extremely short systemic pulmonary collaterals; and balloons have been used to occlude the distal end of Blalock-Taussig shunts prior to attempting coil embolization.

Coil Embolization

Using the modifications outlined above, we attempted to close 104 vessels, including 76 aortopulmonary collateral arteries, 16 Blalock-Taussig shunts, 10 arteriovenous malformations, and 2 venous structures producing cyanosis. Complete occlusion of all vessels was achieved in 76% of cases and subtotal or partial occlusion in a further 20%. Blalock-Taussig shunts were the least likely to be completely closed (65%) as opposed to aortopulmonary collateral arteries, which were closed in 82% of cases. Late follow-up suggested that virtually all vessels with complete or subtotal occlusion remained completely closed on late follow-up and some vessels with partial occlusion progressed to complete closure. Only two cases that were completely or subtotally closed had persistent flow on late follow-up. During this period of time, 10 patients were found to have vessels requiring closure, but with anatomy that has unfavorable for coil embolization.

There were no deaths due to attempted coil embolization. One patient developed severe hemolysis after a deliberate partial embolization of a Blalock-Taussig shunt in an attempt to reduce pulmonary blood flow. Six coils have been inadvertently embolized, five to the lungs and one to the femoral artery. Four of the six were retrieved using catheter techniques through local cutdowns, while the other two have been left and remain without producing pulmonary disability. These results indicate that a large majority of aortopulmonary collateral arteries, Blalock-Taussig shunts, and arteriovenous fistulas can be closed using coil techniques.

Umbrella Closure

Umbrella closure was attempted in 91 patients: 65 with a patent arterial duct, 8 with an intraatrial defect, 8 with ventricular septal defects, and 10 with miscellaneous lesions. Inadvertent embolization to the distal pulmonary arteries occurred in three of the first 10 cases and in two of the subsequent 81. Technical modifications included the use of topical thrombin in high-flow lesions (including the patent arterial duct); balloon occlusion of the site of fixation of the umbrella whenever possible to promote thrombosis; advancement of the long sheath over the guiding wire just prior to release of devices used for ductal closure so as to reduce the chance of snaring the guidewire in the foam; and balloon sizing of most defects to measure the "stretched" diameter rather than its diameter as seen angiographically. Three patients with muscular ventricular septal defects (who had previously undergone surgery or had suffered recent myocardial infarctions) died after placement of the umbrella, although none of the deaths was due, apparently, to closure with the umbrella. No other fatalities occurred.

In the specific subset of patients with a restrictive patent arterial duct, using the recent modifications, we attempted 40 consecutive closures transvenously, 32 of them on an outpatient basis. Complete closure of the duct was achieved in all without complication as judged by auscultation, angiography, or color flow Doppler.

Conclusions

The recent modifications have increased the range of defects that can be successfully closed using transcatheter techniques and have improved the safety of the procedures. Further modifications may allow extension of these techniques to the patient with routine interatrial communications within the oval fossa ("secundum" defects).

II

Imaging in Congenital Heart Disease

2.1

Introduction

P. H. Heintzen

The hands of a cardiovascular surgeon—who is, ideally, a craftsman, artist, and scientist at the same time—are guided by recognizing, judging, and matching images. These images are constructed in his mind, based upon the diagnostic information provided prior to operation, on his experience and on his creative concepts of how best to correct the expected anomaly. The real image of the three dimensional structure then confronts him at the time of the operation. This need for proper imaging, which is both reliable and of high quality, is indispensable for successful cooperation between the pediatric cardiologist and the cardiovascular surgeon.

The rapid evolution of new (and the permanent improvement of old) imaging techniques for the analysis of structure and function of the cardiovascular system mandates that the pediatric cardiologist develop a rationale according to which the specific potential of each of these modalities can be optimally used for arriving at the most direct and comfortable, and yet safe and reliable, way of providing the relevant information about the anatomic abnormality to be corrected and its functional consequences. Imaging, however, should always remain one method within the family of diagnostic procedures, which start with inspection, palpation, auscultation, and proper electrocardiographic recordings. Furthermore, no single method of imaging alone can be expected to answer all the questions or to replace all the other methods. This is particularly true for echocardiography, just because it is such an attractive, valuable, and truly noninvasive method (transesophageal approaches excluded), and which, without question, has revolutionized the rationale of diagnosis in pediatric cardiology.

Sound training in and knowledge of the anatomy, pathophysiology, and hemodynamics of congenital heart diseases, as well as sound information about the history and results of clinical investigations, however, are essential before the echocardiographer even takes the transducer into the hand! The seemingly easy means of obtaining information about the cardiac abnormality could become dangerous if a trend developed for the widespread application of the technique by inexperienced persons.

In this section, therefore, the critical article by Carminati outlines well the potential of cross-sectional echocardiography in the hands of the well-trained cardiologist, stressing the importance of a systematic, segmental approach for analyzing the "basic anatomy" of the atriums, ventricles, and great arteries, which sometimes give a clue also to the "downstream" anatomy. But the major pitfalls and limitations of this method and the frequent need for supplementary information provided by Doppler techniques and/or angiocardiography are emphasized.

It seems to me that there is an even greater potential danger for misusing or overinterpreting the images obtained by the technique of "color coded flow mapping". It starts with the misleading term, "flow" mapping, for what is at best the integrated mapping of velocity by recordings of Doppler shifts. Why not change that labeling to "color coded echo Doppler imaging" (or velocity mapping), at least at the present stage of development of the technique?

With the lack of standardization of the equipment, the different means of processing the signal, the changing philosophy of assigning colors to the complex integrated Doppler signals, we should be very careful with the interpretation and, in particular, with the quantification of the colorful but often ambiguous images.

It can also be said that these critical remarks are equally valid for all methods that currently produce measurements from images. With regard to color-coded echocardiography, Sahn, in his article, provides an excellent overview that shows what can be achieved by an experienced investigator applying the best available technologies. Without doubt, the use of this method adds extremely valuable information to standard cross-sectional echocardiography and facilitates the quantitative analysis of pressure gradients and the evaluation of flow and shunt volumes by pulsed and continuous wave Doppler techniques.

In the chapter concerned with fetal echocardiography, the unique experience of Allan demonstrates what can now be achieved even in prenatal ultrasonic studies. With the appropriate skill and expertise, a high success rate (which is imperative in this field) can be achieved in arriving at the correct diagnosis of cardiac malformations, information which has most important implications. On the basis of the results described in this chapter, one cannot help discussing the question of whether it would be more humane to improve the prenatal diagnostic competence in more centers than to start with new surgical activites, at least before the day-to-day problems of handling the less complex malformations are optimally solved.

The contributions of Ungerleider and Rossi and their colleagues add further information about the broad and useful applicability of echocardiographic techniques before and during corrective surgery for congenital cardiac malformations.

Resonance imaging is the other fascinating "noninvasive," but still, in some ways, experimental technique. But Chung states self-critically in her presentation that it will never replace echocardiography, nor will it—to my belief—even in combination with echocardiography, replace heart catheterization and angiocardiography. We are confronted during a transitional period, therefore, probably with a "diagnostic overkill" by an imaging method before the true place and indications for each of the various methods are found and generally accepted.

At the present time, we are at a stage where the advocates of the various methods try to demonstrate what can be achieved and what is possible from a specific method. This is certainly worthwhile and cannot be replaced by mere theoretical considerations. But what is possible is not necessarily the best, the most convenient, the safest, or the most economic way of obtaining the relevant information for a given patient, or for the group of patients for which the pediatric cardiologist would be responsible.

In any case, if resonance imaging finally becomes the method of choice for preoperative diagnostic of congenital cardiovascular anomalies, the unit for pediatric cardiology, which now houses the facilities for all relevant diagnostic investigation, including heart catheterization, could not afford their own equipment for magnetic resonance and, therefore, would again become dependent on the general radiologist for making the essential decisions.

I believe that resonance imaging will, for the foreseeable future, remain an additional tool in those places where the equipment is available, but it will not be an essential tool required for the solution of our present diagnostic problems. Nevertheless, pioneering activities, such as those documented by Chung, are justified to prove or disprove such predictions. Under these various circumstances, it can be asked if so-called, "invasive techniques" still have a place in the methodologic arsenal of the pediatric cardiologist. As shown in the articles of Fellows and Buersch, the clear answer is: Yes. The indications, nonetheless, have to be adapted continuously to the change in technology, be it the less invasive nature of digital angiocardiography, the progress in the competitive methods or the changing requirements with respect to new diagnostic needs. Digital subtraction angiography is just the tip of the iceberg with respect to the potential of digital functional imaging. In any case, after the usual transition period, digital electronic angiocardiographic imaging techniques employing digital electronics will become the method of choice for the critical, quantitative studies of the dynamic geometric and hemodynamic abnormalities seen in most of the complex cardiovascular malformations needing operation or reoperation. This will certainly be the case for the study of the coronary circulation.

Assessment of Heart Diseases in Children by Cross-Sectional Echocardiography

M. Carminati

Cross-Sectional Echocardiography

Cross-sectional echocardiography is a well-established tool for the diagnosis of congenital heart defects. If the examination follows the precepts of the sequential segmental approach, the "basic anatomy" can be assessed in virtually all patients.[1] The atrial arrangement[2] is usually determined by indirect means (position of inferior caval vein and abdominal aorta with respect to the spine), although the direct visualization of the morphology of atrial appendages is sometimes possible. Both type and mode of atrioventricular connections can be readily diagnosed. In this respect, cross-sectional echocardiography is the best technique for visualizing the internal "crux" of the heart.[3] Identification of ventricular morphology in hearts with biventricular atrioventricular connections is obtained by one or more of the following criteria: position of attachment of the septal leaflets of the atrioventricular valves; the morphology of those valves and their cordal attachments; the arrangement of their papillary muscles and the trabecular patterns of the apical parts of the ventricles.[4]

In cases with univentricular atrioventricular connections, a second rudimentary ventricle is usually present which is anterosuperior with univentricular connection to a dominant left ventricle and posteroinferior when the atrial chambers are connected only to a dominant right ventricle. The position of the rudimentary ventricle is the most reliable echocardiographic guide for identification of the morphology of the dominant ventricle.[3] The great arteries can be recognized by their peripheral branching patterns. The accurate assessment of intracardiac anatomy also includes the identification and description of abnormal relationship. These are particularly frequent in association with abnormal connections, such as seen in so-called "criss-cross" hearts and "superoinferior" ventricles.[5]

A complete evaluation of intracardiac, and particularly extracardiac anomalies, often requires supplementary information provided by Doppler techniques and/or angiocardiography. In some instances, nevertheless, the "downstream" arterial abnormalities (such as aortic arch obstruction) can be anticipated by the arrangement of intracardiac anatomy itself. For example, an

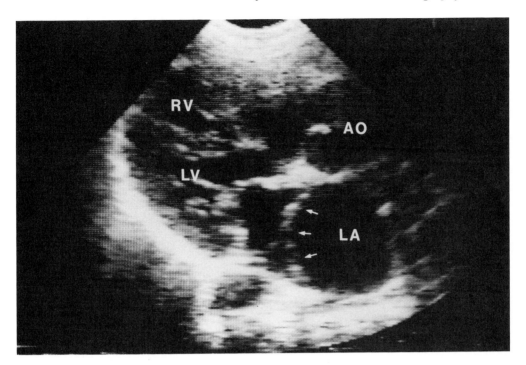

Figure 1. Long-axis parasternal view showing a partition within the left atrium (indicated by arrows) in a patient with pulmonary atresia and ventricular septal defect. The subaortic ventricular septal defect overridden by the aorta is also clearly seen. AO, aorta; LA, left atrium; LV, left ventricle; RV, right ventricle.

interrupted aortic arch is to be anticipated in cases with normal chamber connections and a malalignment ventricular septal defect in which the outlet septum is deviated posteriorly so as to obstruct the subaortic outflow from the left ventricle. Similarly, in cases with discordant ventriculo-arterial connections, aortic arch obstruction is likely if there is a malalignment ventricular septal defect with anterior and rightward deviation of the outlet septum, this lesion again causing some narrowing in the subaortic area.

Coming back to the intracardiac anatomy, any structure that is thin in one plane can be identified angiographically only if the chosen projection is absolutely precise or if the injection of contrast medium produces a clear difference in opacification of blood on the two sides of this structure. In contrast, such thin structures produce a strong reflection of the echo beam.[1] Cross-sectional echocardiography outperforms angiocardiography, therefore, in showing details of the atrial septum, subaortic fibrous shelves, membranes in the left atrium such as found in cor triatriatum (Fig. 1) or supramitral ring;[6] abnormalities of the leaflets of the atrioventricular valves such as clefts,[7] or double orifices.[8] Furthermore, echocardiography is the only technique capable of visualizing structures which are thin in two planes, such as the cordal apparatus of the atrioventricular valves. There is no better tool than echo in the assessment of straddling valves[3,9] or anomalous cordal attachments.

Another field in which cross-sectional echocardiography is particularly useful is represented by intracardiac masses, such as thrombi, vegetations, or cardiac tumors (Fig. 2). Cross-sectional echocardiography, giv-

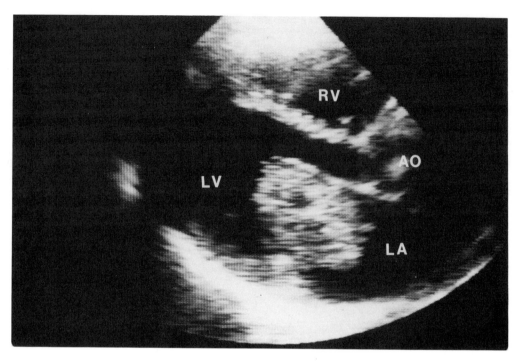

Figure 2. This parasternal long-axis section shows a huge left atrial myxoma which, in diastole, is occupying the mitral orifice AO, aorta; LA, left atrium; LV, left ventricle; RV, right ventricle.

ing sections or slices of tissue, is ideal for the examination of a globular structure like the heart. Problems exist when the structures to be investigated are extracardiac, particularly if they are long and tortuous and not lying in a single plane. The major pitfalls and limitations of echocardiography, therefore, are found in examination of the peripheral branches of the pulmonary arteries, collateral arteries between the systemic and pulmonary circuits, and complex anomalies of the aortic arch. It may also be difficult to visualize all the pulmonary veins, particularly when they drain anomalously with tortuous connection through the posterior and superior mediastinum to the right side of the heart. At present, angiocardiography remains the gold standard for identification of the distribution of the coronary arteries. Nonetheless, a considerable amount of information can now be achieved noninvasively even in this field by use of high-resolution transducers.[10]

References

1. Macartney FJ. Cross sectional echocardiographic diagnosis of congenital heart disease in infants. Br Heart J 1983;50:501–5.
2. Huhta JC, Smallhorn JF, Macartney FJ. Two-dimensional echocardiographic diagnosis of situs. Br Heart J 1982;48:97–108.
3. Carminati M, Valsecchi O, Borghi A, et al. Double inlet ventricle: Cross-sectional echocardiography. In: Anderson RH, Crupi G, Parenzan L, (eds), Double Inlet Ventricle; Anatomy, Diagnosis and Surgical Management. Tunbridge Wells Castle House Publications, 1987, pp 122–32.
4. Sutherland GR, Smallhorn JF, Anderson RH, et al. Atrioventricular discordance; Cross-sectional echocardiographic-morphological correlative study. Br Heart J 1983;50:8–20.
5. Carminati M, Valsecchi O, Borghi A, et al.

Cross-sectional echocardiographic study of criss-cross hearts and superoinferior ventricles. Am J Cardiol 1987;59:114–8.

6. Sullivan ID, Robinson PJ, de Leval M, Graham TP. Membranous supravalvular mitral stenosis: A treatable form of congenital heart disease. J Am Coll Cardiol 1986;8:159–64.

7. Smallhorn JF, de Leval M, Stark J, et al. Isolated anterior mitral cleft. Two-dimensional echocardiographic assessment and differentiation from "clefts" associated with atrioventricular septal defect. Br Heart J 1982;48:109–16.

8. Trowitrsch E, Bano-Rodrigo A, Burger BM, et al. Two-dimensional echocardiographic findings in double orifice mitral valve. J Am Coll Cardiol 1985;6:383–7.

9. Rice MJ, Seward JB, Edwards WD, et al. Straddling atrioventricular valve: Two-dimensional echocardiographic diagnosis, classification and surgical implications. Am J Cardiol 1985;55:505–13.

10. Pasquini L, Sanders SP, Parness I, Colan SD. Diagnosis of coronary artery anatomy by two-dimensional echocardiography in patients with transposition of the great arteries. Circulation 1987;75:557–64.

Applications of Color-Coded Doppler Flow Imaging in Evaluation of Children with Congenital Heart Disease

D. J. Sahn

Introduction

Echocardiography has had its major impact in providing anatomical information for the evaluation of patients with congenital heart disease. The addition of Doppler interrogation has provided noninvasive estimates of the gradients across valves,[1] methods for estimating the amount of blood flow through cardiac chambers,[2] and the amount of blood shunting across septal defects and between the aortic and pulmonary circulation.[3] The dynamic displays available from color flow mapping[4] have further enhanced the appreciation of important aspects of normal and abnormal cardiac flow. While the application of color flow mapping is of importance in extremely complicated forms of congenital heart disease, the amount and the semiquantitative nature of the information on color flow maps (in terms of flow direction and velocity, acceleration, deceleration, turbulence, and the simultaneous imaging of multiple events) can also be illustrated easily using the color flow maps of pa-

tients whose cardiac disease is of a simpler nature.

Atrial Septal Defect

Atrial septal defect, for the most part, represents an easy diagnosis in children and infants, even when the communication is located at sites other than the classical "secundum" defect in the middle of the septum. Subcostal imaging provides a view that is perpendicular to the septum and parallel to the flow from left to right atrium, which is coming towards the transducer. The shunt is basically a flow of low velocity, which, with a good signal-to-noise ratio, is easily imaged. The images obtained demonstrate the size and diameter of the defect. Kyo et al.[5] initially suggested that the maximal flow visualized across an atrial septal defect within the color-encoded area in late systole and early diastole was proportional to the ratio of pulmonary to systemic flow. Our experiments in animals, along with our experience from clinical studies,[6] suggests that the area of shunt indicated by the color flow when the instruments are run at a standardized frequency (4 kHz) and a moderate gain setting is related semiquantitatively to the pulmonary flow minus the systemic flow (that is, the actual amount of flow going across the atrial septal defect after correction for the body surface area of the patients). As such, the color map of flow provides not only visualization of the defect itself but also a semiquantitative estimate of the amount of flow crossing the atrial septum.

The map of flow is also capable of providing information about bidirectional shunts across the atrial septum in newborns where right heart pressures are elevated. An important piece of additional information, which the flow map provides better than either cross-sectional echocardiography or Doppler techniques without the facility of mapping, is the delineation of a fenestrated atrial septum or multiple atrial septal defects. A transcatheter technique has been developed for nonsurgical closure of atrial septal defects using a double umbrella. Patients with fenestration of the atrial septum (that is, multiple holes) are, however not good candidates for such transcatheter closure. The color mapping technique is invaluable, therefore in this setting, since it selects those patient who can be referred for surgery.

Ventricular Septal Defect

Our previous work[6] has shown that, in both animal experiments and clinical experience, color mapping of flow is extremely sensitive for detecting even the smallest interventricular shunts. Shunts between the left and right ventricles are usually of higher velocity than atrial shunts and are usually associated with multiple aliasing and significantly more turbulence. In fact, distortion of the lateral resolution of the ultrasound beam tends to enlarge the anatomical jet, so that defects too small to be seen on cross-sectional echocardiography alone can be recognized with the addition of color mapping. Our experience[7] suggests that such color mapping of flow represents an important means of charting the natural history of ventricular septal defects. It demonstrates the formation of aneurysms as the defects become smaller, even though the size of the ventricular septal defect as judged angiographically remains quite large.

In addition to this ability of color flow mapping to predict the size of these defects, there are other observations that are of significant importance in management. Ludomirsky and associates[8] have shown that the color map achieved is extremely accurate and sensitive for the detection of multiple defects (as in the "Swiss cheese septum"). In some patients, there are so many holes that the surgeon has difficulty in seeing and closing them all. Such infants are, therefore, poor risks for definitive heart surgery, even if they have congestive heart failure because of the combined additive size of the defects. Observations of the gradual acceleration and increasing brightness of flow in the chamber proximal to the hole (that is, the left ventricle, where flow accelerates to go through the ventricular septal defect) are often helpful in verifying the presence of a true septal defect and distinguishing it from false dropout or contamination by swirling or turbulent flow around other areas of the septum.

The true delineation of multiple septal defects in a patient represents an extremely important application of color flow mapping and echocardiography in general, particularly if cardiac catheterization is to be avoided as a requisite before referring such patients to surgery.

Patency of Arterial Duct (Ductus Arteriosus)

A patent duct can represent a serious and important form of congenital heart disease. This is particularly so in premature infants in whom, because of immaturity of the duct and the presence of lung disease, the duct often stays open and imposes an additional volume load on the circulation. Studying the duct noninvasively in these seriously ill and fragile babies has represented an important aspect of cardiac care. Our work, and the work of other groups, has suggested that color mapping of flow provides an important visualization of the position and size of the ductal shunt.[9] Our animal experiments suggested that the size of the shunt can be quickly and easily estimated from the visualization of the turbulent flow coming across the duct from the aorta into the pulmonary arteries. In these experiments,[10] we created in dogs by open-chest surgery a controllable, ductlike communication between the aorta and pulmonary trunk. By measuring the amount of flow through it, we were able to obtain close correlations between the magnitude of the shunt and the maximal area of shunt visualized in the pulmonary trunk. It was the area of maximal systolic flow velocity displayed as turbulence that was most closely correlated, the high quality of the variance "turbulence" display on the Toshiba SSH65A making this area easy to visualize. This provided evidence that the color map display of ductal flow could be used, in premature infants, as a semiquantitative estimate of shunting across the duct. In older children, the actual persistence of the duct itself is often sufficient indication for efforts to be made either at transcatheter closure or surgical ligation, the latter being a simple and safe extracardiac surgical procedure. The technique of color flow mapping[10] has proven to be an extremely sensitive technique for detection of even small ductal shunts.

Other dynamic observations that show the importance of color flow mapping and its ability to show more than one event at the same time are those that suggest that the actual size and positioning of the shunt itself, directed as a high velocity jet back through the duct towards the pulmonary valve, changes the motion and positioning of the leaflets of the pulmonary valve, as would be expected from hydraulic forces. The consequences of this are two fold. In systole, the ductal jet can cause premature closure of part of the leaflets, giving the spurious impression on M-mode echocardiography of pulmonary hypertension. Second, in diastole, the persistence of the ductal jet aimed at the pulmonary valve can distort it in such a way as to produce evidence of valvar insufficiency. This finding, while common in normals, is exaggerated in patients with ductal shunting and is lessened after ligation of the duct.

References

1. Hatle L, Angelsen BA. Doppler ultrasound in cardiology: Physical principles and clinical applications. Philadelphia, Lea & Febiger, 1982.
2. Fisher DC, Sahn DJ, Friedman MJ, et al. The mitral valve orifice method for non-invasive two-dimensional echo-Doppler determination of cardiac output. Circulation 1983; 67:872–7.
3. Valdes-Cruz LM, Horowitz S, et al. A pulsed Doppler echocardiographic method for calculation of pulmonary and systemic flow: Accuracy in a canine model with ventricular septal defect. Circulation 1983;68:597–602.
4. Omoto R. Color Atlas of Real-Time, Two-Dimensional Doppler Echocardiography. Tokyo Shindan-to-Chiryo Co., 1984.
5. Kyo S, Omoto R, Takamoto S, Takanawa E. Quantitative estimation of intracardiac shunt flow in atrial septal defect by real time two-dimensional color flow Doppler. Circulation 1984;70:11–39.
6. Sherman FS, Sahn DJ, Valdes-Cruz LM, et al. Two-dimensional Doppler color flow mapping for detecting atrial and ventricular septal defect. Herz 1987;12:212–6.
7. Hornberger LK, Krabill KA, Sahn DJ, Hagen-Ansert S. Elucidation of the natural history of ventricular septal defects by serial color Dop-

pler flow mapping studies. J Am Coll Cardiol 1987;9:165A (abstract).

8. Ludomirsky A, Huhta JC, Vick W, et al. Color Doppler detection of multiple ventricular septal defects. Circulation 1986;74:1317–22.

9. Swensson RE, Valdes-Cruz LM, Sahn DJ, et al. Real time Doppler color flow mapping for de-tection of patent ductus arteriosus. J Am Cardiol 1986;8:1105–12.

10. Swensson RE, Sahn DJ, Dembitsky W, Elias B. Color Doppler flow mapping of pulmonary ar-tery flow in an animal model of patent ductus arteriosus. J Am Coll Cardiol 1986;9:65A (ab-stract).

Scanning of the Fetal Heart

L. D. Allan

Introduction

In the last eight years, the feasibility and accuracy of fetal echocardiography in specialized centers has become established.[1-4] The complete cardiac scanning technique is time-consuming and requires skilled personnel and high-quality equipment. It is possible, however, to simplify the examination of the heart such that this can be incorporated into a routine obstetric study. Examination of the four-chamber view alone will detect the majority of severe defects, such as mitral, aortic, tricuspid, or pulmonary atresia; double-inlet atrioventricular connection; and atrioventricular septal defects. These defects will occur in approximately two in each thousand live births. From the New England Infant Cardiac Care Program,[5] it can be estimated that about three of each thousand babies present during the first years of life with the most severe forms of congenital heart defect. Ultrasonographers involved in routine screening can readily be taught to obtain, understand, and interpret the four-chamber view. Thus, up to two-thirds of those patients who normally present during infancy to units specializing in pediatric cardiology are identifiable before birth.

Congenital heart disease is complex and varied. But prenatal ultrasound displays in detail the normal and abnormal anatomic features of the fetal heart. A logical approach to heart disease, coupled with rules of orientation, will allow the pediatric echocardiographer to make accurate diagnoses.

Screening

In the screening program, ultrasonographers are taught to obtain a basic four-chamber view of the fetal heart by cutting straight across the fetal thorax just above the diaphragm (Fig. 1). Several crucial features are immediately seen in this section. The normal heart fills about one-third to one-half of the fetal thorax. Its two atriums are of similar size, as are the two ventricles, which also are of similar thickness. The atrial and ventricular septal structures, together with the two atrioventricular valves, meet together at the crux. The deficiency produced by the oval foramen is seen in the atrial septum, but the ventricular septum should be intact.

If doubt exists concerning the details of any of these points, the patient can be referred for further evaluation. Other high-risk groups of mothers who should be selected for specialized fetal echocardiography include those with a family history of congenital heart disease, those with diabetes, those in whom there is evidence of either fetal ar-

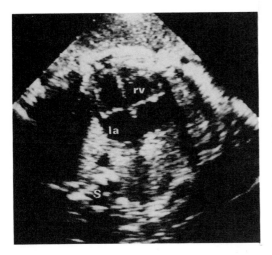

Figure 1. The echocardiogram achieved in four-chamber section shows two ventricles of approximately the same size and two atriums of similar size. The right ventricle lies immediately below the sternum, which is directly opposite the spine. The descending aorta is seen in cross section as a circle lying anterior to the spine. The left atrium lies anterior to the descending aorta. The atrioventricular connection and the two functioning atrioventricular valves can be clearly seen, especially when the image is in motion. S, spine; rv, right ventricle; la, left atrium.

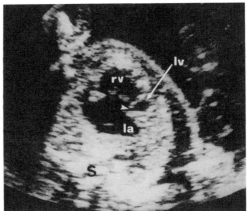

Figure 2. In this case, the left ventricle is much smaller than the right. The mitral valve was absent because of mitral atresia, but there was double-outlet right ventricle with a good-sized aorta. S, spine; la, left atrium; lv, left ventricle; rv, right ventricle.

rhythmias, extracardiac fetal anomalies, or nonimmune fetal hydrops, and those who, during early pregnancy, have been exposed to cardiac teratogens (such as lithium, phenytoin, and steroids).

Typical Findings

An example of an abnormal case readily recognizable by the ultrasonographer on a four chamber view is shown in Fig. 2. Only a small cavity can be seen at the anticipated site of the left ventricle. There is no left atrioventricular valve seen as a patent structure. This is a case of mitral atresia. In this case, both great arteries were of normal size and arose from the right ventricle.

An example of an atrioventricular septal defect with common valve orifice is shown in Fig. 3. Because of the frequent association

of this type of malformation with Down's syndrome, amniocentesis or sampling of fetal blood for chromosomal analysis is indicated when this form of heart disease is identified. Many abnormalities will not be seen on the four-chamber view alone but will require more extensive examination of the rest of the heart to visualize the veno-

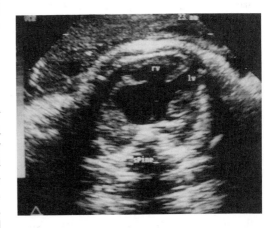

Figure 3. This heart shows a deficiency of the atrioventricular septum at the crux of the heart. This is an atrioventricular septal defect with common valve orifice. Abbreviations as in Fig. 2.

atrial and ventriculo-arterial connections on both sides of the heart.

During our eight-year program, we have studied over 5,000 high-risk pregnancies. An accurate prediction of structural cardiac normality was made in the vast majority of cases. This provides a great deal of reassurance, particularly to mothers who have had a previous child affected. To date, we have predicted correctly the existence of 250 cardiac malformations. We have not made any major false-positive predictions. We overlooked five abnormalities of connection during our learning period but, with greater experience and improved imaging, these errors should not recur. Coarctation of the aorta is a difficult diagnosis and can be missed.[6] In total, 27 minor defects have been missed on the fetal scan in our series. These were anomalies such as small ventricular or atrial septal defects and mild valvar disease. It is important, therefore, that both the patient an the operator are aware of the confidence limits of the technique.

Discussion

The method of selection of patients for fetal echocardiography exposes a more severe spectrum of congenital heart disease than is usually seen postnatally.[7] A high proportion, up to 40%, of the fetuses will have heart disease occurring in association with other extracardiac anomalies. Unusual forms of heart disease are detected, such as pulmonary atresia with a dilated right ventricle and dysplasia of the tricuspid valve. A surprising finding has been the high incidence of spontaneous intrauterine death that has been seen in association with many complex cardiac abnormalities. The severity of the abnormalities detected prenatally is reflected in the outcome (Fig. 4). When parents are faced at an early stage of pregnancy with the prospect that their offspring are afflicted by major structural heart disease, they commonly elect for termination of the pregnancy. This will, of course, depend on

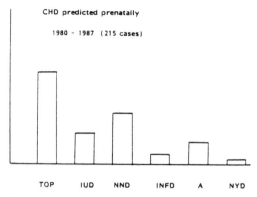

Figure 4. This diagram depicts the outcome of the cases of fetal heart disease seen at Guy's Hospital to the end of 1987. TOP, termination of pregnancy; IUD, intrauterine death; NND, neonatal death; INFD, infant death; A, alive; NYD, not yet delivered.

the type of defect, the likely prognosis, and the wishes of individual parents. It is probable, nonetheless, that a defect such as the hypoplastic left heart syndrome, for which no treatment is generally available at the present time in the United Kingdom and which is universally fatal, could disappear from postnatal practice if prenatal screening methods become widely applied. Where congenital heart disease is anticipated by prenatal diagnosis, delivery of the infant in a unit with pediatric cardiology facilities should give the neonate the best possible chance of survival.

In summary, fetal echocardiography is both possible and accurate in the prediction of structural heart disease from an early stage of pregnancy. The extent of its potential effect on the practice of pediatric echocardiography will depend on the extent of adoption of cardiac screening and on the means of utilization of the information available to doctors and parents in early pregnancy. Such considerations have much individual variation and obviously important ethical aspects. Pediatric cardiac surgery has advanced enormously in the last 20 years, but at the cost of much suffering from experimental techniques performed on newborn babies. Many conditions treated by "corrective" surgery still have such a poor prognosis that termination of pregnancy could be considered a more humane alternative. This is a difficult subject, which should be continually evaluated in terms of medical opinion, social and individual attitudes, and surgical results.

References

1. Allan LD, Tynan MJ, Campbell S, et al. Echocardiographic and anatomical correlates in the fetus. Br Heart J 1980;44:445–51.
2. Lange LW, Sahn DJ, Allen HD, et al. Qualitative real-time cross-sectional echocardiographic imaging of the human fetus during the second half of pregnancy. Circulation 1980;62:799–806.
3. Kleinman CS, Hobbins JC, Jaffe CC, et al. Echocardiographic studies of the human fetus: Prenatal diagnosis of congenital heart disease and cardiac dysrhythmias. Pediatrics 1980; 65:1059–67.
4. Allan LD, Crawford DC, Anderson RH, Tynan MJ. Echocardiographic and anatomical correlates in fetal congenital heart disease. Br Heart J 1984;52:542–8.
5. Allan LD, Chita SK, Anderson RH, et al. Coarctation of the aorta in prenatal life: an echocardiographic, anatomical and functional study. Br Heart J 1988;59:356–60.
6. Fyler DC, Buckley LP, Hellenbrand WE, Cohn HE. Report of the New England Regional Infant Care Program. Pediatrics 1980;65(suppl):376–461.
7. Allan LD, Crawford DC, Anderson RH, Tynan MJ. Spectrum of congenital heart disease seen in prenatal life. Br Heart J 1985;54:523–6.

Cineangiography

K. E. Fellows

Introduction

Cineangiography remains the standard by which other cardiac imaging procedures are measured.[1-3] Modern generators of x-rays and high-resolution imaging chains provide detailed images using cine pulses of only 2.8 msec (stopping any heart motion) in the optimal range of microrads per frame 65–90 kV. These technical factors allow the dose to be as low as 10–20 microrads per frame.[4-6]

Contemporary cineangiography is performed optimally when echocardiography is used prior to the catheterization to provide categorical diagnosis and general anatomic information. This allows tailoring of the cine studies to the fewest injections and shortest times of filming possible. An equally important development has been the use of axially angled projections. These views, which combine standard rotational angles with angulation in the long axis of the patient (45° cranial/45° caudal), provide the best display of cardiac anatomy.

Methods

A complete list of the projections used in contemporary cineangiocardiography is given in Table 1. These include both standard orthogonal and axially angled views.

Table 2 is a list of common congenital heart defects and the projection with which they can be best studied. The concept of axial angulation (angling the x-ray tube–image intensifier tube combination in the long axis of the body) was introduced by Dr. Mac Bargeron of Birmingham, Alabama,[1,3] in order to depict important cardiovascular structures free of superimposition and to eliminate the foreshortening of cardiac structures that is inherent in standard views.

Axially angled views can be produced either by angling the patient on the catheterization table using foam wedges, bolsters, and other nonopaque padding, or by using combinations of x-ray and intensifer tubes that are mounted on special single plane or biplane mechanical structures, thus facilitating not only 360° rotational but also 45° cranial/caudal angulation as well. In a survey (as yet unpublished) made in 1988 of 28 laboratories performing catheterization in North America, 24 (85%) were equipped with mechanical devices for axial angling, indicating the importance of convenience and speed over added cost. The trend now is toward biplane mechanical axial angulation, although it is unclear to me whether it is routinely useful and will justify the extra cost and the installation of cumbersome apparatus. If, in a laboratory with biplane equipment, only one plane angle is available in the axial direction, the other standard x-

Table 1

Glossary of Projections

Frontal	perpendicular to anterior thorax
Lateral	90° off frontal
Right anterior oblique	30° right rotation
Left anterior oblique	70° left rotation
Sitting	frontal + 40–50° cranial angulation
Hepatoclavicular	40° cranial angulation + 40° left obliquity
Long axial oblique	20–25° cranial angulation + 70° left obliquity
Long (right) anterior oblique	20–25° cranial angulation + 30° right obliquity

ray tube–intensifier combination can be used simultaneously at an orthogonal angle to the axial apparatus. When preparing a listing of specific heart defects and the views that optimally display them, such as seen in Table 2, it should be remembered that certain caveats apply. Several important issues need to be considered.

Consideration of Individual Lesions

Atrial Septal Defects

These lesions can be imaged in the long axial oblique projection using an injection in a right pulmonary vein, but why? In most infants and children, echocardiography is better and easier.

Ventricular Septal Defects

Although most defects are imaged best in the long axial oblique view, rarer but surgically difficult defects (such as subpulmonary intraconal or doubly committed subarterial and anterior muscular defects) are best seen in the standard right anterior oblique projection. Both views should be used in all cases.

Atrioventricular Septal Defects

The anatomy of the atrioventricular septum and its deficiency is best seen in the hepatoclavicular view. When the left-to-right ventricular shunt is large, however, and valvar regurgitation is moderate or severe, the standard right anterior oblique view better separates the anteriorly directed shunt from the posterior regurgitation.

Patency of Arterial Duct (Ductus Arteriosus)

This simple lesion can be difficult to visualize because it is often superimposed on the aortic arch in standard lateral and oblique views. The hepatoclavicular and long axial oblique projections eliminate this superimposition.

Tetralogy of Fallot

The diagnosis of this common lesion is made clinically and by ultrasound. The surgeon can see the infundibular anatomy easily, and angiography should be directed at the exclusion of multiple ventricular defects, the depiction of the coronary arterial anatomy, and the demonstration of peripheral pulmonary arterial stenosis. In small children and infants, a biplane left ventricular injection in right anterior oblique and long axial oblique projection will frequently provide all of the information needed.

Tetralogy of Fallot with Pulmonary Atresia ("Pseudotruncus")

Injections made after balloon occlusion of the descending aorta have improved the

Table 2

Anomaly	Principle projection
Secundum atrial septal defect	Long axial oblique (RUL pulmonary vein injection)
Primum atrial septal defect	Hepatoclavicular (LV injection)
VSD, membranous	Long axial oblique (LV injection)
VSD, muscular	
a) Mid/apical	Long axial oblique (LV injection)
b) Anterior	Right anterior oblique (LV injection)
VSD, "AV canal" type	Hepatoclavicular (LV injection)
Complete AV septal defect	Hepatoclavicular (LV injection)
Patent arterial duct	Hepatoclavicular (AO arch injection)
Tetralogy of Fallot	Long axial oblique (LV injection)
	Sitting (RV injection)
Tetralogy with pulmonary atresia (pseudotruncus)	Sitting (ascending and descending Aortic injections)
	Long axial oblique (LV injection)
Common arterial trunk	Hepatoclavicular (truncal valve injection)
	Long axial oblique (LV injection)
Tricuspid atresia	Hepatoclavicular (LV injection)
Complete transposition and DORV	Long axial oblique (LV injection)
Double inlet ventricle	Variable, depending on anatomy, location of hearts, etc. Usually begin with either frontal/lateral of hepatoclavicular views, then additional views as needed
Peripheral PS	
Central	Sitting/lateral (PT injection)
Peripheral (Intrapulmonary)	Frontal/lateral (RPA/LPA injection)

VSD, ventricular septal defect; RUL, right upper lobe; LV, left ventricle; AO, aorta; RV, right ventricle; AV, atrioventricular; DORV, double outlet right ventricle; PS, pulmonary stenosis; PT, pulmonary trunk; PA, pulmonary arteries.

visualization of collateral vessels and pulmonary arteries in this lesion. Although the sitting projection should be used to show the mediastinal segments of the pulmonary arteries, this 45° craniocaudal view superimposes the systemic aortopulmonary collateral arteries and the pulmonary arteries in the lungs. In order to evaluate the number and origin of these collaterals and to exclude peripheral (intrapulmonary) arterial stenoses, appropriate injections should be made in standard frontal and lateral views rather than using axial projections.

Common Arterial Trunk (Truncus Arteriosus)

A retrograde catheter should be used to inject above the truncal valve with the patient positioned to provide the hepatoclavicular view. This not only allows evaluation of truncal valvar insufficiency, but it provides optimum visualization of the pulmonary arterial anatomy.

Tricuspid Atresia

A left ventricular injection in the hepatoclavicular view is so good that rarely is any other view necessary. The only proviso is that the image intensifier should be large enough to include the ventricles, pulmonary arteries, and the aortic arch on the same cine frame.

Double Inlet Ventricle

It is difficult to predict the optimum projections for this anomaly. Usually the initial injection is best done in frontal and lateral views, and subsequent injections decided upon by the information provided in the standard views. Although the hepatoclavicular views is often helpful, because of the frequency in which the heart is right-sided in these patients, the opposite projection ("splenoclavicular" view) must be used.

Coronary Arteries

Injections made after balloon occlusion of the ascending aorta are the easiest means of opacifying the coronary arteries in infants and small children. In tetralogy, the right anterior oblique and long axial oblique projections provide the best display, whereas in complete transposition and double outlet right ventricle, the standard frontal and later projections allow excellent visualization and clear orientation.

Conclusion

Although cineangiography is presently the gold standard for cardiac imaging, developments in cardiac digital angiography, cine magnetic resonance imaging, and cine computed tomography will overtake and replace it in the future. Even then, axial angulation will be employed with those advanced techniques to display optimally most cardiovascular structures.

References

1. Soto B, Coghlan CH, Bargeron L. Present status of axially angled angiocardiography. Cardiovasc Intervent Radiol 1984;7:156–65.
2. Brandt PWT. Axially angiocardiography. Cardiovasc Intervent Radiol 1984;7:166–9.
3. Santamaria H, Soto B, Ceballos R, et al. Angiographic differentiation of types of ventricular septal defects. Am J Roentgenol 1983; 141:273–81.
4. Levin DC, Dunham LR, Stueve R. Causes of cine image quality deterioration in cardiac laboratories. Am J Cardiol 1983;55:171–6.
5. Miller SW, Castrovovo FP. Radiation exposure and protection in cardiac catheterization laboratories. Am J Cardiol 1985;55:171–6.
6. Leibovic SJ, Fellows KE. Patient radiation exposure during pediatric cardiac catheterization. Cardiovasc Intervent Radiol 1983;6:150–3.

Magnetic Resonance Imaging of Congenital Heart Disease
Right Heart Lesions

K. J. Chung and I. A. Simpson

Introduction

Electrocardiographically gated spin echo and cine magnetic resonance imaging have been widely used to assess cardiac anatomy and function. We used this technique for evaluation of infants and children with various congenital heart diseases involving the right heart. We report here our preliminary experience with the applicability and efficacy of this new diagnostic modality.

Patients and Methods

A group of patients, with ages ranging from 6 weeks to 14 years with congenital heart disease involving the right ventricle and pulmonary arteries were studied by magnetic resonance imaging. The body weights varied from 4.2 to 45 kg. The lesions consisted of tetralogy of Fallot, complete transposition, banding of the pulmonary trunk for ventricular septal defect or double-inlet ventricle, pulmonary atresia with intact ventricular septum, tricuspid atresia requiring the Fontan operation, and complex venous anomalies. Patients under 5 years of age were sedated with choral hydrate (80–100 mg/kg) given orally 30 minutes prior to the procedure. This protocol of sedation provided excellent sedation in all patients and produced neither respiratory or circulatory compromise.

Magnetic resonance imaging was performed with a General Electric Signa system operating at a field strength of 1.5 Tesla. For infants weighing less than 20 kg, a 16- or 24-cm cylindrical coil (head or knee coil) was used. Such small coils provide excellent images of the heart and great vessels without interfering with the electrocardiographic gating. They further reduce the potential movement of the babies during the procedure, providing an additional safety feature. Cine magnetic resonance images were obtained using 30° flip angle excitation pulses that allow steady-state magnetic resonance acquisitions with good signal-to-noise ratios and short repetitious time. Gradient-recalled echoes were used for rephasing, allowing short echo time. The gradient reversal is a nonslice selective refocusing technique. Spins excited by initial 30° pulse are refocused even if flow carries them out of the imaging slice. Flowing blood, therefore, is bright on the cine magnetic resonance image. With this technique, high temporal resolution images at multiple levels of the heart can be obtained rapidly for assessment of cardiac function. Furthermore, turbulence associated with valvar disease results in the loss of the bright signal of normal flow. Electrocardiographically gated cardiac imaging using multislice acquisition was initially performed in all patients to localize the optimum slice location and in selective cases, cine imaging was performed. We used several planes to select the optimal ones to demonstrate various cardiac structures. Coronal, axial, and sagittal planes were used for initial localization. Then a software system producing oblique angles was manipulated to obtain the optimum angle for certain areas of interest without changing the position of the patient. For tetralogy of Fallot, sagittal, axial, or 45° sitting-up view was mainly used for visualization of the right ventricular outflow tract and the pulmonary trunk and its branches.

For complete transposition, axial views were used for demonstration of pulmonary venous return, sagittal views for the relationships of the great arteries and both ventricular outflow tracts, and coronal views for the caval venous connections. For pulmonary atresia and banding of the pulmonary trunk, sagittal and axial views provided excellent anatomical details. All three views were used for study of the Fontan procedure and complex venous anomalies.

Results

The quality of the resulting magnetic resonance imaging study was excellent in 81% of the cases, documenting relevant information about all pertinent areas of the heart. Magnetic resonance imaging provided substantive and accurate diagnostic information in another 14% and was nondiagnostic in 5%. The technique was extremely useful for providing information in the areas of the right ventricle and pulmonary trunk (95%) and caval (94%) and pulmonary venous (91%) systems. Poor quality images were mainly the consequence of motion of the patient, marked variation of heart rate, mistriggering of the gating circuit due to interference in the T wave, and flow artifacts produced by prosthetic materials or vascular clips. We compared the results of magnetic resonance imaging in the patients with right heart lesions described here to echocardiography and cineangiography. By utilizing multiple views, the right side of the heart was clearly visualized in 95% of the cases, documenting anatomy similar to the views obtained by conventional angiography. Magnetic resonance imaging was far superior to echocardiography, especially in older children and after surgical repair. Spectral and color flow Doppler echocardiography, however, provided valuable information in regard to right ventricular pressure and the pressure gradient, but did not provide information regarding right ventricular function or peripheral pulmonary arteries. In patients with tricuspid atresia after the Fontan procedure, flow from the right atrium to the pulmonary arteries was seen on coronal and sagittal views in all patients. For complex venous anomalies, magnetic resonance imaging provided better anatomical details than angiography.

Conclusions

Our preliminary experience suggests that magnetic resonance imaging can provide anatomic and functional information equivalent to cineangiography. It can provide dynamic and high-resolution images in any desired plane through the heart and great vessels. It is particularly applicable to small children since it is entirely noninvasive and uses no radiation, yet provides sufficient data for management and, thus far, carries a clean safety record. Its only drawback at the present time is that it cannot, as yet, estimate pressures and shunt magnitude, knowledge of which may be necessary for proper management in certain patients with complex cardiac lesions. Magnetic resonance imaging, however, will not replace echocardiography, which is well established and an important part of a diagnostic sequence for assessing congenital heart disease. With complementary information provided by echocardiography and magnetic resonance imaging, we are now close to providing a noninvasive comprehensive assessment of congenital heart disease without the need for invasive procedures. We believe that these two noninvasive techniques will play an increasingly important role and will become an invaluable part of patient care in children with congenital heart disease.

References

1. Higgins CB. Overview of MR of the heart. Am J Roentgenol 1986;146:907–18.
2. Markiewicz W, Sechtem U, Higgins CB. Evaluation of the right ventricle by MRI. Am Heart J 1987;113:8–15.
3. Higgins CB, Byrd BJ, Farmer DW, et al. MRI in patients with congenital heart disease. Circulation 1984;70:851–60.
4. Didler D, Higgins CB, Fisher MR, et al. Congenital heart disease: Gated MR imaging in 72 patients. Radiology 1986;158:227–35.
5. Chung KJ, Simpson IA, Glass RF, et al. Cine MRI in patients with transposition of the great arteries after surgical repair. Circulation 1988; 77:104–9.
6. Simpson IA, Chung KJ, Glass RF, et al. Cine MRI: A new method for evaluation of anatomy and flow relationship in infants and children with coarctation of the aorta. Circulation 1988;78:142–8.
7. Sechtem U, Pflugfelder PW, Gould RG, et al. Measurement of right and left ventricular volumes in healthy individuals with cine MR imaging. Radiology 1987;163:697–702.
8. Wehrli FW. Introduction to fast-scan magnetic resonance. Milwaukee, Wisconsin, General Electric, 1986.
9. Shellock FG. Biological effects of MRI: A clean safety record so far. Diagn Imaging 1987;9:96–101.

Routine Intraoperative Color Flow Imaging Prevents Surgically Unacceptable Results in Repair of Congenital Heart Lesions

R. M. Ungerleider, W. J. Greeley, J. Philips, and J. A. Kisslo

Introduction

Paralleling the technical advances in cardiac surgery, which have improved results and options for repair of a number of congenital cardiac lesions, has been the increased enthusiasm for the use of intraoperative Doppler echocardiography during cardiac procedures.[1-4] Intraoperative cross-sectional echo using epicardial transducers has been used for the evaluation of congenital heart repairs,[4] but the evaluation of residual shunts and valvar function is limited using this technology. Even the most recently reported studies employing intraoperative color flow imaging[3] during surgery for congenital heart defects reach only "preliminary" conclusions. To determine the usefulness and efficiency of routine intraoperative employment of epicardial Doppler color flow imaging before and after the repair of a variety of congenital cardiac lesions, we studied 140 consecutive patients approached through a median sternotomy at Duke University Medical Center between March 1987 and February 1988.

Patients and Methods

The ages ranged from 1 day to 32 years, with 52 patients (37%) being less than 1 year old and 102 patients (73%) being 3 years of age or under. The smallest patient studied weighed 2.1 kg. One hundred twenty-four (89%) of the operative procedures were for correction as opposed to palliation. The variety of defects encountered are listed in Table 1.

Examinations were performed using a Hewlett-Packard color flow imaging device equipped with a 5-MHz short-focus transducer. The probe for the transducer was cleaned with a commercially available glutaraldehyde solution and then passed over the ether screen into a sterile sheath held by the surgeon. In this manner, the probe could be secured to the surgical side of the drapes and used at any time during the procedure. Data were acquired from the epicardial surface of the heart before the initiation of cardiopulmonary bypass and again at the conclusion of the procedure, usually

Table 1

Duke University Medical Center
Intraoperative Color Flow Imaging

Atrial septal defect	23
Ventricular septal defect (VSD)	20
Tetralogy of Fallot	19
Pulmonary atresia/stenosis	9
Atrioventricular septal defect	18
Complete transposition	5
Corrected transposition	1
Aortic stenosis (+ VSD)	12
Aortic incompetence (+ VSD)	4
Mitral valve + VSD	4
Tricuspid atresia	6
Double inlet ventricle	5
Common arterial trunk	1
Coronary arteriovenous malformations	2
Interrupted arch	3
Totally anomalous pulmonary venous connection	2
Double-outlet right ventricle	3
Other	3
Total	140

after the patient had been weaned from bypass. In some instances, additional data were obtained during periods of rewarming while the patient was still on cardiopulmonary bypass. Routine evaluation included an interrogation of all cardiac chambers and valves as well as the venous inflows and great arterial outflows. Data were analyzed "on-line" in real-time, and decisions were made in each individual case on the basis of the information provided by the Doppler color flow imaging. All images were evaluated by the attending surgeon, cardiologists (echocardiologists), and anesthesiologists. All images were recorded on high-fidelity tape for later review.

Results

The average time of each examination was 3.95 ± 1.96 minutes. There was unquestionably a learning curve in performing these examinations. As experience was gained with the technology, it was found that

an adequate examination could be performed by the surgeon in a relatively short period of time.

The quality of the images obtained from the epicardial surface was exceptional, with excellent resolution produced as compared to images obtained preoperatively by the transthoracic approach. Furthermore, the ability to angle the transducer in various orientations enabled the surgeon to obtain excellent delineation of the anatomic features of each congenital cardiac defect. In the period prior to bypass, it was felt that color imaging had an impact on the operations for 63 patients (45%). In two instances, preoperative diagnoses were changed prior to initiating bypass. In an additional two instances, the planned operation was changed on the basis of the pre-bypass imaging. In 54 patients, Doppler imaging generated information that guided the intracardiac approach or influenced the operative plan. In five patients, the anesthetic management was enhanced by information obtained from the pre-bypass imaging. Routine imaging had its greatest impact in patients undergoing valve repair, particularly in those patients with atrioventricular septal defects. It was also especially useful in delineating the precise location of residual shunts in patients with recurrent ventricular septal defects.

Despite the fact that all patients received preoperative echo Doppler examinations and most patients received preoperative cardiac catheterizations, 32 patients demonstrated 38 previously unsuspected findings. The incidence of finding an unsuspected lesion was not influenced by whether or not the patient had preoperative cardiac catheterization. In certain circumstances, the additional information was invaluable in formulating the operative approach and plan. Predictably, as this study progressed, fewer unsuspected findings were observed, probably because of better preoperative surveillance. In only one case did imaging miss an anatomic feature found during the intracardiac examination of the patient. This was

Table 2

Intraoperative Color Flow Imaging Post-Repair Defects

Degree of defects (patients)	Outcome		
	Reoperated n (%)	Died n (%)	Acceptable n (%)
Tolerable (28)	3 (11)	1 (4)	24 (85)
Concern (7)	4 (57)[a]		3 (43)

[a] 50% survival to acceptable outcome.

in a patient with multiple lesions who was also found to have a divided right atrium at the time of intracardiac exploration. This was easily recognized and dealt with. Later review of the study performed prior to bypass demonstrated that the finding was displayed but was not recognized.

The most significant impact of routine intraoperative Doppler color flow imaging was in the evaluation after repair. In 18 patients (13%), the findings subsequent to the procedure encouraged revision of the operative repair. Twelve of these cases were revised on the basis of the imaging confirming the suspected problems. Of the 12 repairs revised on the basis of imaging alone, six patients had already been weaned from cardiopulmonary bypass and were doing well clinically. In the remaining six patients, imaging was performed during the rewarming period and revisions were performed prior to attempting to wean the patient from the pump. Four of these patients would probably have evidenced no clinical difficulty. This means that 10 patients were at risk for leaving the operating room with suboptimal results had it not been for the routine application of Doppler color flow imaging. Six of these patients had residual shunts, and one had a significant gradient across the repaired site of previous banding of the pulmonary trunk. In two instances, imaging disclosed a technical error that was easily remedied to yield an excellent result. In one case, a ventricular septal defect was shown to be unclosed during rewarming,

thus encouraging the surgeon to complete successful closure.

Eight patients had clinically or anatomically observable evidence for an unacceptable repair. The precise nature of their problem was then clearly disclosed and confirmed by the imaging. In one instance, this was a technical problem with insertion of an aortic allograft that was revised so than the study became acceptable prior to leaving the operating room. Six of these patients had residual shunts or areas of stenosis, such as a stenotic subpulmonary outflow after repair of tetralogy. These also were corrected to provide for a better surgical result.

Although the disclosure of significant residual defects encouraged revision of the repair prior to conclusion of the procedure, 35 patients still left the operating room with some degree of residual defect. This frequency is due largely to the great sensitivity of the technology. Although these defects were considered trivial or "tolerable" in 28 patients (such as leakage aross the suture line closing a ventricular septal defect), seven patients left the operating room with a residual defect that raised some concern for its long-term outcome. The follow-up for these 35 patients is shown in Table 2, indicating that, although it is not necessary to achieve "echoperfect" results, the presence of moderate residual defects may influence the eventual outcome.

Results were also catalogued based upon whether or not imaging raised concern about the nature of cardiac performance at the completion of the procedure. Acceptable operative results (no concerns produced by imaging) were apparent in 105 patients. The remaining 35 patients displayed some form of abnormality, suggesting variable degrees of right or left ventricular dysfunction. The presence of any abnormality detected by imaging after the procedure reduced the chances of a long-term surgically acceptable outcome from 90% to 60%.

Discussion

It was found, overall, that Doppler color flow imaging consistently demonstrated in the working, beating heart the specific anatomic and physiologic features unique to each individual case and helped in directing the most efficient and optimal approach to the intracardiac repair. Routine application of this technique before and after cardiopulmonary bypass provides an appreciation for the nature of the defect being repaired as well as the disclosure of previously unrecognized associated defects. In addition, the evaluation of patients after the repair has been completed can disclose problems which, in many instances, can be remedied so as to yield a more optimal result. As cardiac surgery is performed on younger and smaller patients, with the intent of totally correcting complex intracardiac defects, it is crucial that surgeons find a means of efficiently evaluating their repairs to ensure the most successful outcomes. Intraoperative Doppler color flow imaging can be learned quickly and utilized by the surgeon. As experience is gained, it can become an indispensable tool in the conduct of surgery for complex congenital heart disease.

References

1. de Bruijn N, Clements F, Kisslo J. Intraoperative transesophageal color flow mapping. Initial experience. Anesth Analg 1987;66:386–90.
2. Takamoto S, Kyo S, Adachi H, et al. Intraoperative color flow mapping by real-time two dimensional Doppler echocardiography for evaluation of valvular and congenital heart disease and vascular disease. J Thorac Cardiovasc Surg 1985;90:802–12.
3. Hagler DJ, Tajik AJ, Seward JB, et al. Intraoperative two-dimensional Doppler echocardiography. J Thorac Cardiovasc Surg 1988;95:516–22.
4. Gussenhoven EJ, van Herwerden LA, Roelandt J, et al. Intraoperative two-dimensional echocardiography in congenital heart disease. J Am Coll Cardiol 1987;9:565–72.

Four-Year Experience with Surgery for Congenital Heart Disease Based upon Cross-Sectional Echocardiography

R. I. Rossi, P. Zielinsky, N. Medeiros, J. Bertoletti, N. Daudt,
C. Firpo, I. Castro, J. C. Haertel, F. Lucchese, J. R. Sant'Anna,
P. Prates, and I. Nesralla

Introduction

Since the early stages of surgery for congenital heart disease, cardiac catheterization has been the cornerstone of the preoperative diagnosis. The development of the technique of cross-sectional echocardiography, particularly with the addition of flow analysis with Doppler systems, has dramatically changed this concept. The many advantages of this diagnostic approach have been demonstrated by several authors,[1,2] who have emphasized the excellent morphological correlation and reproducibility of the method. Furthermore, its low cost, negligible morbidity, and ability to be performed at the bedside have transformed its use as the main diagnostic tool for the identification of congenital heart disease. Based upon these facts, we started a prospective study to demonstrate the feasibility and safety of performing surgery for congenital heart disease without prior cardiac catheterization.

Clinical Material

From March 1984 to January 1988, 910 patients with congenital heart diseases required cardiac surgery in our institution. Two hundred thirty-two children (25.5%) were treated solely on the basis of cross-sectional echocardiography. The study group was almost equally divided regarding sex (112 male and 120 female). One hundred ten patients (47.4%) were younger than 1 year (mean 123 ± 121 days) and 122 (52.6%) were older than 1 year (mean: 7.5 ± 6.2 years).

Heart failure was the commonest form of presentation, being detected in 128 patients (55.2%), while severe cyanosis was found in 48 (20.7%). The remaining 56 cases (24.1%) were asymptomatic or had other

Table 1

Surgical Mortality[a]

Procedure	Diagnosis	n	%
Blalock-Taussig shunt	Pulmonary atresia with intact septum	3	2.15
	Tricuspid atresia with severe PS	1	
	Tetralogy of Fallot	1	
Brock + shunt	Pulmonary atresia with intact septum	2	0.86
ASVD repair	Complete AVSD	2	0.86
PT banding and PAD ligation	Muscular VSD + PAD	1	0.43
PT banding	Huge muscular VSD	1	0.43
PT banding; PAD ligation & CoA repair	Perimembranous VSD, PAD, + CoA	1	0.43
Aortic valvotomy	Severe aortic stenosis	1	0.43
Correction of TAPVC	Infradiaphragmatic TAPVC	1	0.43
Norwood	Hypoplastic left heart syndrome	1	0.43
PAD ligation	PAD in severely premature newborn Sepsis	1	0.43
VSD closure	Perimembranous VSD	1	0.43
Total		17	7.31

[a] There were no deaths due to wrong or incomplete diagnosis, $n = 232$ patients in study group. PS, pulmonary stenosis; PT, pulmonary trunk; PAD, patent arterial duct; TAPVC, totally anomalous pulmonary venous connection; VSD, ventricular septal defect; AVSD, atrioventricular septal defect.

clinical findings. Overall in the group, 264 surgical procedures were performed. Palliative operations were exclusively used in the group younger than 1 year, namely Blalock-Taussig shunts ($n = 41, 31.8\%$) and banding of the pulmonary trunk ($n = 12, 9.0\%$). The remaining patients of this group were submitted to definitive operation: ligation of the arterial duct ($n = 31, 23.3\%$); repair of totally anomalous pulmonary venous connection ($n = 10, 7.5\%$); closure of ventricular septal defect ($n = 4, 3.0\%$); correction of atrioventricular septal defect ($n = 1, 0.7\%$); aortic valvotomy ($n = 1, 0.7\%$); Mustard procedure ($n = 1, 0.7\%$) and a Norwood operation ($n = 1, 0.7\%$). In the group older than 1 year, every patient was submitted to definitive procedures. These were closure of atrial septal defect ($n = 48, 36.6\%$); ligation of the arterial duct ($n = 46, 35.1\%$); repair of aortic coarctation ($n = 14, 10.7\%$); correction of atrioventricular septal defect ($n = 6, 4.6\%$); closure of ventricular septal defect ($n = 6, 4.6\%$), repair of abnormal mitral valve ($n = 4, 3.0\%$); repair of partially anomalous pulmonary venous connection ($n = 3$,

2.3%), resection of subaortic stenosis ($n = 2, 1.5\%$), pulmonary valvotomy ($n = 1, 0.8\%$), and correction of totally anomalous pulmonary venous connection ($n = 1; 0.8$).

The surgical mortality was 17 cases (7.3%), which was not significantly different from the overall mortality of surgery for congenital heart disease in our institution in the same period of time ($X^2 = 0.85$). Table 1 summarizes the procedures and diagnosis in those patients who died. The echocardiographic data were misinterpreted in 16 situations. Five defects were missed ("false negatives"), while nine defects were incorrectly diagnosed ("false positives"). These findings are summarized in Table 2. These problems occurred mainly in the early stage of our experience and were part of our learning curve.

Comments

The ideal diagnostic method in pediatric cardiology is expected to provide sufficient information to allow a safe operation

Table 2

Congenital Heart Disease Surgery Based upon Cross-Sectional Echocardiography
$n = 232^a$

False positives		False negatives	
Echo diagnosis	Surgical findings	Echo diagnosis	Surgical findings
Coarctation, VSD, and subaortic stenosis	VSD and subaortic stenosis; no coarctation	VSD and coarctation	VSD, coarctation, and PAD
Coarctation, VSD, and PAD	VSD and PAD; no coarctation	Supravalvar pulmonary stenosis and muscular VSD	Supravalvar pulmonary stenosis, muscular VSD and PAD
Coarctation, ASD, and PAD	VSD and PAD; no coarctation	Secundum ASD (2)	Partially anomalous pulmonary venous connection
Pulmonary atresia with intact septum, PAD	PAD, normal looking pulmonary valve	Absent right AV connection with high pulmonary blood flow and PAD	Absent right AV connection, PAD, and coarctation
ASD (2)	Partially anomalous pulmonary venous connection; no ASD		
Mitral stenosis and ASD	ASD, normal looking mitral valve		
Pulmonary valvar stenosis and ASD	ASD, normal looking pulmonary valve		
TAPVC and VSD	VSD, normal pulmonary venous drainage		
Total 9 (0.38%)		5 (0.21%)	

^{a} Abbreviations as in Table 1.

without increasing the risk to the patients and, preferably, at a low cost. It is clear to us that cardiac catheterization and cross-sectional echocardiography should be complementary in planning the surgical treatment of children with congenital heart defect.[3-7] There are situations in which cardiac catheterization is mandatory prior to operation so as to provide precise surgical indications. It is our current policy to consider invasive studies in the circumstances such as pulmonary atresia with ventricular septal defect when it is essential to study the pulmonary arterial supply; tetralogy of Fallot, when the knowledge of the coronary arterial anatomy and assessment of the pulmonary arterial bed is desirable prior to corrective surgery; multiple ventricular septal defects, where a left ventriculogram is mandatory to visualize the position of the defects; absent right atrioventricular connection and double-inlet ventricle prior to a Fontan procedure, when it is necessary to evaluate the morphology of, and pressure within, the pulmonary arteries. Invasive studies are also considered in pulmonary atresia with intact septum, when one suspects the presence of coronary arterial–ventricular sinusoids in a candidate for right ventricular decompression, in pulmonary hypertension secondary to congenital heart defects and, finally, when there is inadequate or incomplete echocardiographic definition of the anatomy.

On the other hand, based upon the analysis of our data, we believe it is possible to indicate surgical treatment safely using echocardiographic diagnosis alone prior to palliative operations (mainly in neonates), such as banding of the pulmonary trunk, Blalock-Taussig shunts, atrial septectomy, pulmonary valvotomy, and Norwood procedures. In addition, definitive surgery can be indicated without cardiac catheterization for ligation of the arterial duct, repair of aortic coarctation, closure of ventricular septal defects, correction of atrioventricular septal defects, repair of totally anomalous pulmonary venous connection, atrial switches, resection of fixed subaortic stenosis, and repair of deformed mitral or aortic valves.

We conclude, therefore, that both palliative and corrective heart surgery can be performed without additional risk in children based upon cross-sectional echocardiography alone in selected cases. In some situations, cardiac catheterization and angiography are still mandatory prior to operation. The diagnostic problems encountered in this study tended to decrease with improvement of the equipment and experience of the operator.

References

1. Leung MP, Mok CK, Lau KC, et al. The role of cross-sectional echocardiography and pulsed Doppler ultrasound in the management of neonates in whom congenital heart disease is suspected: A prospective study. Br Heart J 1986;56:73–82.
2. Gutgesell HP, Huhta JC, Latson LA, et al. Accuracy of two-dimensional echocardiography in the diagnosis of congenital heart disease. Am J Cardiol 1985;55:514–18.
3. Stark J, Smallhorn J, Huhta J, et al. Surgery for congenital heart defects diagnosed with cross-sectional echocardiography. Circulation 1983; 68(suppl II):129–38.
4. Shub C, Tajik J, Seward JB, et al. Surgical repair of uncomplicated atrial septal defect without "routine" preoperative cardiac catheterization. J Am Coll Cardiol 1985;6:49–54.
5. Lipshultz SE, Sanders SP, Mayer JE, et al. Are routine preoperative cardiac catheterization and angiography necessary before repair of ostium primum atrial septal defect? J Am Coll Cardiol 1988;11:373–8.
6. Talano JV. Doppler echocardiography: Will it help replace the need for cardiac catheterization? Chest 1986;90:3–5.
7. Huhta JC, Glasow P, Murphy DJ, et al. Surgery without catheterization for congenital heart defects: Management of 100 patients. J Am Coll Cardiol 1987;9:823–9.

Digital Subtraction and Functional Angiocardiography

J. H. Bursch

Introduction

Digital image processing today offers a wide spectrum of new diagnostic approaches to the angiographic assessment of congenital heart disease.[1-4] Besides technical advances in high-resolution digital imaging, attaining the diagnostic qualities of conventional film-based angiograms, specific aspects result from postprocessing capabilities utilizing digital subtraction angiography, densito-metric and geometric measurements, as well as the parametric imaging mode for functional studies of the circulation. In this article, I will survey the recent experience from the departments of Pediatric Cardiology and Biomedical Engineering in Kiel.

Selection of Images for Digital Subtraction Angiography

An initial step in the processing of digital angiograms is the selection of pairs of images coinciding with the same cardiac (and respiratory) phase. The fact that young children cannot willingly suspend respiration has been thought a serious limitation for the application of digital subtraction angiography in the pediatric age group. Tech-nical advances and accumulating experience, however, have overcome this methodologic deficiency and now offer a simple and practicable solution. Images are acquired prior to the injection over more than one total respiratory cycle length in order to provide selection of a mask image that will show minimal artifacts when subtracted from any particular contrast image. This interactive process of selection requires about 1 minute, but otherwise facilitates image subtraction under optimal clinical conditions. The overall success rate of high-quality digital subtraction angiography from patients with spontaneous and regular breathing was definitely higher than 90%.

Selective Digital Subtraction Angiography

Subtraction imaging of right and left ventricular angiograms has shown to be profitable for several applications, taking advantage of high-contrast sensitivity. It is possible to decrease the total amount of injection volumes (to ½ or ⅓) and/or to lower the radiation dose down to 10%.[5] With a different intention, conventional volumes of contrast are injected for improved visualization of naturally low-contrasted vascular

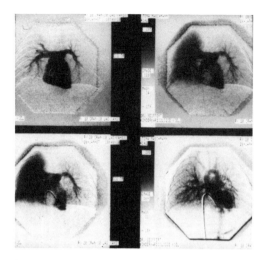

Figure 1. Digital subtraction images for the demonstration of pulmonary vascular and parenchymal opacification. The sequence of images from top left to bottom right corresponds with the temporal course of contrast opacification. The abnormal distribution of contrast in the peripheral lung fields indicates anomalous pulmonary perfusion.

structures, such as small and stenotic vessels with unfavorable flow conditions. In this way, time-consuming catheter manipulation and repeated injections are avoided. Another potential of digital subtraction angiography is imaging of the parenchymal opacification of the lungs and the myocardium.[6] Abnormal pulmonary perfusion can be imaged to provide similar information as pulmonary scintigraphy (Fig. 1).

Intravenous Digital Subtraction Angiography

The injection of contrast medium via a central venous catheter offers comparable contrast resolution as selective angiocardiography.[7,8] Particular use of intravenous digital subtraction angiography has been made for studies in the immediate postoperative state of patients utilizing conventional infusion lines for contrast delivery. A total of about 0.8 ml contrast medium per kilogram of body weight (but no more than 20 ml in adolescents) is injected within 2.5 seconds or less. Particularly significant is the ability to study the morphology of the right and left ventricular outflow tract as, for example, after correction of tetralogy of Fallot or double-outlet right ventricle. Intravenous digital subtraction angiography also detects residual shunts as well as stenotic lesions, such as peripheral pulmonary stenosis or aortic coarctation. Images of the phase of capillary perfusion within the lung are also indicated for the detection of postoperative pulmonary complications such as embolism.

Densitometric Analysis:

Digital systems provide manual outlining of regions of interest in angiographic (subtraction) images. The definition of the regions of interest forms the basis for regional measurements of the contrast mass as, for example, in the ventricular chambers. A particular advantage of densitometry utilizing digital subtraction angiography images (in contrast to videodensitometry of native images) is that structures of nonspecific density (image background) are mostly eliminated, thus causing no disturbing effects on the measurements of the radioopaque indicator (Fig. 2). A numerical value is calculated by summing up all densities (within regions of interest) proportional to the total amount of medium in that chamber. One of the most relevant applications is ventricular densitometry for quantitation of valvar regurgitation[6] with particular emphasis to (postoperative) pulmonary insufficiency. This is applicable to more than half of all patients with valvar regurgitant lesions in the pediatric age group. Ratios of ventricular volumes are calculated from densitometric data of two consecutive cardiac cycles, immediately following injection of contrast. A set of five digital subtraction angiography images is usually processed at the termination of subsequent diastolic and systolic phases. Density ratios represent fractional changes in volume and, thereby, permit de-

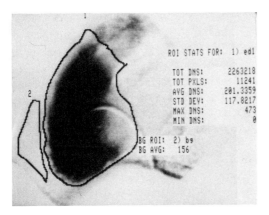

ROI STATS FOR: 1) ed1

TOT DNS: 2263218
TOT PXLS: 11241
AVG DNS: 201.3359
STD DEV: 117.8217
MAX DNS: 473
MIN DNS: 0

BG ROI: 2) bg
BG AVG: 156

Figure 2. Selective right ventricular substraction angiogram in lateral projection for illustration of ventricular densitometry. The ventricular contour was manually traced to the confines of the end-diastolic right ventricular silhouette. Density data are automatically summated with displayed on the monitor (TOT DNS). A second (2) small area is used to measure the averaged background densities (BG AVG) for comparison.

termination of ratios of regurgitant and total stroke volumes as well as ventricular ejection fraction. Digital subtraction angiography systems, in addition, provide geometric analysis of left ventricular volume and analysis of wall motion. At present, computations are only feasible for projections in a single plane, thus producing some limitations as far as the accuracy of determination of volumes is concerned.

Parametric Imaging

The latest advancement in digital angiography relates to the processing of image sequences for analysis of temporal aspects of circulatory flow.[9,10] Temporal changes of densities are calculated from each individual picture element and temporal data are obtained in accordance with the appearance of contrast material at each site. This information is subsequently converted into colors, thus providing a visual aspect of the speed of flow in the angiographic image format. Clinical experience with parametric imaging includes studies of pulmonary and coronary arterial blood flow. In particular, flow distribution has been assessed in the pulmonary arteries as well as the reserve of coronary flow. On a similar basis, the relative volumes of flow through the arterial branches were obtained, providing the potential for evaluation of the effectiveness of systemic-to-pulmonary anastomoses.

References

1. Bogren HG, Bursch JH. Digital angiography in the diagnosis of congenital heart disease. Cardiovasc Intervent Radiol 1984;7:180–8.
2. Heintzen PH, Brennecke R (eds). Digital Imaging in Cardiovascular Radiology. Stuttgart, Thieme, 1983.
3. Heintzen PH. Digital angiocardiography. In: Collins SM, Skorton DJ (eds), Cardiac Imaging and Image Processing. New York, McGraw-Hill, 1985, pp 239–79.
4. Heintzen PH, Bursch JH (eds). Progress in Digital Angiocardiography. Dordrecht, Kluwer Academic Publishers, 1988.
5. Levin AR, Goldberg HL, Borer JS, et al. Digital angiography in the pediatric patient with congenital heart disease: comparison with standard methods. Circulation 1983;68:374–84.
6. Bursch JH, Heintzen PH. The role of digital subtraction angiography in congenital and valvular heart disease. In: Mancini GBJ (ed), Clinical Applications of Cardiac Digital Angiography. New York, Raven Press, 1988, pp 199–217.
7. Brennecke R, Bursch JH, Bogren HG, Heintzen PH. Digital intravenous imaging techniques in pediatric cardiology. In: Mistretta CA, Crummy AB, Strother CM, Sackett JF (eds), Digital Subtraction Arteriography: An Application of Computerized Fluoroscopy. Chicago, Year Book Medical Publ, 1982, pp 133–41.
8. Bursch JH. Digital angiocardiography for assessment of congenital heart disease. In: Friedmann WF, Higgins CB (eds), Pediatric Cardiac Imaging. Philadelphia, WB Saunders, 1984, pp 64–75.
9. Bursch JH, Heintzen PH. Parametric imaging. Radiol Clin North Am 1985;28:183–8.
10. Heintzen PH, Bursch JH, Hahne HJ, et al. Assessment of cardiovascular function by digital angiocardiography. J Am Coll Cardiol 1985;5:150–57.

III

Valvar Disease in Children

3.1

Introduction

R. H. Anderson and G. Crupi

As we have seen demonstrated in the other sections of this volume, remarkable strides have been made in the successful treatment of even the most complex congenital malformations, including lesions such as atrial isomerism (see Part 1, Chapter 3.11). But, as we have also read in the previous section, major problems remain to be overcome in the setting of rheumatic disease of the cardiac valves, a particularly formidable task in the countries of the developing world. In this section, we will find that similar problems confront the surgeon dealing with congenital lesions of the cardiac valves, particularly when they are sufficiently severe to necessitate replacement of the valve. Indeed, the major decision in any child with a lesion of a cardiac valve is whether repair can be achieved or whether the native valve must be sacrificed. This is the major issue to be debated in this section.

The opening chapters are concerned with disease of the mitral valve. Quero Jimenez and his associates discuss the indications for surgery and the potential prognosis after repair, and then the salient pathological features are reviewed by Van Praagh and his colleagues. The trend towards conservative treatment has been unequivocally spearheaded by Carpentier and, in an extensive review, he and his colleagues outline their functional classification of valvar diseases and the results of surgery performed in their own center. The value of the functional approach to diagnosis pioneered by Carpentier is then endorsed by the experience of the group from Padova, who emphasize the long-term results of reparative surgery, having found it possible to preserve the native valve in 31 of 35 patients undergoing surgery for a variety of congenital malformations of the mitral valve.

Not all centers, however, opt for preservation of the mitral valve but continue to search for an optimal prosthetic device. Asano described an experience where the results of repair and replacement are contrasted for surgery on the mitral valve, with repair emerging as the better technique. Harada and his colleagues, however, also from Japan, report an extensive experience of replacement of various valves, mostly mitral, with the St. Jude prosthesis. Their nine-year experience reveals 90.5% actuarial survival and 92.1% calculated free of valve-related events. They conclude that the St. Jude prosthesis is the valve substitute of choice in the pediatric age range. Haàn and his colleagues from Hungary also report an impressive series of long-term results following replacement of diseased valves with mechanical prostheses. Like Harada et al., they conclude that this mode of treatment carries a low incidence of valve-related complications and provides marked long-term functional improvement. But then, in the next chapter, equally impressive results are provided by a collaborative Brazilian investigation into the use of glutaraldehyde-preserved aortic allobioprostheses. The valves were prepared commercially and inserted in 77 patients, 68 in mitral position. There have been only two deaths in this experience encompassing five Brazilian cities. As the authors reasonably conclude, there is surely reason to continue with this clinical trial.

In the final chapters of this section, Todorov and his colleagues from Bulgaria review their experience with surgical treatment of disease of the tricuspid valve in childhood, while Rubay and his associates from Belgium summarize ably the overall dilemmas of the surgeon contemplating replacement of any valve during the period of childhood. They point to the promise of aortic homografts, so graphically demonstrated by the Brazilian cooperation, but describe their own extensive experience of replacement predominantly with mechanical valves. Again they report impressive surgical results, concluding that, when no alternative exists, replacement of valves can be accomplished with a low operative mortality and a satisfactory late survival. The conclusions to be drawn from this section, therefore, are that, if possible, most surgeons would strive to repair the native valve. In this respect, the functional classification of Carpentier has surely proven its worth. But, if replacement is necessary in childhood, excellent results can be obtained with various mechanical prostheses and, if the promise of the Brazilian experience is maintained, also by the use of aortic homografts.

Surgical Indications and Prognosis for Repair of Disease of the Mitral Valve

M. Quero Jimenez, M. J. Maitre Azcarate,
and J. M. Brito Perez

Introduction

Nowadays rheumatic fever and chronic rheumatic heart disease are exceedingly uncommon in our country. During a period of 12 years working in the Medico-Surgical Unit of Pediatric Cardiology in the Hospital Ramon y Cajal (Madrid, Spain) we have seen only three cases of rheumatic heart disease, all of them being referred from abroad. During the same period of time, we have seen 72 cases of congenital disease of the mitral valve. It is the clinical evaluation of the latter lesion that will be outlined in this chapter.

Pathologic Considerations

For the proper understanding of the establishment of sound indications for surgery and to determine prognosis, some general morphologic aspects must first be considered. Congenital disease of the mitral valve may involve the annulus, the leaflets, the tendinous cords, and the papillary muscles. The annulus is seldom involved as an isolated structure, although it is frequently small in congenital obstructive lesions and enlarged in the setting of mitral insufficiency. The pathology of the leaflets is varied. The mural leaflet may be hypoplastic, or the aortic leaflet be the seat of an isolated cleft; the entire tissue may be deficient (often affecting the commissures); the leaflets may prolapse or show perforations, double orifices, or the hammock malformation. The cords may be short, absent, accessory, and/or elongated. The papillary muscles may be abnormally configured as in the complex of the hammock malformations. In deed, the hammock, parachute, and arcade malformations are mixed in nature, so that all three valvar components (leaflets, cords, and papillary muscles) are involved. In our own material, we have studied 72 patients in whom the diagnosis was established by means of echocardiography and/or angiocardiography. The mitral valve was involved in isolation in 26 cases, while there were other associated malformations in 46 patients (Table 1).

Table 1

Pathology of the Mitral Valve and Associated Lesions

Isolated mitral pathology	
Mitral valve prolapse (with severe incompetence)	11
Hammock mitral valve	5
Parachute mitral valve	5
Arcade malformations of mitral valve	2
Congenital perforation	1
Double mitral orifice	2
Total	26
Associated malformations	
Left ventricular and aortic tract pathology	30[a]
Ventricular septal defect	8
Ventricular septal defect and coarctation	2
Patent arterial duct and coarctation	1
Tetralogy of Fallot	2
Double-outlet right ventricle	3
Total	46

[a] In four patients the complete characteristics of the Shone syndrome were present. In 11 patients, aortic coarctation was associated.

Physiopathologic and Clinical Considerations

So as to establish the indications for surgery and to determine prognosis, our 72 patients were analyzed according to the physiopathological nature of the malformation and the degree of its severity (Table 2). The lesion was mainly stenotic in 33 cases (slight in 14, moderate in seven, and severe in 12).

In 25 patients, it was insufficiency which predominanted (slight in 17, moderate in five, and severe in three). In the other 14 patients the malformation was both stenotic and regurgitant, its degree of severity being slight in six patients, moderate in five, and severe in three.

The degree of severity of the malformation was established by combining clinical and physiopathological criteria. We use "slight" to describe patients who are asymptomatic and not requiring any treatment, in whom alterations of myocardial function and/or the pulmonary circulation were nonexistent or mild. "Moderate" disability was used to indicate the appearance of symptoms, that medical treatment may be necessary, and/or that the myocardial and pulmonary circulations are moderately involved. In severely disabled patients, the symptoms are pronounced and/or the myocardium and pulmonary circulation are severely compromised.

Diagnostic Considerations

It is the specific diagnosis of the morphologic and physiopathological situation of each individual patient that determines the indications for surgery and the prognosis. In our 72 patients, diagnosis always was established by means of cross-sectional echocardiography and Doppler studies. In this way, it is possible to demonstrate the parachute

Table 2

The Relationship of Severity to the Functional Malformations of the Valve

	Severity and main classification			
	Slight	Moderate	Severe	Total
Stenosis	14	7	12	33
Insufficiency	17	5	3	25
Both	6	5	3	14
Total	37	17	18	72

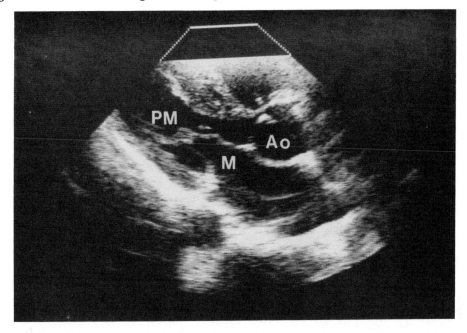

Figure 1a. Left parasternal projection, long axial view, showing a mitral valve with a single papillary muscle. PM, papillary muscle; M, mitral valve; Ao, aortic valve.

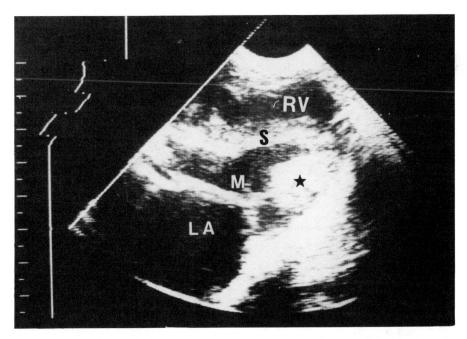

Figure 1b. An arcade malformation of the mitral valve seen in the four-chamber view. The left atrium (LA) appears dilated and the mitral valve (M) inserts in a muscular structure (star) which divides the left ventricle. S, ventricular septum; RV, right ventricle.

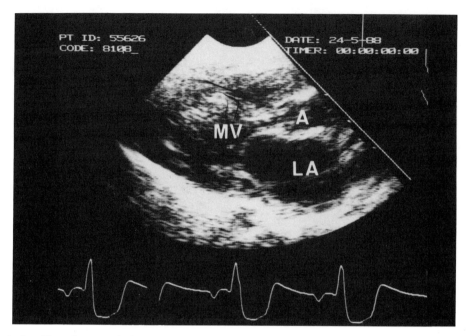

Figure 1c. The characteristic appearance of the hammock malformation of the mitral valve (MV). The left atrium (LA) is dilated. There is associated mild valvar aortic stenosis. A, Aorta.

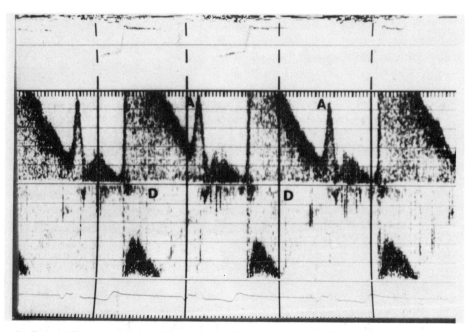

Figure 2. Pulsed-Doppler study of the mitral valve in a case of slight to moderate mitral stenosis. The probe is placed immediately behind the mitral annulus. Note the initially increased diastolic velocity with a posterior slow deceleration slope (D) and a new increased velocity due to atrial contraction (A).

Table 3

Surgical Procedures Used in Pediatric Cardiac Surgery Service of Ramon y Cajal Hospital (Follow-up: 3 months to 10 years)

	Cases	Procedure	Mortality
Mitral stenosis			
Isolated parachute mitral valve	2	Prosthesis	1
Parachute mitral valve and subaortic stenosis	2	Prosthesis	1
Hammock mitral valve and aortic coarctation	1	Prosthesis	0
Restricted opening (limited to the postero-medial commissure) + aortic coarctation	1	Commissurotomy	0
Mitral insufficiency[a]	10	Prosthesis—5 Annuloplasty—5	1 1
Combined mitral malformation	2	Prosthesis	0
Total	18	Prosthesis—12 Reconstructive surgery—6	4 (22%)

[a] Among the five patients with a prosthesis, one had aortic stenosis and another one with insufficiency required an aortic prosthesis as well. In the subset of patients with mitral annuloplasty, one of them had supraaortic stenosis and another one was associated with an aortic stenosis at the valvular level.

deformity (Fig. 1a), the arcade malformation (Fig. 1b), or the hammock lesion (Fig. 1c). Double orifice can also be diagnosed. The degree of stenosis can be assessed by studying the maximal velocity of the diastolic flow of blood across the mitral valve (Fig. 2). Valvar insufficiency is depicted optimally by means of color echocardiography. When it has been determined to insert a prosthesis, it is most important to measure the region of the atrioventricular junction in which the prosthesis is to be inserted.

Surgical Options

After having determined the pertinent morphologic, physiopathologic, and clinical situation, the surgical options are reconstructive[1-5] versus replacement.[6-10] In our patients, the indications for surgery were established on the basis of severe symptomatology and/or evidence of pulmonary hypertension. Cases with mild to moderate symptomatology are followed carefully, particularly if it is thought that a prosthesis may be needed. With those considerations in mind, surgery has been performed to date in 18 of our 72 patients (Table 3). All were below the age of 6 years. A prosthesis was inserted in 12 cases and repair was carried out in six. Fourteen survived, and all are asymptomatic after a period of follow-up ranging from 3 months to 10 years. Only three of them have needed medical treatment. Moderate degrees of valvar disease may be treated surgically when bypass surgery is being carried out for other associated lesions. Such cases have not been included in this study. Repair should be performed whenever possible. The proportion submitted to repair and valvar replacement varies from one center to another. In our unit, replacement predominates in the proportion of 2:1. The long-term prognosis for congenital malformations of the mitral valve is still uncertain despite undeniable recent advances. In our opinion, nonetheless, those with only a mild to moderate degree of impartment should have surgery delayed for as long as possible.

References

1. Antunes MJ, Colsen PR, Kinsley RH. Mitral valvuloplasty: A learning curve. Circulation 1983;68:1170–5.
2. Carpentier A, Branchini B, Cour JC, et al: Congenital malformations of the mitral valve in children: Pathology and surgical treatment. J Thorac Cardiovasc Surg 1976;72:854–66.
3. Carpentier A, Chauvaud S, Fabiani JN et al: Reconstructive surgery of mitral valve incompetence: Ten-year appraisal. J Thorac Surg 1980;79:338–48.
4. Cosgrove DM, Chavez AM, Lytle BW, et al: Results of mitral valve reconstruction. Circulation 1986;74:(Suppl 1)82–7.
5. Chauvaud S, Perier P, Touati G, et al: Long-term results of valve repair in children with acquired mitral valve incompetence. Circulation 1986;74:1104–9.
6. Borkon AM, McIntosh CL, Von Rueden TJ, Morrow AG: Mitral valve replacement with Hancock bioprosthesis: Five to ten years follow-up. Ann Thorac Surg 1981;32:127–37.
7. Borkon AM, Soule L, Reitz BA, et al. Five year follow-up after valve replacement with the St. Jude Medical valve in infants and children. Circulation 1986;74:1110–5.
8. Bortolotti U, Milano A, Mazzucco A, et al: Alterazioni strutturali delle bioprotesi di Hancock applicate in età pediatrica. G Ital Cardiol 1980;10:1520–25.
9. Daliento L, Nava A, Fasoli G, et al. Dysplasia of atrioventricular valves associated with conduction system anomalies. Br Heart J 1984;51:243–51.
10. Gallucci V, Bortolotti U, Milano A, et al. Isolated mitral valve replacement with the Hancock bioprosthesis: A 13-year appraisal. Ann Thorac Surg 1984;38:571–8.

Surgical Pathology of Malformations of the Mitral Valve

R. Van Praagh, K. A. Chacko, and B. O'Connor

Introduction

We undertook this study in an effort to attain a better understanding of the surgically relevant pathologic anatomy of congenital anomalies of the mitral valve.

Material

We reexamined 45 postmortem cases. Congenital stenosis was seen in 26 cases (58%), while congenital regurgitation was found in 13 (29%). These were combined stenosis and regurgitation of congenital origin in two (4%), and a double orifice of the valve was observed in four (9%). In the latter four cases, the double orifice was thought to be physiologically insignificant. Hence, of these 45 cases, 41 (91%) were considered to be physiologically and clinically significant and, hence, of surgical importance. For the purposes of this surgically oriented presentation, attention will be focused on the first two groups only.

Findings

Congenital Mitral Stenosis

Typical congenital mitral stenosis[1] with obliteration of interchordal spaces and reduction of the interpapillary muscle distance (Fig. 1A) was found in eight of the 26 cases (31%). One of these had vegetations consistent with old bacterial endocarditis. As expected for typical congenital mitral stenosis, there were two papillary muscles in each case.

A parachute deformity of the valve occurred in eight cases (31%). All the tendinous cords were inserted into the posteromedial papillary muscle group in seven of these eight cases with two separate atrioventricular valves (Fig. 1B). All the cords inserted into the anterolateral papillary muscle group in the remaining case, which also had separate atrioventricular valves. In parachute mitral valve with a divided atrioventricular canal, it is the anterolateral papillary muscle group that is typically absent (Fig. 1B). The papillary muscle groups, however,

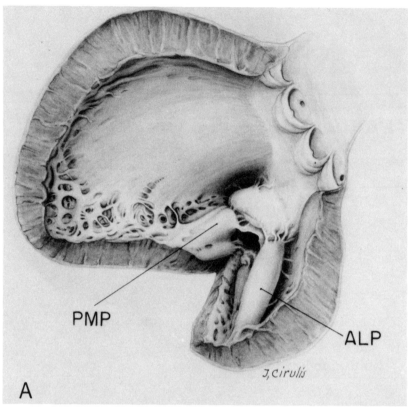

PMP

ALP

J. Cirulis

A

Figure 1. Congenital mitral stenosis. (A) Typical congenital mitral stenosis. The left ventricle and ascending aorta have been opened to show reduced interpapillary muscle distance and obliteration of intercordal spaces. ALP, anterolateral papillary muscle; PMP, posteromedial papillary muscle. (B) Parachute mitral valve (MV). The left ventricle and ascending aorta are opened to show that all the tendinous cords insert into the large PMP, the ALP being absent, the small valvar orifice opens eccentrically into the left ventricular wall. (C) Fusion of the papillary muscle groups, a forme fruste of the parachute valve, with marked reduction of the interpapillary muscle space (IPMS), and intercordal obliteration except at the anterolateral commissure (ALC). FR, fibrous ridge. (D) Left atrial view of double orifice mitral valve (DOMV) with a central subdividing strand. ASD 2°, atrial septal defect within the oval fossa; LA, left atrium, LV, left ventricle; PV's pulmonary veins; and S 1°, primary atrial septum. (E) A double orifice, seen from within the opened left ventricle, showing a prominent muscular ridge (R) subdividing the orifice into a main posteromedial orifice (POr) and an accessory anterolateral orifice (AOr). The ridge is confluent with the anterolateral muscle. Note the multiple muscular ventricular septal defects (VSD's). (F) Supramitral stenosing ring (SMR) seen from its left atrial aspect. LAA, left atrial appendage. (Reproduced with permission from Ruckman and Van Praagh[1] and from Bano et al.[2]).

may both be present but fused together (Fig. 1C).

A diminutive mitral valve in the setting of a hypoplastic left ventricle was found in four cases (15%). This constellation is the typical form of congenital mitral stenosis found in association with the hypoplastic left heart syndrome, the other findings usually being aortic atresia with a small-chambered and thick-walled left ventricle together with endocardial fibroelastosis. Clinically and surgically, this anatomic type is not relevant to congenital mitral stenosis.

The mitral valve had a dual orifice by

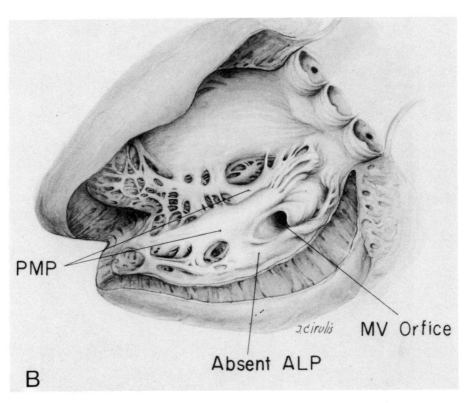

B

PMP

Absent ALP

MV Orfice

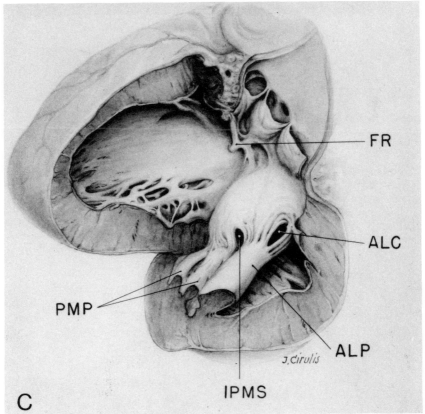

FR

ALC

PMP

IPMS

ALP

C

Figure 1. (*continued*)

93

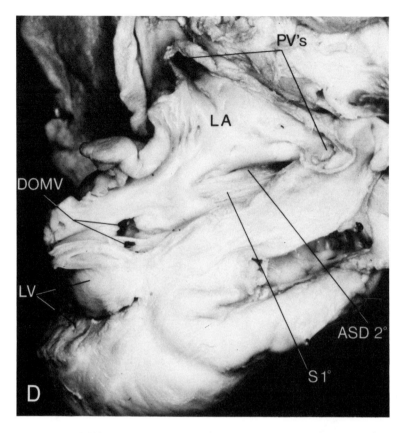

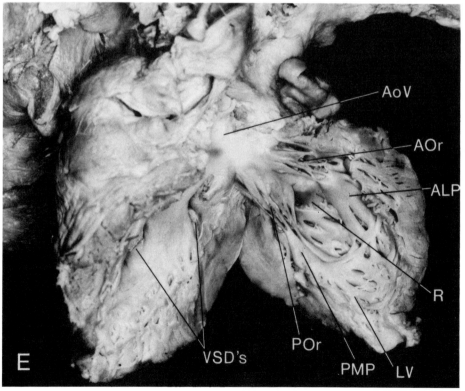

Figure 1. (*continued*)

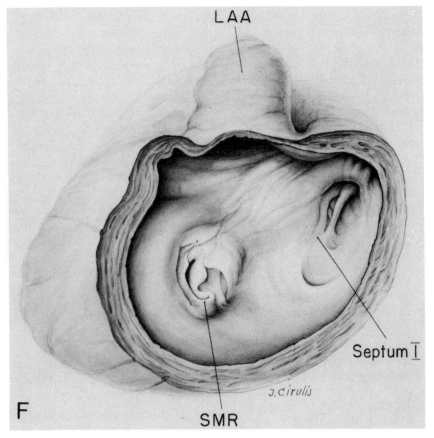

Figure 1. (*continued*)

virtue of a central fibrous strand (Fig. 1D) in three cases (12%), this being an infrequent and little-known form of congenital mitral stenosis. Two papillary muscles are present, but they may be abnormally close together and fused at their bases.[2] In one case (4%), a double-orifice was due to an accessory anterolateral orifice and a subdividing muscular ridge (Fig. 1E). This rare form of congenital stenosis is produced by the muscular ridge being confluent with the anterolateral papillary muscle (Fig. 1E). Both papillary muscles are present, but one is malformed.

Direct insertion of the leaflets of the valve into the crest of the muscular ventricular septum occurred in one case (4%). The mitral valve did not attach via tendinous cords to the papillary muscles. This anomaly is very rare. Completing this group was a solitary example of a stenosing supravalvar ring within the left atrium (Fig. 1F).

Congenital Mitral Regurgitation

Typical congenital regurgitation was found in four cases (31%). There was upward hooding of intercordal leaflet tissue, some obliteration of intercordal spaces, tethering of the leaflets by thick and short cords, and an inability of the leaflets to coapt. An isolated cleft was observed in four cases (31%). Only mild regurgitation appeared to have been present in most of these.

Marked underdevelopment of the anterolateral papillary muscle was found in two cases (15%). The aortic leaflet of the mitral valve was asymmetrical, being triangular instead of the anticipated semicircular shape.

Congenital perforation of the mural leaflet was found in one case (8%). This perforation, in the absence of subjacent tensor apparatus, could have been patched, there by avoiding replacement of the value.

Congenital prolapse, with the typical "hemorrhoidal" appearance, occurred in one case (8%). A double orifice with severe regurgitation through the accessory anterolateral orifice was found in one case (8%). Three papillary muscles were present in the left ventricle. The regurgitant accessory orifice could have been patched.

Arrangement of the Papillary Muscles

Of the 26 cases with valvar stenosis, two papillary muscles were found in 14 cases (54%); the muscles were fused in three (12%); a solitary papillary muscle was seen in eight (31%), and there was absence of both papillary muscles in one case (4%). When the valve was regurgitant, two papillary muscles were seen in 10 of the 13 cases (77%); there was marked underdevelopment of the anterolateral papillary muscle group in two (15%); and three papillary muscles were seen in one case (8%). In cases with congenital regurgitation (as opposed to stenosis), there were no cases with fusion of the papillary muscles, or with only one papillary muscle or absence of both papillary muscles.

Discussion

For full understanding of the morphology of the mitral valve, it is important to note that the mitral valve is a canal with an inlet [that may be abnormal, as in stenosing mitral ring, (Fig. 1F)], a middle portion (thickened leaflets), and an outlet (the cords and intercordal spaces, papillary muscles, and the ventricular myocardial architecture).

Any part of the canal can be malformed. A ring within the tendinous cords appears to result in an orifice.[2] This applies to the normal valvar orifice and to accessory orifices in valves with dual orifices.

An inverse relationship exists between the leaflet tissue of the valve and the tendinous cords.[2] Where leaflet tissue normally is maximal (for example, at the center of the aortic leaflet of the valve), tendinous cords are minimal. In contrast, where leaflet tissue normally is minimal (as at the commissures), cords are maximal. The inverse relationship is seen as one progresses from the center of the aortic leaflet to either commissure.

The tension apparatus is of fundamental importance in understanding anomalies of the valve. The tension apparatus is the "sinner." The mitral valve leaflets are the "sinned against" (the "victim"). Echocardiographic attention preoperatively should be focused not only on the leaflets, but above all on the tension apparatus that makes these anomalies comprehensive.[1-3] Similarly, intraoperative surgical diagnosis should be focused not only on the leaflets, but above all on the subjacent tensor apparatus. It is here that the real anomaly usually resides. This is where surgical valvoplasty should be focused. Needless to say, the annulus of the valve and its leaflets are important, but one should never forget that "most of the woe lies below"!

References

1. Ruckman RN, Van Praagh R. Anatomic types of congenital mitral stenosis: report of 49 autopsy cases with consideration of diagnosis and surgical implications. Am J Cardiol 1978; 42:592–601.
2. Bano-Rodrigo A, Van Praagh S, Trowitzsch E, Van Praagh R. Double-orifice mitral valve: A study of 27 postmortem cases with developmental, diagnostic, and surgical considerations. Am J Cardiol 1988;61:152–60.
3. Freed MD, Keane JF, Van Praagh R, et al. Coarctation of the aorta with congenital mitral regurgitation. Circulation 1974;49:1175–84.

Classification of Congenital Malformations of the Mitral Valve and Their Surgical Management

A. Carpentier, S. Chauvaud, and S. Mihaileanu

Introduction

Congenital malformations of the mitral valve still pose a difficult surgical problem. The lesions are complex and frequently associated with other congenital malformations. Echocardiography now makes possible, however, the recognition of these lesions in most cases prior to undertaking any operation. In this article, we will outline the functional classification we have developed for these lesions and discuss the appropriate surgical treatment.

Functional Classification

In spite of multiple anatomic features, it is also possible to classify congenital lesions of the mitral valve from a functional aspect. The malformations are classified according to whether there is valvar incompetence, stenosis, or both. Then, from the echocardiographic findings, it is possible to know prior to surgery if the motion of the leaflets is normal, prolapsed, or restricted. The papillary muscles can be either normal or abnormal. When more than one anomaly is present, it is the primary lesion that is used for classification.

The aim of surgery is to restore normal function rather than normal anatomy of the mitral valve. Four basic techniques are used and are easily reproducible: remodeling of the annulus, resection and suture of the leaflets, shortening of the tendinous cords,[1] and fenestration of fused cordal support.

Congenital Mitral Valve Incompetence

Normal Leaflet Motion

Annular Dilatation

Pure and isolated annular dilatation can be congenital. The dilatation mainly affects the mural (posterior) leaflet and not the aortic (anterior) leaflet. This anomaly can always be treated with reconstructive surgery. Annuloplasty by means of a prosthetic ring is possible in most of the cases. If the operation is performed on patients having a body weight less than 10 kg, it is preferable to avoid the use of a prosthetic ring since this can create stenosis at a later age. In this situation, valvar incompetence can be corrected by means of rectangular resection and suture of the edges of the leaflet along with annular plication. The resection should be electively performed in the areas of indentation of the mural leaflet.

Cleft Leaflet

This condition affects the aortic leaflet. In this respect, those so-called "clefts" found in atrioventricular septal defects have not been included in this analysis. The valvar apparatus is normal except for the cleft that separates the aortic leaflet into two hemileaflets. Abnormal tendinous cords are often attached to the free edges of the cleft. The orifice may be dilated but the paired papillary muscles are normal. In most cases, recreation of the leaflet can be performed by direct suture. When the edges are rolled and retracted, however, a pericardial patch is necessary to fill the gap between the two hemileaflets.

Deficiency of the Leaflet

Localized agenesis of the leaflet tissue is usually localized to the mural leaflet. The free edge of the defective area is usually free of tendinous cords. Surgical correction is obtained by rectangular resection of the corresponding part of the leaflet and suture of the free edges.

Prolapsed Leaflet

In this condition, the free edge of one or both leaflets overrides the plane of the atrioventricular orifice during systole. It is a functional definition that excludes the billowing mitral valve without valvar incompetence. A billowing valve may become prolapsed if cordal rupture or elongation occurs.

Elongated Cords

Cordal elongation usually involves all the tendinous cords arising from one of the papillary muscles. Elongated cords have been described in Marfan's syndrome and can be associated with Barlow's syndrome. Cordal elongation is treated by shortening the cords. Dilatation of the annulus is corrected by a prosthetic ring.

Elongated Papillary Muscles

Elongation of the papillary muscles is usually associated with anomalous origin of the left coronary artery from the pulmonary trunk, but this condition may exist in the absence either of other intracardiac malformations or coronary arterial anomalies. The papillary muscle involved is thin, flattened, and elongated. It has a fibrotic appearance with a pale or yellowish color. Elongation of a papillary muscle is corrected by the technique of muscle shortening. The papillary muscle is buried in the left ventricular wall.

Absent Cords

Absence of one or several tendinous cords attached to the free edge of the leaflet leads to prolapse of the corresponding portion of the leaflet. When the leaflet is totally devoid of cordal support, correction is obtained by means of resection and suture. When secondary cords are present on the ventricular surface, the free edge of the leaflet can be sutured to the secondary cords.

Restricted Leaflet Motion with Normal Papillary Muscles

Commissural Fusion

One or both commissures can be fused. The tendinous cords are short in this setting, while the papillary muscles are normally developed or hypertrophied and adherent to the commissure. The valvar tissue between the cords is thin and multiperforated, a condition that is different from rheumatic disease. Valvar incompetence is due either to limitation of the motion of the aortic leaflet, annular dilatation, or both. Commissurotomy and splitting of the papillary muscle is advised. But commissurotomy is difficult because incision into the abnormal commissural tissue may create commissural incompetence. The use of a prosthetic ring, concentrating the plication at the commissure, usually corrects the residual valvar incompetence.

Short Cords

Reduction of the length of the cords leads to limitation in the motion of the leaflets. The cords are not fused, and they are well individualized. The papillary muscle is often hypertrophied and may create an associated stenosis. Surgical correction includes fenestration of the papillary muscle in order to restore the mobility of the leaflets. Annular remodeling is carried out to restore the appropriate size of the annulus.

Restricted Leaflet Motion with Abnormal Papillary Muscles

Parachute Mitral Valve

All the tendinous cords are attached to a single papillary muscle. The intercordal spaces are often obliterated by abnormal valvar tissue leading to an associated stenosis. Valvar incompetence is due to associated lesions such as clefts, hypoplasia of the tissue of the leaflets, short cords, or annular dilatation. The implantation of the parachute papillary muscle is always in the lower half of the left ventricle. Treatment is achieved by splitting the single papillary muscle, fenestration of intercordal spaces, and remodeling of the annulus.

Hammock Mitral Valve

In this condition, the muscular subvalvar apparatus is implanted high in the posterior wall underneath the mural leaflet. All the cords are attached on this muscular formation. The valvar orifice is obstructed by intermixed cords leading to an associated valvar stenosis. Incompetence may be due to various causes such as clefts, hypoplasia of the aortic leaflet short cords, and annular dilatation. Surgical treatment is especially difficult. Techniques involve fenestration of the intercordal spaces, splitting of the muscular tissue, mobilization of the hammock from the left ventricular wall, and remodeling of a deformed annulus.

Papillary Muscle Hypoplasia and Agenesis

Poor development of one or both papillary muscles leads to valvar incompetence. The tendinous cords are short, and the mobility of the leaflet is impaired Underdevelopment of the tissue of the leaflets in the vicinity of the abnormal papillary muscle is present. The most frequent anomaly is hypoplasia of the anterolateral muscle associated with hypoplasia of the corresponding half of the leaflet. Correction of the valvar insufficiency is obtained by an annuloplasty incorporating a prosthetic ring. The annulus is reshaped by reducing the angle of the commissure in order to compensate for the lack of valvar tissue.

Congenital Mitral Valve Stenosis

With Normal Papillary Muscles

Papillary Muscle and Commissural Fusion

The two papillary muscles are attached to the commissure. The leaflet tissue at the commissure is fused. The tendinous cords are absent. The central orifice of the mitral valve is between the two papillary muscles. This anomaly is corrected by commissurotomy, fenestration of the papillary muscles, and removal of secondary cords.

Excess Valvar Tissue

The valvar apparatus is otherwise normal except for the obstruction of intercordal spaces by anomalous leaflet tissue. The abnormal tissue is often thin, very similar to valvar tissue. Cordal fenestration and removal of excess tissue leads to relief of the obstruction.

Supravalvar Ring

The ring is a circumferential, discontinuous ridge of fibrous tissue. It is attached partially on the valvar tissue below the annulus and also on the atrial wall slightly above the annulus. It leads to a limitation in the motion of the leaflet as well as narrowing of the valvar orifice. The supravalvar ring may be the only malformation with a normal mitral valve underneath. But more often, the supravalvar ring is associated with a parachute mitral valve, subvalvular aortic stenosis, and aortic coarctation; the combination is often called the Shone syndrome. Surgical treatment consists of resection of the fibrous tissue, taking care not to injure the tissue of the leaflets.

With Abnormal Papillary Muscles

Parachute Mitral Valve

All the cords are attached to a single papillary muscle. The stenosis results from obliteration of the intercordal spaces by excess valvar tissue and restriction in the motion of the leaflets by short cords. The parachute is corrected by splitting the papillary muscle and fenestration of the intercordal spaces.

Table 1
Mitral Valve Incompetence in 108 Patients

Normal leaflet motion
Annular dilatation (7)
Cleft leaflet (15)
Leaflet defect (3)
Prolapsed leaflet
Elongated cords (22)
Elongated papillary muscle (10)
Absent cords (4)
Restricted leaflet motion
With normal papillary muscle
Commissural fusion (15)
Short cords (4)
With abnormal papillary muscle
Parachute valve (10)
Hammock valve (14)
Papillary muscle hypoplasia and
agenesis (4)

Number of patients is in parenthesis.

Hammock Mitral Valve

The papillary muscles are absent and replaced by a muscular formation that is implanted high and posteriorly in the left ventricle. The muscular apparatus is the cause of the obstruction. Tendinous cords of the anterior leaflet cross the central orifice toward the hammock and participate to the obstruction. The functional orifice is, in effect, the multiple spaces between the cords. In severe cases, the orifice is reduced to a fibrous diaphragm with scattered holes. Surgical treatment is difficult. The goal is to create two separate papillary muscles by splitting the hammock valve. Removal of the secondary cords is necessary.

Clinical Results

Congenital Mitral Valve Incompetence

From 1979 to 1987, 108 patients (Table 1) under 12 years of age underwent operation for congenital valvar incompetence following the techniques of Carpentier.[2] The

Table 2

Congenital Mitral Valve Incompetence

		Valve repair (%)	Hospital death (%)	Reoperation (%)
Normal leaflets	25	100	4	0
Prolapsed leaflets	36	94.5	11.1	8.8
Restricted motion				
Normal muscles	19	79	16	12
Abnormal muscles	28	89	18	4

period of follow-up is between 18 months and 10 years with a mean of 8.5 years.

Twenty-five patients with normal motion of the leaflets underwent operation at a mean age of 5.3 years (range, 0.7–12 years) (Table 2). Repair of the valve was always possible. The hospital mortality was 1/25 (4%); 83% of the patients (20/24) are in functional class I of the New York Heart Association and 16% are in class II. No patient has required reoperation and no thromboembolic events have occurred.

Thirty-six patients with prolapsed leaflets underwent operation (Table 2). Their ages ranged between 1 and 12 years, with a mean of 4.5 years. Repair was possible in 94.5%. The hospital mortality was 11.1%; 88% of the patients are in class I and 12% in class II. No thromboembolic events occurred. Three patients (8.8%) needed reoperation because of mitral valvar incompetence.

Operations were performed on 19 patients with restricted motion of the leaflets and normal papillary muscles (Table 2). Their ages ranged between 0.5 and 12 years, with a mean of 4.2 years. Repair was achieved in 79% of the cases. The hospital mortality was 16%. Thromboembolism occurred in 6%. Of the survivors, 69% are in functional class I, 19% in class II, and 12% in class III. Reoperation was necessary in 12%. There were 28 patients with restricted leaflet motion and abnormal papillary muscles, ranging in age between 0.8 and 12 years with a mean of 5.2 years (Table 2). Valve repair was possible in 89%. Hospital mor-

tality was 18%. Thromboembolism occurred in 8%. Of the survivors, 74% are in class I, 13% are in class II, and 13% in class III. Reoperation was required in one patient (4%).

Congenital Mitral Valvar Stenosis

There were 20 patients with normal papillary muscles (Tables 3 and 4) requiring an operation with ages ranging between 0.5 and 12 years and a mean of 5.2 years. Valve repair was possible in 85%. The hospital mortality was 20%. Thromboembolism occurred in 6%; 88% of the surviving patients are in class I and 12% in class II. No reoperation has been performed.

Fourteen patients needed an operation in the setting of abnormal papillary muscles (Tables 3 and 4). The ages ranged between 0.4 an 12 years, with a mean of 4.5 years. Valve repair was possible in 86%. Thromboembolism was present in 20% of the pa-

Table 3

Mitral Valve Stenosis in 34 Patients

With normal papillary muscles
    Papillary muscle commissural fusion (10)
    Excess valvar tissue (5)
    Supravalvar ring (5)
With abnormal papillary muscles
    Parachute mitral valve (5)
    Hammock mitral valve (9)

Number of patients is in parenthesis.

Table 4

Congenital Mitral Valve Stenosis

		Valve repair (%)	Hospital death (%)	Reoperation (%)
Normal muscles	20	85	20	0
Abnormal muscles	14	86	29	20

tients. All thromboembolic events occurred after replacement of the mitral valve with a mechanical prosthesis. Of the survivors, 70% are in class I, 10% in class II, and 20% in class III. Reoperation has been performed in 20%. Mortality in the perioperative period is due mainly to pulmonary arterial hypertension with fixed vascular resistance. This results from severe valvar stenosis and from associated anomalies such as patency of the arterial duct, and ventricular septal defect.

References

1. Carpentier A. Cardiac valve surgery: "The french correction." J Thorac Cardiovasc Surg 1983;86:323–37.
2. Carpentier A, Chauvaud S, Fermont L. Congenital mitral valve incompetence. Surgical management and long term results. In: Doyle EF, Engle MA, Gersony WM, et al. (eds), Abstract Second World Congress of Pediatric Cardiology. New York, Springer-Verlag, 1985, p 20.

Long-Term Results after Repair of Congenital Malformations of Mitral Valve

V. Gallucci, G. Stellin, A. Mazzucco, U. Bortolotti, M. Rubino,
A. Milano, and G. Faggian

Introduction

The surgical treatment of congenital malformations of the mitral valve still represents a therapeutic challenge. For the most part, this is because of the young age at presentation and the high incidence of associated complex cardiac anomalies. Problems related to the use of most of the currently available mechanical and bioprosthetic valves in the pediatric age group [1-3] justify the generalized trend towards reparative surgery.[4,5] Since information on the results of surgical treatment of dysplasia of the mitral valve in children is still limited, in this article we present the result of a review of our experience with this subject.

Material and Methods

Patient Population

A total of 35 consecutive patients underwent surgery because of congenital dysplasia of the mitral valve between March 1972 and December 1987. There were 14 males and 21 females with a median age of 6 years. The range was from 5 months to 15 years. Five patients were under 1 year of age. Valve malformations associated with atrioventricular septal defects, hypoplasia of the left heart, and univentricular atrioventricular connection were excluded.

The indications for operation were based on the preoperative symptoms (chronic congestive heart failure, exertional dyspnea, retarded growth, and repeated lung infections), on the presence of increased pulmonary arterial pressure, and on the presence of associated intracardiac lesions.

Preoperative cardiac catheterization was performed in all cases. It failed, however, to reveal the mitral valvar malformation in four, in whom it was observed during surgery (supravalvar membrane in two, isolated cleft of the aortic leaflet in one, and a hammock valve in one). The peak systolic pulmonary arterial pressure was markedly increased in 12 children. The mitral valve malformations were classified according to the concept of Carpentier and his col-

Table 1

Classification of Cases with Mitral Valve Incompetence

Normal motion of the leaflet (9 cases)	Annular dilatation (1) Leaflet defect (1) Cleft leaflet (6) Accessory orifice and commissural leaflet (1)	
Prolapsed leaflet (4 cases)	Elongated cords (3) Absent cords (1)	
Restricted leaflet motion (5 cases)	Normal muscles Abnormal muscles	Short cords (2) Parachute valve (1) Hammock valve (17) PM hypoplasia (1)

Number of patients is in parenthesis. PM, papillary muscle.

leagues.[4] Incompetence was subdivided into: nine cases with normal motion of the leaflets, four cases with prolapse of the leaflets, and five cases with restricted motion of the leaflets (Table 1). Stenosis was divided into: nine cases with normal papillary muscles, and seven cases with abnormal papillary muscles (Table 2). When more than one lesion was present, the malformation was classified according to the primary defect. Associated cardiovascular defects were present in 71% of the cases, the most common being lesions of the left heart and ventricular septal defect.

Surgical Technique

Standard moderately hypothermic cardiopulmonary bypass was employed in all

Table 2

Classification of Cases with Mitral Valve Stenosis

Normal papillary muscles (9 cases)	Commissural fusion (4) Supravalvar ring (5)
Abnormal papillary muscles (7 cases)	Parachute valve (7)

Number of patients is in parenthesis. PM, papillary muscle.

cases. Particular care was taken to inspect the entire apparatus of the mitral valve and to assess both its competence and coaptation of the leaflets by injecting cold saline solution into the left ventricular cavity. When needed, annular dilatation was treated by insertion of a Carpentier ring or, more recently, by means of a commissural annuloplasty similar to the one described by Kay, et al.[6]

Results

In 31 cases (88%) it was possible to preserve the native valve. In four cases (12%), after at least one attempt to reconstruct the native valve, it was excised and replaced with a tilting disc prosthesis. There were five hospital deaths, four after conservative surgery and one after replacement of the valve, giving an overall mortality rate of 14.2% (70% CL 8.3–23.7). The causes of death were excessive bleeding due to coagulopathy in two cases and a low output syndrome in two. One of these patients died intraoperatively after repeated attempts to preserve a severely dysplastic hammock valve. Another died on the second postoperative day, with signs of pulmonary vascular obstructive disease, which was histologically proven to be of grade 4 at autopsy. The last patient died three weeks after surgery with mediastinitis and septic shock. There was only one late death. This occurred in a 6-year-old child, who died suddenly at home 26 months after surgery, being in chronic congestive heart failure following replacement of the mitral valve and resection of an associated subaortic fibrous shelf.

Three children required reoperation 2, 22, and 24 months after the initial procedure, respectively. In all of them the mitral valve had been previously repaired, using a Carpentier ring annuloplasty in two and a commissural annuloplasty in the other. A further reconstruction was unsuccessful in all, and the valve was eventually replaced with a mechanical prosthesis.

Clinical long-term follow-up was obtained in all 29 survivors for periods of 4 months to 15 years after surgery. All but two children are asymptomatic. Of these, one has been recently discharged after reoperation performed to resect a subaortic fibrous shelf and to reconstruct further the mitral valve because of recurrent stenosis. The second has signs of persistent cardiomegaly with moderate valvar incompetence. Three years previously he had undergone repair of a severely malformed parachute-type valve together with resection of a supravalvar membrane. Reinvestigation for further treatment has been refused by the parents.

Cross-sectional echocardiographic and Doppler studies were performed at the time of the follow-up examination in all patients treated conservatively. Among those who were asymptomatic, 13 have no signs of valvar regurgitation or stenosis. A trivial to mild residual valvar incompetence is present in seven while, in two, a moderate degree of regurgitation or stenosis persists. The peak pulmonary arterial pressure is within normal limits in all. The five children in whom a prosthetic valve was inserted are free of symptoms. No embolic episodes were reported in the whole series, while no hemorrhages occurred in those receiving sodium warfarin.

Discussion

There is only a very limited experience published in the surgical literature of the long-term effectiveness of surgical repair of congenital malformations of the mitral valve.[4,5] This disease has been treated more frequently by replacement of the valve with a prosthesis in order to avoid any residual valvar dysfunction. Because of the unfavorable flow patterns of the small-sized prostheses, however, along with the tendency of young children to outgrow the valve in a short time, the difficulty of an appropriate anticoagulation therapy, and the accelerated degeneration of biological valve substitutes, we believe that reconstruction of the native valve should always be attempted, especially in infants and young children. Nevertheless, in those cases in which the whole valvar apparatus appears severely malformed and if, after an initial attempt at reconstruction, a satisfactory result cannot be achieved, a prompt replacement of the valve is recommended. Our current policy for valve replacement in the mitral position is to utilize a tilting disc or a bileaflet mechanical prosthesis. The latter is usually preferred when a valve of small size is required because of its superior hemodynamic performance. Thus far neither early nor late thromboembolic episodes have been observed in the entire series. In agreement with others,[4,5] we believe there is no need for anticoagulant therapy after any type of valvoplasty. Although our six children in whom a mechanical valve was inserted are treated with sodium warfarin, despite the higher risk of anticoagulation in the pediatric population, no significant hemorrhages related to anticoagulation have occurred so far.

Among the 24 patients who underwent reconstruction of the mitral valve, 22 are asymptomatic. This further confirms the validity of the conservative treatment, despite the possible presence of a residual hemodynamic impairement.

Two children underwent reoperation after valvar annuloplasty with a Carpentier ring. In both of them, scar tissue produced by the sutures securing the ring itself might have limited a proper growth of the annulus as well as adequate motion of the leaflets. Currently, when annular dilatation is present, it is repaired by plicating the mural leaflet at one or both of the commissures. This does not require the use of foreign prosthetic material and, in our hands, had proved to be very effective even in the long term.

In conclusion, our data suggest that conservative treatment of malformations of the mitral valve in the pediatric population, even in the presence of severe valvar dysplasia, is the treatment of choice. Our results thus far encourage us to attempt reparative surgery whenever possible, in order to avoid or delay replacement of the valve with a prosthesis.

References

1. Borkon AM, Soule L, Reitz BA, et al. Five year follow-up after valve replacement with the St. Jude medical valve in infants and children. Circulation 1986;74(Suppl I):110–15.
2. Elliott MJ, de Leval M. Valve replacement in children. World J Surg 1985;9:568–78.
3. Milano A, Vouhe PR, Baillot-Vernant F, et al. Late results of left-sided cardiac valve replacement in children. J Thorac Cardiovasc Surg 1986;92:218–25.
4. Carpentier A, Branchini B, Cour JC, et al. Congenital malformations of the mitral valve in children. Pathology and surgical treatment. J Thorac Cardiovasc Surg 1976;72:854–66.
5. Lessana A, Viet TT, Ades F, et al. Mitral reconstructive operations. A series of 130 consecutive cases. J Thorac Cardiovasc Surg 1983;86:553–61.
6. Kay JH, Zubiate P, Mendez MA, et al. Mitral valve repair for significant mitral insufficiency. Am Heart J 1977;96:253–62.

3.6

Surgical Treatment of Disease of the Mitral Valve in Children

K. Asano

Introduction

Fifty patients less than 20 years of age with disease of the mitral valve have undergone surgery in our institute over the period 1966–1986. The surgical techniques and their results are discussed in this article.

Classification and Materials

The diseases were classified into three groups. The first was made up of 17 patients with mitral regurgitation in the absence of any other intracardiac anomaly. The second group of 30 patients consisted of those with regurgitation in the setting of an associated intracardiac anomaly. The third group of three patients was those with mitral stenosis. The ages ranged from 1 to 20 years with a mean of 7.7 ± 6.0 years. Those with valvar stenosis or regurgitation in association with another lesion were younger than those having pure valvar regurgitation (5.6 ± 5.4 years and 4.7 ± 3.5 years vs 11.8 ± 5.5 years respectively). Diseases of the mitral valve due to rheumatic carditis and infective endocarditis were excluded.

Pathological Findings and Associated Anomalies

In 10 of the hearts, the lesion present was a cleft in the aortic leaflet of the valve. Short cords were found in two cases while a floppy valve was observed in 30. The valve was flail in three and the cause unknown in the other. Most had dilatation of the mitral annulus. Congenital stenosis was found in only three patients, one with a dysplastic valve and the others with commissural fusion and short tendinous cords (Table 1). There were no patients with abnormal papillary muscles.

Thirty-five patients had associated intracardiac anomalies or other valvar lesions. Severe regurgitation of the tricuspid valve was found in three of the patients with mitral regurgitation but no other congenital lesion. The congenital lesions in the 30 patients with regurgitation were ventricular septal defects in 18, atrial septal defects in five, ventricular septal defect with patency of the arterial duct in one, isolated patency of the duct arteriosus in one, and complicated lesions in another four. The remaining patient, a 6-year-old girl, had annuloaortic ectasia. Pulmonary hypertension of more than 70 mmHg peak systolic pressure was found in

Table 1

Operative Procedures

					Procedure				
Findings	PMAP	BMAP	Ring	Suture of cleft	Suture of cleft + PMAP	Chordoplasty	OMC	MVR	Total
Cleft of aortic leaflet				4	5			1	10
Short cords	1							1	2
Double orifice								1	1
Floppy valve	12	1	1			1		15	30
Flail valve	2							1	3
Unknown MR								1	1
Dyplastic valve								1	1
Commiss. fusion with short cords							2		2
Total	15	1	1	4	5	1	2	21	50

PMAP, posterior mitral annuloplasty; BMAP, bilateral MAP; OMC, open mitral commissurotomy; MVR, mitral valve replacement.

17 of the patients in this group. Two of those with mitral stenosis had an associated atrial septal defect or pulmonary stenosis with tricuspid regurgitation.

Surgical Techniques

The most frequently used technique was a unilateral annuloplasty at the more regurgitant commissure. The suture needle was passed through the posterior part of the annulus, taking a larger bite than taken anteriorly so as to bring the posterior annulus toward the commissure. One baby was treated with a bilateral annuloplasty because of a marked dilatation of the annulus, while another baby was treated only by shortening the elongated cords so as to avoid leaving the valve stenotic. Clefts, when present, were sutured and, if necessary, unilateral annuloplasty was added. Severe floppy valves, flail aortic leaflet, and short cords in older children were all treated with replacement of the valve. Replacement was frequently performed earlier in our experience but, later, this was limited to special cases in which difficulties were encountered during attempted repair. Two patients with mitral stenosis were repaired by commissurotomy with cordopapillotomy and the other had replacement of the mitral valve (Table 1).

Surgical Results

Overall hospital mortality was 10% and late mortality 12%. Only 6.9% of the patients undergoing repair died, in contrast to 14.3% of those having replacement of the mitral valve. All six late deaths were in those undergoing valvar replacement. Among the 45 survivors, four patients underwent reoperation, one of them after commissurotomy and the others after valvar replacement. One of the latter died immediately after the reoperation.

Long-term survivors were all in New York Heart Association class I or II. Twenty-five of 26 patients who underwent repair revealed none or mild (grade 2/6) systolic murmurs. The cardiothoracic ratios were sharply decreased in most patients, either

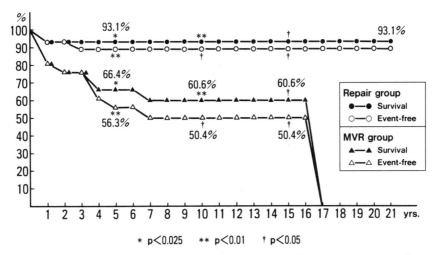

Figure 1. Actuarial survival rates and event-free rates from deaths and reoperations: repair versus mitral valve replacement (MVR).

after repair or replacement of the valve. The actuarial survival and the event-free rates from deaths and reoperations of the groups undergoing repair and valvar replacement group are shown in Figure 1. There were significant differences both in survival and event-free rates between the two groups.

Discussion

Various techniques have been used for repair of mitral regurgitation, mostly chosen according to the intraoperative findings. There are, however, troublesome problems following surgical treatment. Thus complete control of mitral regurgitation may leave a critical stenosis, particularly in small children. Use of annular ring techniques with nonabsorbable materials or replacement of the valve may disturb the growth of the mitral annulus in growing patients. Mitral regurgitation, therefore, should be repaired as far as possible with techniques such as unilateral annuloplasty, since the long-term re-

sults are most encouraging in patients treated in this fashion. Replacement of the valve should be reserved for special cases when technical difficulties are encountered during attempted repair.

In another series, 68 patients with atrioventricular septal defect have undergone surgery in our institute over the same period of time. Some of these patients treated with ordinary techniques of repair not infrequently developed congestive failure due to residual regurgitation across the atrioventricular valve in the period of follow-up. Recently, therefore, we devised a new method of total circular annuloplasty using absorbable suture material (Vicryl). This has now been used in six patients with separate valve and three with a common valve. Follow-up studies by means of angiocardiography and echocardiography demonstrated that this method had decreased regurgitation across the atrioventricular valve without incurring either significant or progressive valvar stenosis. It is suggested that this type of annuloplasty might also be applicable to repair of mitral regurgitation in children.

Nine-Year Experience with St. Jude Medical Prosthesis in Children

Y. Harada, Y. Imai, H. Kurosawa, M. Kawada, K. Ishihara, and S. Fukuchi

Introduction

In this article, we discuss our nine-year experience using the St. Jude medical prosthesis in children. We prefer to repair valvar lesions in children whenever possible. When prosthetic replacement is unavoidable, however, the St. Jude medical prosthesis is our choice for the pediatric age group.

Patients Treated

Since 1979, we have implanted the prosthesis in 48 children. There were 22 boys and 26 girls. Their ages at operation ranged from 4 months to 15 years with the average age being 7 years. Of the 48 children, 16 cases were less than 5 years of age. Four late deaths occurred among those under 2 years of age. Twenty-eight children underwent replacement of their mitral valve. The replacement was performed as a primary procedure in five, after valvoplasty in eight, as a part of an intracardiac repair in four, and because of malfunction of porcine xenografts or valvar thrombosis in 11. Reoperation accounted for about 70% of all our experience with replacement of the mitral valve.

The aortic valve was replaced in 15 children. In 13, patch enlargement of the ventriculo-aortic junction was performed as an additional procedure in all but two using the Konno or Nicks procedure. Double valvar replacement was carried out in two patients. In one, the aortic and mitral valves were replaced using the Manouguian procedure. The mitral and tricuspid valves were replaced in the other because of calcific degeneration of porcine xenografts. We have needed to replace the left-sided tricuspid valve in three children with discordant atrioventricular connection. No operative death has occurred so far.

The size of prosthesis placed in aortic position ranged from 21 to 25 mm, whereas that in atrioventricular position ranged from 19 to 31 mm. The use of larger prostheses in the aortic position was made possible in all cases by means of liberal use of the patch enlargement of the ventriculo-aortic junction. A prosthesis larger than 25 mm in diameter could be used in all children in atrioventricular position except for four. These four were all under 5 years of age, and will be candidates for reoperation in the future because of somatic growth.

The period of follow-up, comprising 201

ACTUARIAL FREE RATE

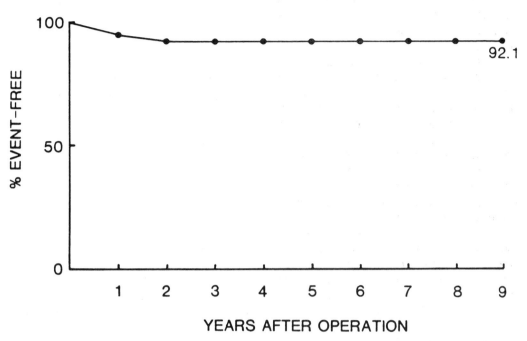

Figure 1. The actuarial curve showing the proportion of patients free of valve-related complications.

ACTUARIAL SURVIVAL CURVE

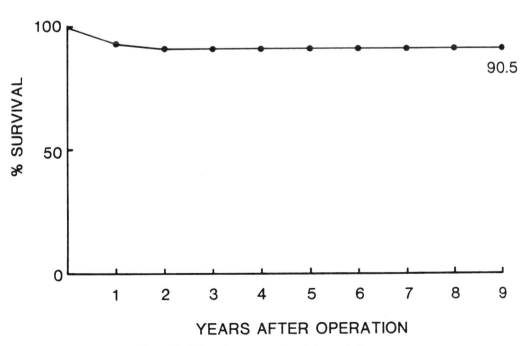

Figure 2. The nine-year actuarial survival curve.

patient-years, ranges from 1 to 9 years, with an average of 4.2 years. Anticoagulation was instituted in all 48 children, 39 being treated with warfarin, whereas the nine operated in the last two years have received a regimen of aspirin combined with dipyridamole.

Three valve-related complications have occurred, one due to thromboembolism and the other two from valvar thrombosis. The thromboembolism caused a cerebral thromboembolic event that resolved spontaneously. One of the thromboses resulted in sudden death, while the other led to successful re-replacement of the valve, again using the St. Jude medical prosthesis. All these complications occurred in children on warfarin who underwent valvar replacement. There were no instances of hemorrhage related to anticoagulation, endocarditis of the prosthetic valve, or primary valvar failure. The linearized rates of thromboembolism and thrombosis are 0.5 and 1.0% per patient-year, respectively. The actuarial rate free from all valve-related complications at nine years is 92.1% (Fig. 1).

As already indicated, four late deaths occurred, all in children less than 2 years of age at operation. One was due to valvar thrombosis and the others from complications unrelated to the valve. The interval from the operation ranged from five to 18 months. The actuarial survival rate at nine years is 90.5% (Fig. 2).

Discussion

We have shown that the St. Jude medical prosthesis is the cardiac valve substitute of choice for use in the pediatric age group. Anticoagulation using aspirin and dipyridamole is warranted in some selected patients in whom this prosthesis has been inserted.

Late Results of Valvar Replacement with Mechanical Prostheses Below the Age of 15 years

A. I. Haàn, E. Koncz, K. Kadar, L. Bendig, A. Fehér,
and M. Lengyel

Introduction

In this chapter, we review our experience over 13 years in 43 children in whom attempts to preserve the native heart valve were unsuccessful or impossible. Because of this, it was necessary to replace the valve with mechanical prostheses.

Material and Methods

From 1975 until January 1988, 16 female and 27 male patients ranging in age from 5 to 15 years with a mean of 11 years, underwent prosthetic valvar replacement using a mechanical prosthesis at the Hungarian Institute of Cardiology. The aortic valve was replaced in 22 patients with a mean age of 11.8 years, the mitral valve in 13 with a mean age of 10.7 years, the tricuspid valve in two with a mean age of 12 years, the aortic and mitral valves in three with a mean age of 11 years, and the mitral and tricuspid in the remaining three with a mean age of 8.3 years. The St. Jude medical valve was used in 28 patients: seven were inserted in mitral, 17 in aortic, and four in tricuspid positions. The Bjork-Shiley valve was inserted 11 times, six in mitral, four in aortic, and one in tricuspid position. Sorin valves were inserted six times in mitral, three times in aortic, and once in tricuspid position. One patient had the aortic valve replaced by a Carbomedics prosthesis. Miscellaneous procedures were performed in addition to valvar replacement in 13 patients (30%). Fifteen patients (34.8%) had undergone 19 previous cardiac surgical interventions. The underlying pathological cause for replacement of the valves was congenital in 26 instances (60.5%), rheumatic in 12 (27.9%), infectious endocarditis in four (9.3%) and iatrogenic in one (2.3%).

The operative technique included standard cardiopulmonary bypass with a bubble oxygenator, moderate hypothermia, cardioplegic arrest and topical cooling with 4°C iced saline. Long-term anticoagulation was achieved with warfarin in all but five patients having replacement of the aortic valve in whom aspirin was used. Regular follow-up was made by our cardiologists including physical examination and the usual noninvasive diagnostic methods. A cumulative follow-up period of 144.2 patient-years was analyzed to evaluate the valve-related mortality and morbidity. The late follow-up ranged from two months to 13 years. Two patients were partially lost to follow-up after three years (96% complete). Actuarial survival was determined by the Kaplan-Meier method.

Results

Ten of the patients had undergone a previous repair of the valve one week to 10 years (mean 52 months) before the valvar replacement (Fig. 1). The average time between valvotomy and replacement of the aortic valve ranged from 3 to 10 years (mean 6.8 years). The range was significantly lower when repair of the aortic valve had been at-

tempted (one week to one month). The result was also less favorable in the case of attempted repair of the mitral valve (range one month to one year). Two patients had had prior replacement of the mitral (Liotta) or aortic (Carpentier) valves with bioprostheses two to six years previously. The indication for reoperation was severe tissue degeneration and calcification, partly caused in the first case by infection with *Staphylococcus epidermidis*. Concomitant operative procedures were performed in 13 patients in addition to the valve replacement.

Preoperatively six patients were in functional class IV of the New York Heart Association criteria, 20 were in class III, 15 were in class II, and two were in class I. All the survivors are now in functional class I except for one who is in class II. All are in sinus rhythm, and only four patients require cardiac medication.

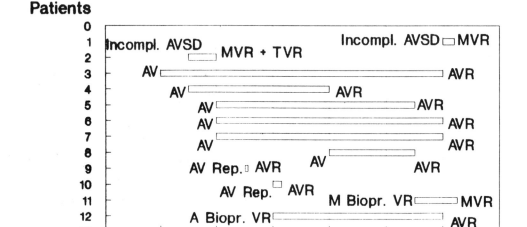

AV: Aortic valvotomy
AV Rep.: Aortic valve repair
AVR: Aortic valve repl.
MVR: Mitral valve repl.
TVR: Tricusp. valve repl.

Late Results of MPVR Below 15
Hungarian Institute of Cardiology
Budapest

Figure 1. Intervals between prior valve operations and valvar replacement with a mechanical prosthesis (MPVR).

ACTUARIAL SURVIVAL

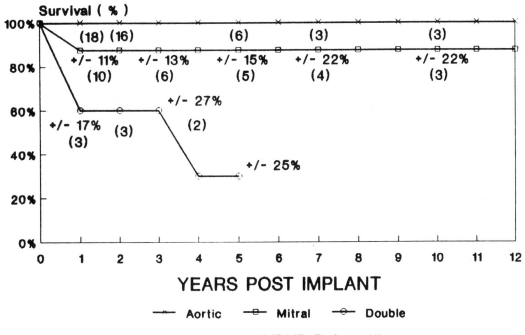

Late Results of MPVR Below 15
Hungarian Institute of Cardiology
Budapest

Figure 2. Actuarial survival curves following replacement of aortic, mitral and double valves (including early and late deaths).

Early Death

Three patients (7%) died during the postoperative period following the initial operation. There was no early mortality for those having replacement of the mitral and aortic valves. The death rate, however, was 50% in those having replacement and the tricuspid valve (together with repair of associated anomalies) and 33% in those having a double replacement. Both latter patients had previously undergone open heart procedures. Nonvalvar causes were responsible for the three hospital deaths. Preoperatively, all these patients had been in class IV of the New York criteria. There were two late deaths (overall mortality 11.6%). One

was valve-related due to intracerebral bleeding following warfarin anticoagulation. The cause of the other death was noncardiac, aortic dissection occurring in a patient with Marfan's syndrome who had had replacement of the aortic valve. It occurred more than three and a half years after the implantation. There was no late death after replacement of the aortic valve, and no operative death occurred among the 12 children undergoing surgery because of rheumatic heart disease. The type of valve inserted did not influence the mortality. Actuarial survival at 10 years was 100% after replacement of the aortic valve, 89% after mitral, and 30% following double valvar replacement (Fig. 2).

Thrombosis as a valve-related complication occurred in the tricuspid valve three years after implantation in a patient who had two St. Jude valves implanted. The cause was obvious failure of long-term warfarin therapy. The drug abruptly became unavailable in a "developing" country. The thrombosed valve was successfully replaced. We have not experienced any other thromboembolic or hemorrhagic complications.

No patient has required repeated iron therapy. Another valve-related complication occurred in one patient in terms of a hemodynamically unsignificant grade II leak across an aortic prosthesis.

There was no incidence of postoperative prosthetic valvar endocarditis, and no structural failure was detected. The need to place a larger prosthesis because of somatic growth has only recently occurred.

Discussion

Although preoperative functional status in class IV, concomitant operative procedures, reoperation, and multiple valvar replacements have all increased the operative risk, we have found that valve replacement using mechanical prostheses in childhood carries a low incidence of valve-related complications and provides a marked functional improvement over a long period of follow-up.

References

1. Ilbawi M, Idriss FS, DE Leon SY, et al. Valve replacement in children. Ann Thorac Surg 1987;44:398–403.
2. Borkon MA, Soule L, Reitz BA, et al. Five year follow-up after replacement with the St. Jude medical valve in infants and children. Circulation 1986;74(suppl I):110–15.
3. Spevak PJ, Freed MD, Castaneda AR, et al. Valve replacement in children less than 5 years of age. J Am Coll Cardiol 1986;8:901–8.
4. Robbins RC, Bowman FO, Malm JR. Cardiac valve replacement in children: A twenty-year series. Ann Thorac Surg 1988;45:56–61.
5. Elliott MJ, deLeval M. Valve replacement in children. World J Surg 1985;9:568–78.
6. Williams WG, Pollock JC, Geiss DM, et al. Experience with aortic and mitral valve replacement in children. J Thorac Cardiovasc Surg 1981;81:326–33.
7. Bradley LM, Midgley FM, Watson DC, et al. Anticoagulation therapy in children with mechanical prosthetic cardiac valves. Am J Cardiol 1985;56:533–35.
8. Schaffer MS, Clarke DR, Campbell DN, et al. The St. Jude medical cardiac valve in infants and children: Role of anticoagulant therapy. J Am Coll Cardiol 1987;9:235–9.
9. Verrier ED, Tranbaugh RF, Soifer SJ, et al. Aspirin anticoagulation in children with mechanical aortic valves. J Thorac Cardiovasc Surg 1986;92:1013–20.

3.9

Glutaraldehyde-Preserved Aortic Allobioprostheses in Children

M. A. Meier, E. Buffolo, I. S. Casagrande, C. A. Salles,
J. C. de Andrade, J. T. Mendonca, and J. W. Neto

Introduction

Use of valvar bioprosthesis is mandatory whenever anticoagulation is contraindicated. In underdeveloped countries, for socioeconomic reasons, the control of anticoagulation therapy is difficult and onerous. The problem becomes crucial if the patient is the pediatric age group. The porcine xenograft was thought to be the solution until it became clear that these bioprostheses were susceptible to degeneration and required replacement after a relatively short time.[1-4] In consequence, the initial enthusiasm for this type of bioprostheses declined, and the search for the ideal valvar substitute in children proceeded.

The longest surviving tissue valves reported in the literature are the homologous aortic valve, either in the fresh or preserved state.[5,6] Early in our experience, we operated upon a small group of patients using homologous valve preserved in etilic alcohol. Despite the high incidence of reoperation within a period of five years, a few patients had surprisingly long survival times

A multicenter study from Sao Paulo, Belo Horizonte, Aracaju, Maceio and Rio de Janeiro, Brazil.

free of reoperation. One patient did not require reoperation until 16 years after the implant. Based on this experience, and also on other reports concerning the use of the homologous aortic valve,[7] we decided to undertake a trial with glutaraldehyde-preserved and stent-mounted allobioprostheses in children. The results are described in this article, in which we share our hopes and apprehensions in the pursuit of a good valvar substitute for children.

Allobioprostheses

The valves are processed by an industrial laboratory with a long experience in manufacturing porcine bioprostheses. The human aortic valves are procured under sterile conditions, 6–12 hours after death, from 12- to 36-year-old males and females, and placed in cold, balanced electrolyte solution. Excess tissue is trimmed, and the valves are fixed with glutaraldehyde under a very low pressure over a period of three to four weeks. If the valve then passes a series of tests, it is mounted on a flexible stent made of a acetalpolymer and a dacron ring. The result is a very low profile prostheses

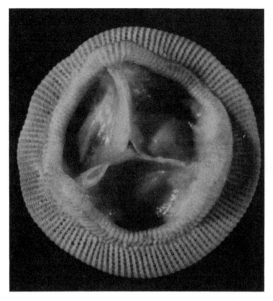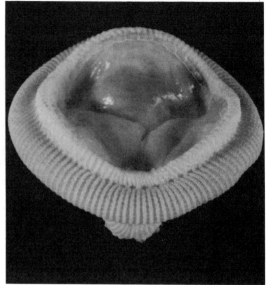

Figure 1. The allobioprosthesis viewed from its superior and inferior aspect.

with good hydrodynamics (Fig. 1). Flow studies in the experimental setting revealed extremely low pressure gradients across the valves sized 21–31 mm. The prostheses are stored in formolaldehyde and are refrigerated. The valves were made available for our study in aortic and mitral models and sizes ranged from 21 to 31 mm.

Patients and Methods

Our series of 77 patients underwent surgery below the age of 15 years, from the period between September 1984 and August 1987. There were 37 boys and 40 girls, whose ages ranged from 5 to 15 years, with a mean of 10.8 ± 2.4 years. Twelve patients were in functional class II, 47 in class III, and 18 in class IV (using the grading system of the New York Heart Association).

Mitral regurgitation was the primary hemodynamic lesion, being found in 33 patients. Mitral stenosis was seen in 19, aortic regurgitation in five, and combined aortic and mitral regurgitation in nine. Eleven patients underwent surgery to replace previously implanted bioprostheses, which degenerated in a short time (mean of 19.4 months), and one had undergone a previous reconstruction of the mitral valve.

The mitral valve was replaced in 63 patients, the aortic valve in five, while the aortic and mitral valves were replaced in the other five. Five patients received the allobioprostheses in the mitral position and mechanical prostheses in the aortic position. Other cardiac procedures were performed in six patients, namely tricuspid annuloplasty in two and closure of an atrial septal defect in four. The operations were performed with cardiopulmonary bypass in 1.2–1.4 $L/m^2/min$, hemodilution, a disposable bubble oxygenator, and crystalloid cardioplegia.

One patient died immediately after the operation (mortality rate of 1.3%) and one in the late postoperative period after an interval of seven months. Two patients needed reoperation: one with rupture of the leaflets after 22 months, and the other with calcification and rupture of the leaflets after 28 months. Both survived the reoperation.

Follow-up after 10–46 months (with a total period of 171.2 years) shows that 97.1

± 2.3% of the patients are free from failure of the allobioprosthesis. These results are far superior to the results that we obtained previously with mechanical valves and xenografts in the same age group.

Discussion

There are some data to suggest that free homografts sterilized with antibiotics and preserved in nutrient medium offer more satisfactory results than the use of presently available bioprosthetic valves.[8] This type of implant has not thus far enjoyed widespread application because of the complex logistics for procurement, sterilization, and storage. A secondary disadvantage of homograft valves is the more demanding surgical technique needed for their implantation as compared to prosthetic devices. To overcome these problems, we developed the idea of utilizing the same technology generated in the manufacturing of porcine bioprostheses to produce an allobioprostheses of comparable quality and availability. The great advantage of bioprostheses in children is the quality of life in terms of freedom from embolism, anticoagulation, and noise. Another advantage, at least in our experience, is the fact that problems, if they occur, usually manifest themselves slowly, giving time for the institution of corrective measure. With mechanical valves, the accidents are acute and reoperations are performed under critical circumstances.

We realize that our experience is too small and too short in duration to be truly significant, but, if we compare these results with our results obtained with either mechanical valves or reconstruction of valves in children, there is surely reason to persevere with this clinical trial.

References

1. Berry BE, Ritter DG, Wallace RB, et al. Cardiac valve replacement in children. J Thorac Cardiovasc Surg 1974;68:705–14.
2. Oyer PE, Miller DC, Stinson EB, et al. Clinical durability of the Hancock porcine bioprostheses valve. J Thorac Cardiovasc Surg 1980;80:824–33.
3. Curcio CA, Commerford PJ, Rose AG, et al. Calcification of glutaraldehyde-preserved porcine xenografts in young patients. J Thorac Cardiovasc Surg 1981;81:621–5.
4. Kutsche LM, Oyer PE, Shumway NE, Baum D. An important complication of Hancock mitral valve replacement in chldren. Circulation 1976;60(suppl I):98–103.
5. Barratt-Boyes BG. Long term follow-up of patients receiving a free-hand antibiotic sterilized homograft aortic valve. In: Rabago G, Cooley DA (eds), Heart Valve Replacement. Mt. Kisco, New York, Futura Publishing Co., 1987, pp 167–79.
6. Ross DN. Aortic valve replacement. Br Heart J 1971;33:39–46.
7. O'Brien MF, Stafford GE, Gardner MAH, et al. A comparison of aortic valve replacement with cryopreserved and fresh allograft valves, with a note on chromosomal studies. J Thorac Cardiovasc Surg 1987;94:812–20.
8. Barratt-Boyes BG. Long term follow-up of aortic valvar grafts. Br Heart J 1971;33:60–71.

Surgical Treatment of Lesions of the Tricuspid Valve in Childhood

A. Todorov, S. Lasarov, N. Arnaudov, V. Pilosof, N. Slavkov,
S. Lambreva, M. Vitanova, A. Tschirkov, and D. Velitschkova

Introduction

In childhood heart disease, the tricuspid valve can be affected in isolation as a main lesion, as it is with Ebstein's malformation. It can also be part of a complex congenital malformation, as in an atrioventricular septal defect, ventricular septal defect with straddling valve, or a malformed valve within a hypoplastic right ventricle or in the setting of pulmonary atresia with intact ventricular septum.[1] In rare cases, bacterial endocarditis affecting the right heart in children may also be an indication for surgery of the tricuspid valve.[2] In this article, we summarize our experience in the surgical treatment of lesions of the tricuspid valve as a solitary or primary lesion, excluding corrective surgery within the frame of an hypoplastic right ventricle, straddling valve, and atrioventricular septal defect.

Materials and Methods

During the period January 1985 until December 1987 at the National Heart Center, Sofia, 12 children (11 girls and one boy) with a mean age of 10.3 years (range from 4.9 to 16 years) underwent surgery on the tricuspid valve (Table 1). Ten children exhibited Ebstein's malformation of the tricuspid valve. One child of 12 years presented with an advancing valvar regurgitation due to bacterial endocarditis complicating the course of closure of a small perimembranous ventricular septal defect. The last child, age 9 years, underwent surgery because of the intimate involvement of the tricuspid valve in adipose cellular degeneration of the right ventricle. All children were diagnosed on the basis of the clinical data and routine clinical investigations (electrocardiogram, phonocardiogram, x-ray) as well as with Doppler and cross-sectional echocardiography. The children all underwent catheterization with intracardiac electrocardiography and cineangiography.

Surgical treatment was performed according to the usual technique of extracorporeal circulation using moderate hypothermia (28°C), bicaval cannulation, and with cold and chemical cardioplegia for the majority of the cases. The competence of the tricuspid valve was tested hydraulically after

Table 1

Patient Characteristics

Patient	Sex	Age at presentation	Diagnosis	Age at operation	Procedure	Follow-up	Complications
NMC	F	4 y	EM	5 y	TrVr-IS 27	3 y 2 mo	Gradient 20mm
ZST	F	5 mo	EM + PS	6 y	Hardy + PV comm.	2 y 6 mo	—
MPE	F	6 mo	EM	11 y	Hardy	2 y	Recurrent Trins = TrVr-JS 29
KDT	F	3 y	EM + ASD	16 y	TrVr-IS 31 + ASD closure	2 y	—
KNV	F	3 y 6 mo	EM	10 y	TrVr-IS 31	2 y	PM insertion
ZNZ	F	3 y 5 mo	EM + VSD + ASD + PS	13 y	TrVr-IS 31 + VSD/ASD closure + PV comm	1 y	—
ISD	F	2 y	EM + ASD	10 y	TrVr-IS 31 + ASD closure	1 y	—
GHD	F	2 y	EM + ASD	10 y	TrVr-IS 31 + ASD closure	1 y 2 mo	—
KHS	F	9 y	EM + FO	13 y	TrVr-IS 31 + FO closure	1 y 2 mo	—
IMO	M	1 mo	EM + FO	6 y	TrVr-IS 31 + FO closure	1 y 1 mo	—
AAM	F	10 y	VSD + BE + vegetations	14 y	TrVr-IS 31 + VSD closure	1 y 4 mo	—
THS	F	4 y	Adipose cell degeneration of RV	9 y	TrVr-IS 27	6 mo	—

EM, Ebstein's malformation; TrVr, tricuspid valve replacement; PS, pulmonary stenosis; ASD, atrial septal defect; VSD, ventricular septal defect; FO, foramen ovale; BE, bacterial endocarditis; IS, Ionescu-Shiley.

plastic repair. Single buttressed sutures were used on the septum and a continuous suture for the rest of the valvar annulus when it was necessary to replace the valve. All replacements were performed with the low-profile Ionescu-Shiley model of pericardial bioprosthesis. The follow-up of all the children took place in the National Center with regular outpatient check-ups and cross-sectional echocardiography every six months. The children who underwent replacement of the valve were anticoagulated for a period of six months postoperatively.

Results

Before operation all patients were followed-up for a mean period of 8.3 years. Within this period, three patients developed congestive heart failure, declining from class III to IV of the New York Heart Association, and demonstrated marked cardiomegaly and regurgitation across the tricuspid valve. Four children manifested increasing cyanosis along with a progressive valvar regurgitation. The child with the tumor in the right ventricle remained asymptomatic during a period of five years before operation.

The children with Ebstein's malformation presented clinically at a mean age of 1.9 years ±1.5, with a range of 1 month to 4 years. Seven of them had associated cardiac lesions: an atrial septal defect within the oval fossa in five, pulmonary valvar stenosis in one, and a small ventricular septal defect, valvar pulmonary stenosis, and an atrial septal defect in the other. Additional rhythm disturbances were observed in two patients: one with an atrial flutter and one with supraventricular tachycardia.

Destruction of the leaflets with thrombotic deposits on the edge of the ventricular septal defect and the leaflets were found at operation in the child with bacterial endocarditis. The anterior papillary muscle along with the anterosuperior and inferior septal leaflets were included in the tumor mass of the child with adipose cellular degeneration of the right ventricle.

Apical displacement and dysplasia of the septal leaflets were the salient features in all the patients with Ebstein's malformation, along with different sizes of the atrialized right ventricular wall. Additional severe changes in the anteroseptal and mural leaflets were found in four patients. An attempt at plastic repair of the valve was made in four cases, in whom the anatomy seemed appropriate. It was successful in two, and abandoned in favor of valve replacement in the other two after repeated hydraulic tests and re-repairs.

Overall, 10 valves were replaced, leaving the coronary sinus in the atrium above the prosthesis. Closure of an atrial septal defect was also performed in five patients, while pulmonary valvar commissurotomy and closure of a ventricular septal defect or pulmonary valvar commissurotomy and closure of atrial septal defect were additional procedures in two other patients.

Valvar replacement resulted in complete atrioventricular block in one patient, requiring later insertion of a pacemaker.

There were neither hospital nor any late deaths.

All but two patients showed improvement in their functional status and/or cyanosis. In nine of the 10 children receiving a valvar prosthesis (all of "adult size"), there was no gradient across the prosthesis as assessed by Doppler echocardiography at a mean period of 24.8 months after the operation. There was only one child with deteriorating function of the prostheses (a gradient of 20 mm) three years after the implantation of a 27-mm Ionescu-Shiley device. There was one late failure of repair which necessitated replacement two years after the initial surgery.

Discussion

Until 1974, the operative treatment of Ebstein's malformation gave most disappointing results, particularly in children below the age of 15 years in whom there was 50% hospital mortality.[3] Poor prognostic factors, however, make surgical treatment unavoidable in Ebstein's malformation. There are marked cardiomegaly, severe cyanosis, congestive heart failure, and an early clinical manifestation of the lesion.[4] Treatment in infants still remains an unsolved problem.[5] In our series, 60% of the affected children demonstrated congestive heart failure and/or increasing cyanosis. Heart failure and cyanosis were absent in two children. In these patients, nonetheless, the presence of obvious anatomical changes together with dysfunction of the valve and signs of cardiomegaly were sufficient reasons for earlier operative intervention.

The controversy between plastic repair and valvar replacement in Ebstein's malformation is mainly due to the great variability in the anatomy of this malformation. After the introduction of plastic repair by Hardy and his colleagues in 1964,[6] better results were reported with this technic.[7,8] Both the improvements of the technique of replacement, and the recent availability of better valve substitutes, however, have allowed the option of taking a more flexible approach when plastic repair is impossible.[9,10]

Although early calcification of the bioprostheses used in childhood is well recognized, convincing data for fast deterioration of these prostheses in tricuspid position is lacking. The hemodynamic advantages and the possibility of safely avoiding the need for long-term anticoagulation seem to justify the use in children of low-profile pericardial bioprostheses in tricuspid position.

References

1. Kirklin JW. Ebstein's malformation. In: Kirklin JW, Barratt-Boyes BG (eds), Cardiac Surgery. New York, John Wiley & Sons, 1986, pp 899–909.
2. Stern JH, Sisto DA, Strom JA, et al. Bioprosthetic tricuspid valve replacement for endocarditis in addicts. In Bodnar E, Yacoub M (eds), Biologic and Bioprosthetic Valves. USA, Yorke Medical Books, 1986, 560–1.
3. Watson H. Natural history of Ebstein's anomaly of tricuspid valve in childhood and adolescence. An international cooperative study of 505 cases. Br Heart J 1974;36:417–27.
4. Radford DJ, Graff RF, Nelson GH. Diagnosis and natural history of Ebstein's anomaly. Br Heart J 1985;54:517–22.
5. Kumar AJ, Fyler DC, Miettinen OS, Nadas S. Ebstein's anomaly. Clinical profile and natural history. Am J Cardiol 1971;28:84–9.
6. Hardy KL, May JA, Webster CA, et al. Ebstein's anomaly. A functional concept and successful definitive repair. J Thorac Cardiovasc Surg 1964;48:927–40.
7. Danielson GK, Fuster V. Surgical repair of Ebstein's anomaly. Ann Surg 1982;196:499–503.
8. Schmidt-Habelmann P, Meisner H, Struck E, et al. Results of valvuloplasty for Ebstein's anomaly. Thorac Cardiovasc Surgeon 1981;29:155–7.
9. Barbero-Marcial, Verginelli G, Awad M, et al. Surgical treatment of Ebstein's anomaly. Early and late results in twenty patients subjected to valve replacement. J Thorac Cardiovasc Surg 1979;78:416–22.
10. Bove SL, Kirsh MM. Valve replacement for Ebstein's anomaly of the tricuspid valve. J Thorac Cardiovasc Surg 1979;78:229–32.

Results and Long-Term Follow-Up of Valve Replacement in 61 Children

J. E. Rubay, T. Sluysmans, P. Jaumin, A. Vliers, M. Goenen,
A. Matta, Y. Kestens-Servaye, and C. H. Chalant

Introduction

When unavoidable, valvar replacement in children using prostheses presents a unique set of problems because of their growth, the restrictive hemodynamics of small valves, and the potential complications of anticoagulation. In addition, the ideal prosthesis for use in children should have an extended functional life. Recognition of accelerated calcification of porcine bioprostheses has prompted reevaluation of the use of mechanical valves.[1,2] This retrospective study reviews our experience with replacement of valves in children in order to assess the survival rates and the valve-related complications.

Patients and Methods

From December 1968 through December 1987, 61 patients younger than 14 years of age (mean ± standard deviation: 9 ± 3.1 years) underwent replacement of one or more cardiac valves. Congenital lesions were present in 49 patients (80%) and were heterogeneous. Rheumatic disease was seen in nine (15%) and infective endocarditis in three (5%) (Table 1).

Thirty-three patients (54%) had had previous cardiac operations. Thirty patients had isolated replacement of the aortic valve, 15 patients had isolated replacement of the mitral valve, and eight patients had combined aortic and mitral replacements. Among the seven patients who had replacement of the tricuspid valve, two had corrected transposition so that the morphologically tricuspid valve was the systemic atrioventricular valve. One patient had replacement of both the mitral and tricuspid valves. Fifty-seven mechanical and 16 bioprosthetic valves were inserted.

The majority of prostheses were of adult size, but some small devices were implanted (Starr-Edwards No. 1 in five patients, Bjork-Shiley 17 or 19 in eight patients, St. Jude medical 19 in four patients and Sorin 19 in one patient). Three patients sustained major ischemic changes during insertion of the prosthesis, which had to be replaced during the procedure. Concomitant procedures were performed in 30 children (49%).

Children receiving mechanical prostheses were prescribed permanent anticoagulation. Two patients were lost to fol-

Table 1

Indications for Valve Replacement

	Patients (n)
Aortic position	
Rheumatic heart disease	1
Endocarditis	1
Congenital	28
Isolated AS	20
Associated AR	8
+ Common arterial trunk	2
+ Marfan syndrome	1
+ Larsen syndrome	1
+ Miscellaneous	4
Mitral position	
Rheumatic heart disease	4
Endocarditis	2
Congenital	12
AVSD	5
Corrected transposition	2
DORV	1
Miscellaneous	4
Aortic and mitral position	
Rheumatic heart disease	4
Endocarditis	0
Congenital	4
AS + MS	2
AR + MR	1
TGA	1
Tricuspid position	
Congenital	
Ebstein's malformation	5

AS, aortic stenosis; AR, aortic regurgitation; AVSD, atrioventricular septal defect; DORV, double outlet right ventricle; MS, mitral stenosis; MR, mitral regurgitation; TGA, complete transposition.

low-up. In the other patients, follow-up encompassed 330 patient-years with a mean interval of 6.3 years.

Results

There were three early deaths (5%) and 10 late deaths (Table 2). The cumulative survival rate was 83% ± 6% at 5 years and 72% ± 8% at 10 years for the whole group (Fig. 1). Excluding the right-sided valvar replacements, the overall 10-year probability of survival was 72% ± 8%. All the survivors are in class I of the New York Heart Association except three who are in class II.

Cross-sectional echocardiography disclosed a left ventricular ejection fraction higher than 80% in all but three patients. Doppler echocardiographic studies were performed in nine patients after replacement of the aortic valve and in three after replacement of the mitral valve and revealed normal peak gradients.

There were five deaths, directly related to the replacements, one early and four late (Table 2). Seven patients were found to have had thromboembolic episodes; the linearized rate was 2.1 per 100 patient-years. These were considered major in two patients—one after replacement of the aortic and the other after mitral valve replacement (0.6 per 100 patient-years). Both occurred early after operation (less than 30 days postoperatively). The actuarially determined thromboembolic-free survival (± standard error) after replacement of the aortic valve is 79% ± 13% at 10 years and 82% ± 11% at 10 years after replacement of the systemic atrioventricular valve. Hemorrhagic complications of anticoagulation occurred in five patients, with a major event occurring in one patient early after the operation. The linearized rate was 1.5 per 100 patient-years.

Four patients developed endocarditis, and two of those died. Reoperation was needed in 11 patients. The only cause for reoperation in the group of patients with a bioprosthetic valve was primary tissue failure, which occurred in nine valves. Somatic growth was the main cause for replacement of mechanical valve, which occurred in three patients. A paravalvar leak occurred in one patient, thrombosis in another, and endocarditis in a third.

Discussion

When unavoidable, replacement of heart valves in infants and children by prostheses requires consideration of several variables that are unique to this age group.

Table 2

Details of Deaths of Children with Valve Replacement

Diagnosis	Age	Operation	Beat time to death	Cause
EARLY				
DORV, MR	3 y	MVR, BS21	DO	Hypo LV
TGA, SA-VVRg	6 y	SA-VVRp, SJ27	DO	PHTA
AS	13 y	AVR, BS19	1 day	myocardial infarction
LATE				
Endocarditis	10 y	AVR, BS17	1.5 months	Endocarditis
Endocarditis	7 y	MVR, HC25	2 months	Sepsis, lymphoma
AS	7 y	AVR, BS19	2.5 months	Technical failure
AS	14 y	AVR, SE7	8 months	LVF
AR + MR	10 y	AVR, BS21 + MVR SE1	44 months	Endocarditis
Corrected transposition	14 y	SA-VVRp, C31	55 months	RVF
Ebstein's malformation TI	9 y	TVR, HC31	62 months	Arrhythmia
MR	11 y	MVR, HC29	65 months	? Cause
Larsen disease, AR	5 y	AVR, BS27	84 months	Aortic dissection
AR	13 y	AVR, BS23	88 months	? Cause (sudden)

DORV, double outlet right ventricle; MR, mitral regurgitation; MVR, mitral valve replacement; BS, Bjork-Shiley prosthesis; DO, day of operation; LV, left ventricle; TGA, complete transposition; SA-VVRg, systemic atrioventricular valve regurgitation; SA-VVRp, systemic atrioventricular valve replacement; SJ, St. Jude medical prosthesis; PHTA, pulmonary hypertension; AS, aortic stenosis; AVR, aortic valve replacement; HC, Hancock prosthesis; SE, Starr-Edwards prosthesis; LVF, left ventricular failure; AR, aortic regurgitation; RVF, right ventricular failure; TI, tricuspid incompetence; TVR, tricuspid valve replacement.

The major ones are the choice and durability of the valve, the need for anticoagulation, and the effect of growth.

There is no doubt that bioprostheses should no longer be used in children because accelerated calcification and degeneration occur in these valvar substitutes.[1] Encouraging results of the use of fresh antibiotic sterilized aortic homografts[3] together with the increasing availability of these prostheses are likely in future to lead to an increased application of this technique. At present, nonetheless, most cardiac surgeons would opt for mechanical prostheses as the valve substitute of choice in children.

As we have shown, satisfactory early and late results can be achieved when these are inserted in aortic position. This procedure can usually be delayed until an adult-sized valve can be inserted. The mean age of our patients was 10.6 years. In younger children, or in children with aortic stenosis

not amenable to repair, enlargement of the ventriculo–aortic junction may allow insertion of an adequate-sized prosthesis.[4] The operative mortality is low (3% in our series) and is comparable to the rates observed by others.[5] Satisfactory late survival can be achieved whatever the type of mechanical prosthesis inserted. The overall incidence of late thromboembolic events is low (0.5 per 100 patient-years). The usual finding of sinus rhythm and a high cardiac output, with high velocity of blood across the aortic orifice may be a partial explanation for these satisfactory findings.

At present, there is no satisfactory valvar substitute for use in the mitral position. Every effort should be made, therefore, to preserve the native mitral valve. Operative mortality is relatively high (12%) for replacement in mitral position and may be due to the younger age of the patients (a mean of 8.5 years in our series) and the higher incidence of underlying major congenital

• ESTIMATED PROBABILITY OF SURVIVAL ───────

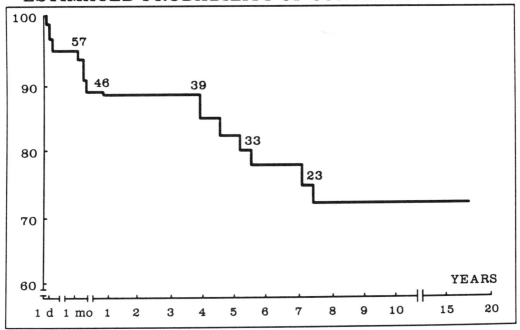

Figure 1. Actuarial survival curve (Kaplan-Meier) for all recipients of valvar prostheses. The curve includes the operative mortality. The 5-year survival rate is 83% ± 6% and survival rate at 10 years is 72% ± 8.

cardiac disease. Late survival, however, is satisfactory. The overall incidence of late thromboembolic events is 1.0 per 100 patient-years. Interestingly, the risk of thromboembolism after replacement of the mitral valve appears to be substantially less in children than in adults. Perhaps the relatively low incidence of atrial fibrillation in children accounts for some of this difference. The mechanism of thromboembolism is also different between the patients with replacement of the aortic and mitral valves, the former being associated with development of fibrin thrombi and the latter with thrombi composed of platelets.[6] As do most investigators,[7,8] we recommend long-term anticoagulation mainly because thromboembolic episodes tend to be time related and are thus likely to occur during longer periods of follow-up.

Among our five patients with Ebstein's malformation who underwent valvar re-

placement with a bioprosthesis, two are free of any complication in the short term follow-up. One died as a consequence of the underlying disease, and the other two had percutaneous balloon dilatation of a stenotic xenograft and replacement of the valve at nine years, respectively.

The problem of "outgrowing" the prosthesis deserves some comment. It seems likely that any prosthetic valve inserted in a child with congenital mitral stenosis will require replacement as a result of somatic growth.[9] Of the few children who received small prostheses (Starr-Edwards No. 1), some may require reoperation. One of these children underwent reoperation 11 years after the first implantation. For stenotic aortic lesions, enlargement of the ventriculo–aortic junction usually allows insertion of a prosthesis of adequate size.[4,10] Among the patients who received small prostheses (Bjork-Shiley 17, and 19, St. Jude medical

19), only one has required a reoperation. Since most of the patients in this study have yet to complete their growth, however, frequent and regular clinical and Doppler echocardiography assessment is mandatory to detect any inadequacy of the valves.

We conclude from our experience that replacement of valves in children can be accomplished with a low operative mortality and satisfactory late survival. Yet, it is still a major procedure that should not be undertaken lightly. At present, in our opinion, mechanical valves offer the best prognosis, despite the small risk of anticoagulation.

References

1. Geha AS, Laks H, Stansel HC Jr. Late failure of porcine valve heterografts in children. J Thorac Cardiovasc Surg 1979;78:351–61.
2. Williams DB, Danielson GK, McGoon DC, et al. Porcine heterograft valve replacement in children. J Thorac Cardiovasc Surg 1982; 84:446–50.
3. Barratt-Boyes BG, Roche AHG, Subramanian R, et al. Long term follow-up of patients with antibiotic sterilized aortic homograft valve inserted freehand in the aortic position. Circulation 1987;75:768–77.
4. Konno S, Imai Y, Iida Y, et al. A new method for prosthetic valve replacement in congenital aortic stenosis associated with hypoplasia of the aortic valve ring. J Thorac Cardiovasc Surg 1975;70:909–17.
5. El Makhlouf A, Friedli B, Oberhansli I, et al. Prosthetic heart valve replacement in children. J Thorac Cardiovasc Surg 1987;93:80–5.
6. Pumphrey CW, Fuster V, Chesebro JH. Systemic thromboembolism in valvular heart disease and prosthetic heart valves. Mod Concepts Cardiovasc Dis 1982;51:131–36.
7. Schaff HV, Danielson GK, Didonato RM, et al. Late results after Starr-Edwards valve replacement in children. J Thorac Cardiovasc Surg 1984;88:583–9.
8. Elliott MJ, de Leval M. Valve replacement in children. World J Surg 1985;9:568–78.
9. Friedman S, Edmunds H Jr, Cuaso CC. Long term mitral valve replacement in young children. Influence of somatic growth on prosthetic valve adequacy. Circulation 1976; 57:981–6.
10. Piehler JM, Danielson GK, Pluth JR, et al. Enlargement of the aortic root or annulus with autogenous pericardial patch during aortic valve replacement. Long term follow-up. J Thorac Cardiovasc Surg 1983;86:350–8.

IV

Rheumatic Heart Disease

4.1

Introduction

S. John

In many Third World countries, rheumatic disease still occupies pride of place as the greatest killer among lesions affecting the heart. While I concede that prophylaxis should be the key for prevention of rheumatic valvar disease, surgery becomes mandatory once the disease is established. Prophylaxis, in any case, is intertwined inexorably with economic factors and, therefore, its implementation in the countries where it is most needed becomes an arduous task. In these countries, the young are often affected, and, in those patients, the disease is followed by disability and death. The disease often involves the mitral valve in isolation or in association with other valves, the process of disease leading to various degrees of valvar deformation. The choice of treatment, therefore, varies from closed mitral commissurotomy to replacement of single or multiple valves. As an introduction to this section, in this article I will review briefly the extensive experience gained in Velore, India, in the surgical treatment of rheumatic disease of the heart in the young.

Mitral Stenosis

Stenosis of the mitral valve, when seen in young patients in India, is a unique entity characterized by its short duration and the rapid progression of symptoms. Between 1956 and September 1987, 5,014 patients seen at Velore underwent closed mitral valvotomy, of whom 1,265 were below the age of 20 years. The youngest patient was 6 years old, and there was a marked male preponderance. All patients prior to operation were in classs III or IV of the grades established by the New York Heart Association, and 96% were in sinus rhythm. Mild mitral incompetence occurred postoperatively in 18%. Severe mitral regurgitation necessitated emergency replacement of the valve in two subjects (0.3%). Overall, however, an excellent valvotomy was achieved in 96.5%. The overall hospital mortality (Fig. 1) was 3.39%; during the last 10 years, this has fallen to 0.85%.

In those subjects having advanced valvar dysfunction with significant regurgitation across the mitral or aortic valves, we have resorted to replacement of the diseased valve or valves. Our results in such young patients over the last two decades[1] lend support to this aggressive management as the favored technique. In the setting of severe regurgitation, we prefer the certainty of hemodynamic correction to the possibility of later progression of the disease after failure of attempted repair.

Mitral Incompetence

The presence of severe mitral incompetence necessitates replacement of the

HOSPITAL MORTALITY

OVER ALL   43/1265 :: 3.39%

LAST TEN YEARS

1978 – 1988 APRIL   4/469 :: 0.85%

Figure 1. Results of closed mitral valvotomy.

valve even in the young subject. Selection of the ideal prosthesis for the child and adolescent poses a dilemma. In our center, 195 patients below the age of 20 have undergone valvar replacement. Of these, 65% were in class IV of the grading of the New York Heart Association. Only four patients had stenosis as the dominant lesion, and two of those had previously undergone valvotomy. An associated shunt at the atrial level was found in 15. There was an overall hospital mortality of 9.7%, but only three deaths have occurred among the 92 patients (3.2%) undergoing surgery in the last five years. An embolus-free survival curve of 94.7% was seen at an interval of 18 years, with an actuarial survival curve of 71.2% during the same time frame. In view of its known low incidence of thromboembolism and long-term durability, we have used the Starr-Edwards ballvalve prosthesis in about 85% of our patients. Notwithstanding the need for anticoagulation and the prospects of pregnancy, the results with this prosthesis are promising in this age group.

Discussion

Rheumatic heart disease continues to be a major cause of morbidity and mortality in the Third World. Closed mitral valvotomy is here to stay, and we continue to be devoted advocates of this operation for mitral stenosis. Where advanced valvar dysfunction is evident, nonetheless, replacement of the valve becomes imperative. We are of the firm opinion that reparative procedures have very little or no place in the treatment of severe valvar dysfunction following rheumatic disease. Furthermore, Chauvaud and his colleagues[2] have reported a reoperation rate of about 25% using reparative techniques over a period of 10 years. In view of the acknowledged advantage of its long-term durability and increased resistance to thromboembolic events, the Starr-Edward prosthesis must be considered the device of choice. Operative mortality has been very low with this valve and, in recent years, has been almost comparable to the results of the reparative procedures reported by Chauvaud et al.[2] The patients have been 95% free of embolic events, even at the end of a period of 15 years. Our overall late mortality of 0.44–1.18% for replacement of solitary or multiple valves, respectively, contrasts very strikingly with the higher figures reported by several other investigators. Currently we are investigating the use of aspirin as the sole drug for anticoagulation with favorable results to date.

References

1. John S, Bashi S, Jairaj PS, et al. Mitral valve replacement in the young patient with rheumatic heart disease. Early and late results in 118 subjects. J Thorac Cardiovasc Surg 1983; 86:209–16.

2. Chauvaud S, Perier P, Touati G, et al. Long term results of valve repair in children with acquired mitral valve incompetence. Circulation 1986;74:1104–9.

Morphological Determinants of Successful Balloon Valvoplasty in Chronic Rheumatic Valvar Disease

G. Thiene, M. Turri, L. Daliento, U. Bortolotti, and V. Gallucci

Introduction

Rheumatic fever is still by far the leading cause of dysfunction of cardiac valves even in Western countries.[1] In the last decade, our experience with the surgical pathology of mitral valvar disease has shown that more than 80% of the excised valves exhibited evidence of rheumatic disease (Table 1), but less than 1% of the patients were under 20 years of age (Table 2).

Mechanical dilatation of stenotic valves by closed commissurotomy, introduced in 1923 by Cutler and Levine[2] for the mitral valve and in 1952 by Bailey[3] for the aortic valve, was long considered the only effective means for managing mitral stenosis. It remains the treatment of choice in some environments, especially in countries with limited resources. Extremely good results by means of closed mitral valvotomy were reported by John, et al.[4] in 3,724 patients operated in Velore, India, from 1956 to 1980. The survival at 24 years was 84%, and rates of thromboembolism and restenosis ranged only from 0.03% to 0.16%, and 0.42% to 1.14% per year, respectively.

Balloon Valvotomy

Balloon valvoplasty for treatment of rheumatic valvar stenosis[5-7] was introduced with the aim of achieving the same effect as closed mitral commissurotomy by means of the expansive force of the balloon. Although the efficacy of this procedure is controversial,[8] its application has been extended from chronic inflammatory to calcific degenerative disease. It can now, therefore, be considered an alternative to surgical therapy in patients either with acquired aortic or mitral stenosis.[9] The technique is particularly attractive because of its simplicity, ease of performance and low mortality. Its efficacy in terms of hemodynamic results, however, has been questioned, while the risk of harmful or life-threatening complications in left-side heart valvoplasty has been stressed.[10-13]

Advantages of Balloon in the Young

Conservative treatment by balloon valvoplasty in young people with rheumatic valvar stenosis has several apparent advan-

Table 1

Surgical Pathology of Mitral Valve Disease: Department of Cardiovascular Surgery, University of Padova (1981–1986)

Etiology	n	%
Rheumatic	379	82.6
Floppy	51	11.1
Ischemic	11	2.4
Endocarditis	11	2.4
Other	7	1.5
Total	459	100.0

mechanical devices be implanted. This constitutes a particularly undesirable setting in young women who may wish to become pregnant. Moreover, unlike closed surgical valvotomy, there is no need for thoracotomy, only a few days of hospitalization are required, the procedure does not necessitate blood transfusion, and it can be repeated several times. As stated by Inoue et al.,[5] who first applied this technique, balloon valvoplasty in rheumatic valve disease is the equivalent of commissurotomy without thoracotomy.

tages over surgical replacement of the valve[14] in view of the following factors. First, valve prostheses are prohibitively expensive in Third World nations, where rheumatic valve disease still constitutes a major disaster. Interestingly enough, 25% of the surgical population of John, et al.[4] were less than 20 years old. Second, the surgical anatomy in the young is more favorable than in adults because of the suppler leaflets and a lower incidence of calcification of the stenotic valves. Third, because of the mismatch between prosthesis and heart with growth, reoperation is often necessary. Hence, fourth, there is the operative risk of repeated interventions. Fifth, there is the known propensity for accelerated dystrophic mineralization when bioprostheses are employed as valvar substitutes. Sixth, there is the need for chronic anticoagulation therapy should

Mechanisms of Valvotomy

The role of percutaneous balloon valvoplasty has been well established in children and young adults with a variety of congenital or acquired disorders,[6,15] and the precise mechanism by which relief of obstruction is achieved has been investigated both in autopsied material[10,12] and during operations for valvar replacement.[3] Stenotic (or predominantly stenotic) valves are the lesions that may benefit from balloon valvuloplasty. Commissural fusion is one of the hallmarks of postrheumatic mitral or aortic stenosis, and commissural splitting appears to be the main mechanism by which relief may be achieved. This may be accomplished with particular efficacy at the aortic level, where only fusion of the commissures and rigidity of the cusps account for stenosis (Fig. 1). At the mitral valve, however, because of its peculiarly complex anatomy, stenosis at commissural level is rarely an isolated finding. A reduced orificial diameter is, in most cases, also the consequence of obliteration of intercordal spaces due to cordal fusion, a substrate which cannot be relieved by balloon valvoplasty alone.[16] When used in the setting of mitral disease, however, no injury to the subvalvar structures was observed after balloon valvoplasty (Fig. 2).

Table 2

Surgical Pathology of Rheumatic Mitral Valve Disease: Department of Cardiovascular Surgery, University of Padova (1981–1986)

Specimens (n)	477
Sex	317 female, 160 male (2:1)
Age (years):	range 13–70
	mean 51.7 ± 10.5
	patients < 20 years: 4 (0.8%)

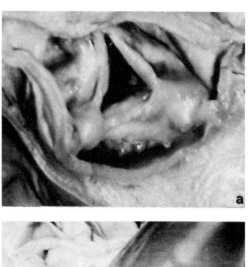

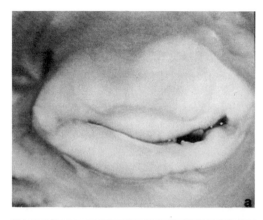

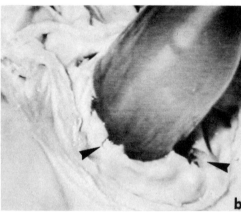

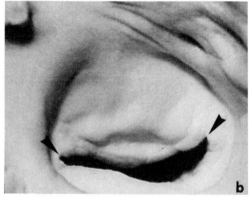

Figure 1. In rheumatic disease of the aortic valve, stenosis is due to fusion of two commissures (a). The same valve is shown during expansion of a balloon (b). Note the splitting of the previously fused commissures (arrows).

Figure 2. Rheumatic stenosis of the mitral valve also is due to commissural fusion (a). Note the fish-mouth orifice. After balloon valvoplasty (b), the orifice is enlarged because of commissural splitting (arrows).

Discussion

Contraindications to balloon valvoplasty are valvar regurgitation and, in the case of mitral stenosis, predominant subvalvar disease or left atrial thrombus with the risk of embolization. It has been demonstrated that the presence of extensive calcific deposits, classically considered a contraindication to closed commissurotomy, did not prevent favorable results, since fracturing of nodular calcific deposits by balloon valvoplasty may also occur.[10]

Balloon valvoplasty of stenotic rheumatic valves is, by definition, a palliative procedure. Since restenosis is very common after surgical valvotomy, it most likely also will limit the success of balloon valvoplasty. Even if stenosis should recur after balloon valvoplasty, however, reapplication of this procedure is not hindered because pericardiotomy and scarring of the chest wall are avoided. In children with rheumatic and stenotic cardiac valves, therefore, balloon valvoplasty may be of great help in deferring replacement of the valve until the child has become an adult.

Acknowledgments: Supported by the National Council for Research, Target Project "Biomedical Technology," Rome, Italy.

References

1. Community control of rheumatic heart disease in developing countries. A major public health problem. W.H.O. Chron 1980;34:336–45.
2. Cutler EC, Levine SA. Cardiotomy and valvulotomy for mitral stenosis: Experimental observations and clinical notes concerning an operated case with recovery. Bost Med Surg J 1923;188:1023–30.
3. Bailey CP. The surgical treatment of mitral stenosis. Dis Chest 1949;15:377–97.
4. John S. Bashi V, Jairaj PS, et al. Closed mitral valvotomy: Early results and long-term follow-up of 3724 consecutive patients. Circulation 1983;68:891–6.
5. Inoue K, Owaki T, Nakamura F, Miyamoto N. Clinical application of transvenous mitral commissurotomy by a new balloon catheter. J Thorac Cardiovasc Surg 1984;87:394–402.
6. Lock JE, Khalilullah M, Shrivastava S, et al. Percutaneous catheter commissurotomy in rheumatic mitral stenosis. N Engl J Med 1985;313:151–8.
7. Babic UU, Pejcic P, Djurisic Z, et al. Percutaneous transarterial balloon valvuloplasty for mitral valve stenosis. Am J Cardiol 1986;57:1101–4.
8. Messmer BJ. Personal view: Balloon, where do you fly? Eur Heart J 1987;8:1170–1.
9. Rahimtoola SH. Catheter balloon valvuloplasty of aortic and mitral stenosis in adults: 1987. Circulation 1987;75:895–901.
10. Kaplan JD, Isner JM, Karas RH, et al. In vitro analysis of mechanism of balloon valvuloplasty of stenotic mitral valves. Am J Cardiol 1987;59:318–23.
11. Beekman RH. Percutaneous balloon valvuloplasty: Long-term studies are needed. J Am Coll Cardiol 1987;9:732–3.
12. McKay RG, Lock JE, Safian RD, et al. Balloon dilatation of mitral stenosis in adult patients: post-mortem and percutaneous mitral valvuloplasty studies. J Am Coll Cardiol 1987;9:723–31.
13. Robicsek F, Harbold NB. Limited value of balloon dilatation in calcified aortic stenosis in adults: Direct observations during open heart surgery. Am J Cardiol 1987;60:857–64.
14. John S, Bashi S, Jairaj PS, et al. Mitral valve replacement in the young patient with rheumatic heart disease. J Thorac Cardiovasc Surg 1983;86:209–16.
15. Petit J, Leriche LH, Piot JD, et al. Valvuloplastie mitrale endoluminale chez l'adulte jeune et l'enfant. Arch Mal Coeur 1987; 8:1261–7.
16. Acar J, Vahanian A. La valvuloplastie mitrale percutanee: Nouvelle therapeutique du retrecissement mitral. Arch Mal Coeur 1987;7:1101–4.

Conservative Surgery of Acquired Mitral Valvar Incompetence in Children

S. Chauvaud, S. Mihaileanu, and A. Carpentier

Introduction

The surgical management of mitral valvar incompetence in children remains controversial. The long-term results of valvar replacement point to several drawbacks related to the different types of valvar prosthesis.[1,2] In addition, anticoagulation therapy after replacement with mechanical prostheses still remains an unsolved problem in children. On the other hand, the high rate of early calcification of bioprostheses in children seems to be a contraindication to the use of this type of valvar substitute.[1] In this chapter, therefore, we will describe our experience with conservative treatment of mitral regurgitation.

Clinical Material

Eighty-nine consecutive children under 12 years of age underwent surgical correction. Their ages ranged from 2 to 12 years, with a mean of 8.3 ± 2.5 years; 45 were male. The main cause of valvar incompetence was rheumatic fever (94%). The other causes were infectious endocarditis (4.5%) and Barlow's syndrome (1.5%). There are characteristic features of acquired mitral valvar incompetence in children. Thus, 91% were in sinus rhythm and incompetence of the tricuspid valve was rare (13.5%). No patient with disease of the aortic valve was included in this study.

Classification

Normal Leaflet Motion (5.6%)

With this variant, the free edge of the leaflets remained below the plane of the annulus during systole and opened normally during diastole. The incompetence was due to annular enlargement and/or its deformation.

Prolapsed Leaflet (83%)

With this pattern, one or both leaflets were overriding the plane of the annulus during systole. The prolapse was due to elongation of either the cords or the papillary muscles. Annular enlargement was always present but was a secondary lesion. This group included 28 patients (31.4%) with mixed lesions, namely prolapse of the aortic ("anterior") leaflet and restricted motion of the mural ("posterior") leaflet.

Restricted Leaflet Motion (11%)

In this final group, the leaflets were thickened and cords were fused, leading to impaired motion of the leaflets. Some degree of mitral stenosis was present in these patients due to commissural fusion.

Surgical Techniques

Prosthetic Ring Annuloplasty

This technique is based on a precise measurement of the valvar apparatus so as to restore an optimal orificial area and a normal annular shape. Ring annuloplasty was used in 78 patients (88%). Attempts were made to avoid the use of a prosthetic ring in growing children. Commissuroplasty was performed in 11 children.

Shortening of Tendinous Cords

Cordal elongation of the aortic leaflet was corrected by cordal shortening. The cords were buried in the anterolateral papillary muscle (30 patients), the posteromedial muscle (32 patients), or both (14 patients).

Leaflet Resection and Suture

Nineteen patients with a prolapsed mural leaflet were treated by quadrangular resection and suture associated with plication of the corresponding part of the annulus; 17 patients with prolapse of the aortic leaflet underwent a triangular resection. This technique has now been replaced by transposition of tendinous cords from the mural to the aortic leaflet.

Cordal Fenestration and Resection

Thick and fibrotic cords were fenestrated or resected. Commissural fusion was treated by commissurotomy and splitting of the papillary muscles.

Leaflet Enlargement

Fibrosis of leaflet tissue was responsible for retraction of the leaflets. Widening of the surface area was achieved by means of an autologous pericardial patch treated with glutaraldehyde. Enlargement of the aortic leaflet was performed in three patients and of the mural leaflet in a further three. Tricuspid valvar incompetence was treated with a prosthetic ring annuloplasty in 12 patients.

Anticoagulation Therapy

Anticoagulation was used for two months after surgery. Thereafter, it was discontinued if the patient was in sinus rhythm. Indefinite anticoagulation was advised in the presence of atrial fibrillation.

Results

The hospital mortality was 2.3% (two patients). Both deaths were related to postoperative low cardiac output. Of the surviving patients, 86% were in NYHA class I or II after repair of the mitral valve repair, 12.5% in class III, and 1.5% in class IV. The actuarial survival rate at five years was 95.05 ± 2.32% and at 10 years was 89.96 ± 8.3%. The late deaths were due to intracerebral hemorrhage, bacterial endocarditis, sudden death, and reoperation in one case each. The incidence of valve-related death was 2.8 ± 1.9 at five years and 5.4 ± 3.2% at 10 years. The linearized rate was 0.5 ± 0.3% per patient-year.

Two embolic events occurred. A transient hemiplegia was observed one week after operation while an amaurosis was seen in an arrhythmic patient not receiving anticoagulation therapy. At five years, 99 ± 0.8%, and at 10 years 98 ± 19%, of the patients were free of any thromboembolic event. The linearized rate of thromboembolism was 0.3 ± 0.2% per patient-year. Twelve patients underwent reoperation. The actuarial risk of reoperation at five years was 13.4 ± 4.3%, and at 10 years, 21.6 ± 7%.

The causes of reoperation were recurrent mitral valvar incompetence in three; mitral valvar stenosis in two; detachment of the prosthetic ring in two; unrecognized prolapse of a leaflet in two; endocarditis in one; and annular dilatation not treated by a prosthetic ring in two. One patient died after reoperation.

Discussion

On an actuarial basis, 69 ± 6.8% of the patients were free of valve-related mortality and morbidity after a period of 10 years. The linearized rate of complication was 3 ± 0.8% per patient-year. Our results confirm that, at 10 years, repair of the mitral valve according to the techniques pioneered by Carpentier carries a low incidence of valve-related death and thromboembolic complication for acquired mitral valvar incompetence in children.

The reoperation rate is reasonable and compares favorably in terms of long-term mortality and morbidity with replacement of the mitral valve.[2,5] The major problem of valvar repair in children is its long-term viability. Reoperation may be necessary because of inadequate repair, recurrent rheumatism, endocarditis, or secondary failure. It is noteworthy that six of 12 reoperations were related to technical factors. These can be avoided and should be considered representative of our learning curve.

References

1. Attie F, Kuri J, Zanoniani C, et al. Mitral valve replacement in children with rheumatic heart disease. Circulation 1981;64:812–7.
2. Sade RM, Ballenger JF, Hohn AR, et al. Cardiac valve replacement in children: Comparison of tissue with mechanical valve. J Thorac Cardiovasc Surg 1979;78:123–7.
3. Carpentier A. Cardiac valve surgery—the "French correction." J Thorac Cardiovasc Surg 1983;86:323–37.
4. Chauvaud S, Perier P, Touati G, et al. Long term results of valve repair in children with acquired mitral valve incompetence. Circulation 1986;74:1104–9.
5. John S, Bashi V, Jairaj P. Mitral valve replacement in the young patient with rheumatic heart disease: Early and late results in 118 subjects. J Thorac Cardiovasc Surg 1983;86:209–16.

Reconstructive Surgery for Rheumatic Mitral Valvar Disease in Children

R. Sequeira De Almeida, E. J. Ribeiro, S. L. Bassi,
P. R. Brofman, and D. R. Loures

Introduction

The surgical management of rheumatic mitral valvar disease is a complex subject and remains controversial. Its complexity is due to the severity of the mitral valvar lesion, the involvement of other valves and, especially, the age at which these patients present with the disease. In developing countries, disease of the mitral valve is one of the commonest lesions caused by rheumatic fever. This disease very often affects children in a way that produces early and severe damage to the valve; thus, the only form of treatment is surgical. The controversy relates to the decision concerning repair versus replacement. Should we replace the valve by a prosthesis, or should we attempt to repair the native valve? If we opt for replacement, we will surely encounter problems such as the hazards of anticoagulation after replacement with a mechanical prosthesis or the high rate of calcification of leaflets in bioprostheses inserted in children and young adults. If we decide to repair the mitral valve, we are left with other problems. Precise preoperative anatomical and perioperative functional assessment is difficult. Also, the technical ability of the surgeon var-

ies markedly, and the long-term results in the pediatric age group remain uncertain.

Recently, however, the long-term results of repair in children with rheumatic mitral valve disease[1,2] suggest a superiority over replacement of the valve. In this article, we describe our experience at the Servico de Cirurgia Cardio-Vascular-Hospital Evangelico de Curitiba—Brazil with reconstructive surgery for rheumatic disease of the mitral valve in childhood.

Patients and Methods

Between February 1980 and February 1988, 108 patients under the age of 18 years with rheumatic disease of the heart underwent surgical correction of their valvar lesion. Seventy-two patients (66.6%) underwent repair of the mitral valve, and they constitute our study group. Their ages ranged from 5 to 18 years, with a mean of 13.82 ± 0.32 years. There were 41 girls (56.9%) and 31 boys. Five children were less than 10 years of age, 36 were 10–15 years old, and 29 were between 15 and 18 years old. Rheumatic fever was the cause of all lesions observed that were diagnosed by

Table 1

Proposed Functional Classification for
Rheumatic Disease of the Mitral Valve

Mitral insufficiency due to:	
Annular dilatation and deformation	6 patients
Cleft in mural and/or aortic leaflets	4 patients
Mitral insufficiency due to annular deformation with:	
Cordal elongation	10 patients
Cordal rupture	9 patients
Mitral insufficiency and stenosis due to annular deformation with thickening of free margin of leaflet:	
With commissural and/or cordal fusion and cordal elongation	8 patients
With commisural and/or cordal fusion and cordal rupture	4 patients
Mitral stenosis due to:	
Commissural fusion	26 patients
Commissural and cordal fusion with retraction of papillary muscles	5 patients

clinical history or at the time of surgery by means of the anatomical findings. Sixteen patients (22.2%) presented 19 associated lesions, with tricuspid insufficiency in seven, aortic insufficiency in eight, tricuspid stenosis in two, and an atrial septal defect in the other. Only one patient was in New York Heart Association functional class I. Nineteen patients were in class II (27.7%), 41 patients (56.9%) were in class III, and 10 (13.8% were in class IV. Sixty-nine patients (95.8%) were in sinus rhythm, and only three (4.2%) showed atrial fibrillation. The mean cardiothoracic ratio was 0.61 ± 0.01. Sixty-four patients (88.8%) underwent catheterization, which showed a mean pulmonary arterial pressure of 37.60 ± 1.91 mmHg and a mean pulmonary wedge pressure of 22.42 ± 1.12 mmHg. We have used, for the purposes of categorization, the functional classification of Carpentier modified according to Dr. E. J. Ribiero. The categorization was based on the echocardiographic, angiographic, and surgical findings (Table 1). The surgical management was similar for all patients. Operations were performed using cardiopulmonary bypass with moderate systemic hypothermia (25°C). Intermittent aortic cross-clamping was used until 1987 when the St. Thomas cardioplegic solution was used for myocardial protection. A prosthetic ring was used in 41 patients which was closed in 19 cases and open in the rest. The ring varied in size from 24 to 32 mm. All associated lesions were treated at the same time as the mitral valve repair: a De Vega annuloplasty was performed in 17, and repair of aortic insufficiency was accomplished in six of eight. The valve was replaced in the other two. Valvotomy was possible in the two cases of tricuspid stenosis, and the solitary case of aortic stenosis was successfully repaired. The atrial septal defect was closed by direct suture.

Results

The hospital mortality was 1.38% (1/72). Death in this child was due to left ventricular failure associated with residual mitral insufficiency. The period of follow-up ranged from six months to 8.5 years, with a mean period of 3.34 ± 0.24 years. The long-term data were obtained from our routine outpatient clinic. Five patients were lost at follow-up between two and 3.5 years postoperatively. Thirteen reoperations (18.3%) were required from four days to 66 months after the initial procedure (mean 32.21 ± 6.95 months). Replacement of the valve was performed in each case. Reoperation was needed in nine cases because of new episodes of rheumatic fever within a mean period of 45.2 months. A technical error was responsible for failure of the repair in the other four, which was diagnosed within a mean period of three months after the repair. The prostheses used at replacement were mechanical in nine patients and bioprostheses in four. There were two late deaths, both occurring after replacement of

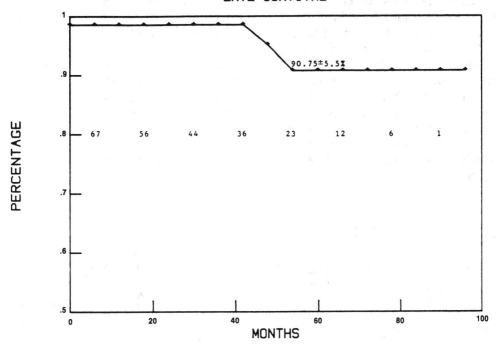

Figure 1a

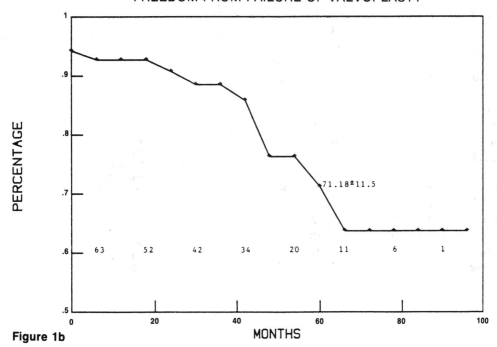

Figure 1b

Figure 1. Actuarial curves of the 72 patients with rheumatic disease of the mitral valve: (a) late survival, including hospital mortality; (b) freedom from failure of valvoplasty.

the valves due to low cardiac output. Long-term follow-up showed that 75.3% (52/69) of the patients were in functional class I, 21.7% (15/69) were in class II, and 2.9% (2/69) were in class III. The long-term actuarial survival rate at five and eight years was 90.7 ± 5.5%, and the freedom from failure of the repair was 71.2 ± 8.0% at five years and 63.7 ± 10.1% at the end of eight years. The actuarial curves for late survival, including hospital mortality and freedom from failure of repair are shown in Fig. 1.

Discussion

Several studies[3-5] have emphasized the need for surgical repair rather than replacement for congenital disease of the mitral valve, but only a few reports have been published on the treatment of rheumatic mitral valvar disease in childhood.[1] The classification we have used has been developed to complement that evolved by Carpentier and his colleagues.[6] We believe that their categorization ignores an important morphologic variant of valvar dysfunction characterized by annular deformation and cordal elongation or rupture associated with commissural and/or cordal fusion and thickening of the free margin of the leaflets. This particular lesion seems to be the most difficult to handle and the one that requires a much longer period of analysis at the time of repair. In our experience, this is the group that had the highest incidence of reoperations due to technical errors during the repair.[7]

Our results are similar to those obtained by Chauvaud et al.,[1] both in terms of late survival and freedom from failure of the valvoplasty, and they are superior at the end of seven years to the survival reported by

Milano et al.[8] after replacement of the mitral valve with either biological or mechanical prostheses, respectively.

The major problem we encountered is that, despite our best efforts, a large number of our patients, due either to social–economic problems or inadequate social assistance, would not continue prophylactic treatment to prevent recurrences of rheumatic fever after repair of their valves. Nine of the 13 reoperations (69.2%) were due to new episodes of rheumatic fever.

References

1. Chauvaud S, Perier P, Touati G, et al. Long-term results of valve repair in children with acquired mitral valve incompetence. Circulation 1986;74(suppl I):104–9.
2. Brofman P, Barbero-Marcial M, Loures D, et al. Reparacao cirurgica da valva mitral em pacientes jovens. Arq Bras Cardiol 1987;49(suppl I):160–8.
3. Carpentier A, Branchini B, Cour JC, et al. Congenital malformations of the mitral valve in children. Pathology and surgical treatment. J Thorac Cardiovasc Surg 1976;6:854–66.
4. Almeida RS, Elliott MJ, Wyse RK, et al. Surgery for congenital abnormalities of the mitral valve, at the Hospital for Sick Children, London from 1969–1983. J Cardiovasc Surg 1988;30:95–9.
5. Stellin G, Bortolotti U, Mazzucco A, et al. Repair of congenital malformed mitral valve in children. J Thorac Cardiovasc Surg 1988;95:480–5.
6. Carpentier A, Chauvaud S, Fabiani JN, et al. Reconstructive surgery of mitral valve incompetence. Ten year appraisal. J Thorac Cardiovasc Surg 1980;79:338–48.
7. Ribeiro EJ, Ferreira MJA, Escorsin M, et al. Cirurgia conservadora da valva mitral em adultos. Arq Bras Cardiol 1987;49(suppl I):164–71.
8. Milano A, Vouhe PR, Baillot-Vernant F, et al. Late results after left-side cardiac valve replacement in children. J Thorac Cardiovasc Surg 1986;92:218–25.

Replacement of Mitral Valve in Childhood with Preservation of Tendinous Cords and Papillary Muscles

C. A. Curcio and S. L. Cronjé

Introduction

Clinical and experimental evidence suggests that preservation of the papillary muscles and tendinous cords during replacement of the mitral valve has a beneficial effect on global postoperative left ventricular function.[1-4] David and colleagues[5,6] have developed a technique for this procedure and have reported good clinical and hemodynamic results in a group of patients who received a porcine bioprosthesis. We have used a similar technique with only minor modifications, replacing the mitral valve in children and adolescents mostly with a St. Jude medical prosthesis.

Materials and Methods

Fourteen children underwent replacement of the mitral valve with preservation of the papillary muscles and tendinous cords. The patients were 6–18 years old with a mean age of 12.6 years. There were seven boys and seven girls. Eleven patients had mixed valvar disease of rheumatic origin, two had pure rheumatic mitral regurgitation, and one mitral regurgitation due to infective endocarditis. The latter had also a ventricular septal defect and severe aortic regurgitation. Significant rheumatic aortic regurgitation was present in five other patients; three patients had active rheumatic pancarditis. A compromised left ventricle with an ejection fraction less than 30% was present in eight patients. All were in functional class IV or more of the New York Heart Association. Isolated replacement of the valve was carried out in eight patients. In the other six, both the mitral and aortic valves were replaced. The ventricular septal defect was closed in the patient with this lesion.

Operative Technique

All the operations were performed on conventional cardiopulmonary bypass using moderate systemic hypothermia and myo-

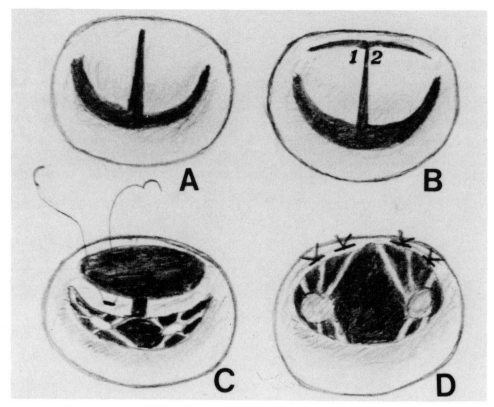

Figure 1. The technique of insertion of the valve. Procedure involving the aortic leaflet.

cardial protection with crystalloid cardioplegia. The tendinous cords and papillary muscles were preserved in all the patients (Figs. 1 and 2). The aortic leaflet is split in the middle (Fig. 1A). The midline incision is then continued parallel to the annulus on both sides (Fib. 1B). Tension on the corners of the leaflets with forceps (Fig. 1B) permits visualization of the ventricular aspects of the two hemileaflets, and the portion of the aortic leaflet receiving cordal insertions is excised under direct vision. Once the central portion of the leaflet has been excised (Fig. 1C), the commissural edges, still anchored to the tendinous cord, are resuspended to the annulus with a few interrupted stitches (Fig. 1D). The same procedure is applied to the mural leaflet when this leaflet is thick and redundant, as is the case in most instances of mixed mitral valvar disease. The leaflet is split in the middle and the incision

is continued parallel to the annulus on both sides (Fig. 2A). Part of the leaflet is excised, taking care to preserve at least the primary tendinous cords (Fig. 2B). The commissural edges of the leaflet, together with the anchored cords, are resuspended to the annulus (Fig. 2B,C). When the mitral valve has been prepared in this fashion, a St. Jude medical prosthesis is implanted using interrupted stitches (Fig. 2D).

Results

One patient having replacement of both aortic and mitral valves died of varicella pneumonia three weeks after the operation (7.1% operative mortality). A postmortem study confirmed the diagnosis of varicella pneumonia with diffuse consolidation of both lungs. Both prosthetic valves were well

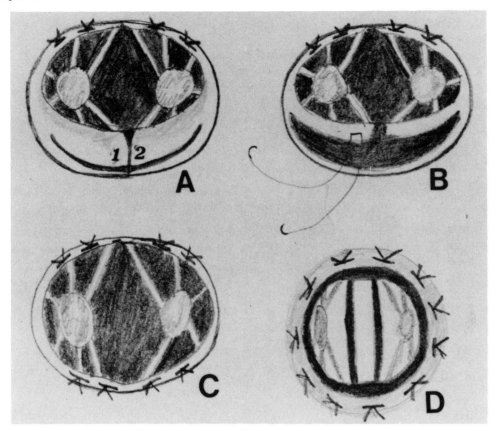

Figure 2. The technique of preparation of the mural leaflet during insertion of the valvar prosthesis.

seated and unimpeded in their function. This was also the patient with the ventricular septal defect, which was well closed.

The remaining 13 patients had an uncomplicated postoperative course characterized by a ready hemodynamic recovery and minimal or no need for inotropic support. No cases of malfunction of the prostheses were recorded early postoperatively as assessed clinically and by cinefluoroscopy. The patients who survived the operation were all discharged from the hospital in functional class II of the New York Heart Association.

Discussion

Replacement of the mitral valve in childhood with preservation of the tendi-nous cords and papillary muscles is a safe procedure with the prostheses used in this study. The beneficial effects of this procedure on the left ventricular performance in adults has been observed by several investigators.[1,2,6] Lillehei and associates[1] preserved the tendinous cords during replacement of the mitral valve with a Starr-Edwards prosthesis and reported decreased mortality and lower incidence of left ventricular dysfunction. More recently, improved left ventricular function using this approach has been confirmed by the extensive experimental and clinical work of David and his colleagues.[3-7] These observations are concordant with our clinical impression.

In our series, in spite of the generally poor preoperative hemodynamics, the advanced pathology, and the severely compromised left ventricle in most of the patients, there was a more prompt post-operative recovery and less need for inotropic support than in patients submitted to conventional valvar replacement. Furthermore, there was no morbidity or mortality related to the valvar surgery.

We conclude that replacement of the mitral valve with preservation of the papillary muscles and tendinous cords is a safe procedure during childhood and may have a beneficial effect on postoperative left ventricular performance. The procedure is recommended for patients undergoing valvar replacement for chronic mitral regurgitation, especially in the presence of poor left ventricular function.

References

1. Lillehei CW, Levy MJ, Bonnabeau RC: Mitral valve replacement with preservation of papillary muscle and chorade tendineae. J Thorac Cardiovasc Surg 1964:47:532–43.

2. Miller DW Jr, Johnson DD, Ivey TD: Does preservation of posterior chordae tendineae enhance survival during mitral valve replacement? Ann Thorac Surg 1979;28:22–8.

3. David TE, Uden DE, Strauss HD: The importance of the mitral apparatus in left ventriculare function after correction of mitral regurgitation. Circulation 1983;68(suppl II):76–82.

4. Hansen DE, Cahill PD, Derby GC, Miller CD: Relative contribution of the anterior and posterior mitral chordae tendineae to canine global left ventricular systolic function. J Thorac Cardiovasc Surg 1987;93:45–55.

5. David TE. Mitral valve replacement with preservation of chordae tendineae: Rationale and technical consideration. Ann Thorac Surg 1986;41:680–2.

6. David TE, Burns RJ, Bacchus CM, Druk MN. Mitral valve replacement for mitral regurgitation with and without preservation of chordae tendineae. J Thorac Cardiovasc Surg 1984;88:718–25.

7. Spence PA, Peniston CM, David TE, et al. Toward a better understanding of the etiology of left ventricular dysfunction after mitral valve replacement: An experimental study with possible clinical implications. Ann Thorac Surg 1986;41:367–71.

Valve Replacement Using Mechanical Prostheses in Children

M. J. Antunes

Introduction

In our experience, the performance of mechanical prostheses in children has been demonstrably superior to that of bioprostheses. The incidence of complications related to the valve, however, with special emphasis of thromboembolic events, was at least as significant as in adults. We are unable to support the concept, therefore, that anticoagulation may not be essential in younger patients. A large number of young patients with rheumatic carditis seen in the Third World require replacement of their diseased valves. In our unit, 21.4% of the patients belonging to Third World types of population were 15 years old or younger. Many patients were so severely ill that they required emergency replacement of the diseased valve during the active phase of the disease.

In the past, we had found that only 19% of such patients were alive and free of complications seven years after implantation of a bioprosthesis in the mitral position.[1] The accelerated calcification of porcine prostheses preserved in glutaraldehyde has been confirmed by several authors.[2,3] Hence, since 1980, we have preferred to use mechanical prostheses for replacement of

diseased valves. In this article, we describe the performance of these prostheses implanted in children, with special relevance to events directly relating to the use of this type of prostheses.

Patients and Methods

From May 1980 through April 1985, 182 black children, 15 years old and younger, had replacement of their aortic and/or mitral valves in our unit in Johannesburg (Table 1). We have analyzed only patients with rheumatic valvar disease. There were 99 valves inserted in mitral position, 24 to replace the aortic valve, while both valves were replaced in 59 patients. The mean age of all patients was 12.5 years. There was a predominance of females in those having replacement of the mitral valve and of males in the group with both valves being replaced, while the distribution of sexes was even in those needing replacement of the aortic valve. In all three groups there was a vast predominance of regurgitant lesions, either in isolation or in association with stenosis. Thirty-two patients (17%) had had previous valvar surgery. Only 7% of the patients were in atrial fibrillation, all but two in those

Table 1

Clinical Data

	MVR	AVR	DVR	Total
Patients	99	24	59	182
Age (years)				
Mean	11.9	13.0	12.7	12.5
Range	4–15	9–15	6–15	4–15
Sex (% M/F)	43/57	50/50	66/34	52/48
Lesion (%)				
Stenosis	9	4	10	9
Regurgitation	43	79	73	57
Mixed	23	13	7	17
Previous surgery (%)	25	4	10	17
Active rheumatic carditis (%)	34	33	56	41
Infective endocarditis (%)	9	—	14	9
Emergency surgery (%)	28	54	49	38
Atrial fibrillation (%)	10	4	17	7

AVR, aortic valve replacement; DVR, replacement of aortic and mitral valves; MVR, mitral valve replacement.

needing replacement of the mitral or both aortic and mitral valves. Medtronic-Hall (88%) and St. Jude medical prostheses were used in all patients. Altogether, 242 prostheses were implanted. Of the patients, 41% had active carditis at the time of the procedure and 38% underwent their operation on an emergency basis.

All patients were anticoagulated with warfarin sodium controlled according to a prothrombin index of 25–40% of normal. In the last four years of the study, dipyridamole (given in doses of 100 mg thrice daily) was also administered to all patients. Compliance was poor in more than half the patients. Because of the logistical problems related to the characteristics of the population, 34 patients (18.7%) were lost to follow-up. The remainder were followed up for a cumulative period of 579.5 patient-years, with a range from three to eight years (mean 4.9 years).

Results

Twelve patients (6.5%) died early. The mortality for replacement of the mitral, aor-

tic, and both valves was 3.0%, 12.5% and 10.2%, respectively ($p < 0.01$). There was no difference in the mortality between patients with regurgitation and those with stenotic lesions, but the mortality of procedures performed on an emergency basis (11/47 cases; 23.4%) was higher than that of elective replacement (1/136; 0.6%; $p < 0.01$). Patients operated on with active carditis had a higher operative mortality (7/75; 9.3%) than those without (5/107; 4.6%; $p < 0.05$).

Twenty patients died late (4.8% per patient-year). The incidence of late mortality for replacement of the mitral valve (3.1% per patient-year) and of the aortic valve (2.8%

Table 2

Causes of Late Mortality

	n	% per patient-year
Cardiac		
Valve-related		
Non-valve-related	6	1.0[a]
	8	1.4
Noncardiac	1	0.2
Unknown	13	2.2
TOTAL	28	4.8

[a] Adjusted figure, 1.9% per patient-year (see text).

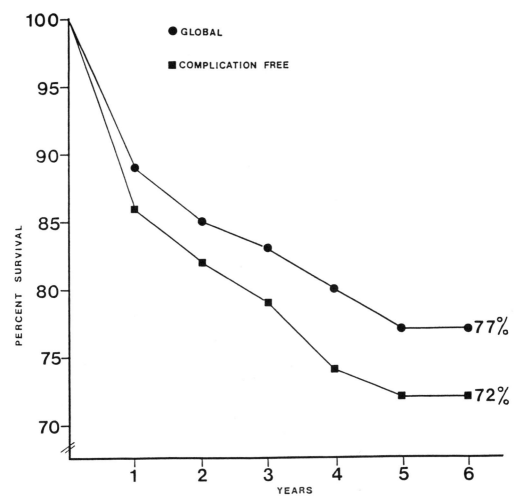

Figure 1. Actuarial global survival and complication-free survival of children with mechanical valvar prostheses.

per patient-year) was lower than that for replacement of both valves (10.0% per patient-year; p < 0.01). The causes of late mortality are summarized in Table 2. They were related to the prosthesis in six cases (1.0% per patient-year). The cause of death could not be ascertained in 13 patients (46%). In order to avoid major distortions in the figures, the mortality of unknown causes was redistributed to all other groups in percentages identical to those where the deaths were of known cause. Actuarially, 77 ± 4% of the patients were alive at five years (Fig. 1), but freedom from mortality related to the pros-

thesis was 95 ± 2%. Twenty-two patients (3.8% per patient-year) needed reoperations during the period of follow-up. Thrombotic obstruction and endocarditis of the prosthetic valve (eight cases each) and periprosthetic leaks (five cases) were the main reasons for reoperation. The incidence of reoperation was similar for those having replacement of the mitral and aortic valves (2.8% per patient-year) but lower than in those having replacement of both valves (6.7% per patient-year; p < 0.05). In actuarial terms, 84 ± 4% of the patients were free from reoperation at five years (Fig. 2).

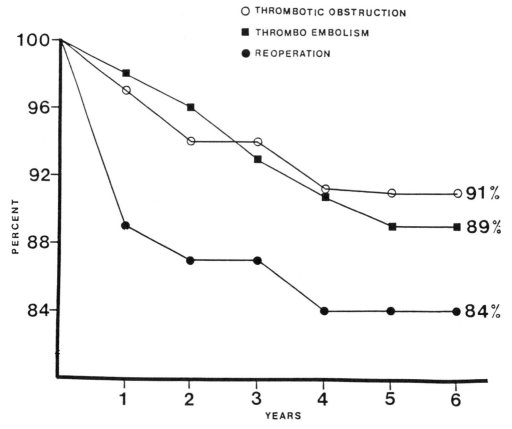

Figure 2. Actuarial probability of freedom from reoperation, prosthetic valve thrombosis, and systemic thromboembolism in the same group of patients.

The incidence of thrombosis on the prosthetic valve was 1.6% per patient-year. For replacement of the mitral valve, it was 1.1% per patient-year, for the aortic valve 1.4% per patient-year, and for replacement of both valves it was 2.7% per patient-year ($p < 0.05$). Thrombosis was fatal in 22% of the cases involved (0.4% per patient-year). Major systemic thromboembolic events occurred in 11 patients (1.9% per patient-year). One patient had two episodes. No known fatal cases were registered. Actuarially, after five years, freedom from thrombotic obstruction of the prosthesis and from systemic thromboembolism was 91 ± 3% and 89 ± 3%, respectively (Fig. 2).

Prosthetic valvar endocarditis occurred in eight patients (1.4% per patient-year), all of whom needed reoperations. One died

(12.5%) and another one required a second reoperation. Two patients had fatal hemorrhages related to anticoagulation (0.3% per patient-year). Five patients (0.9% per patient-year had bland periprosthetic leaks of hemodynamic significance, all requiring reoperation, and one patient (20%) died. Actuarial freedom from all mortality and morbidity related to the prosthesis after five years was 72 ± 5% and freedom from failure of the prosthesis was 80 ± 4%. The linearized incidence of the latter was 4.7% per patient-year.

Discussion

The choice of a prosthesis for replacement of diseased cardiac valves is influenced by the type and characteristics of the population. Porcine bioprostheses, once accepted as the best substitute for these young patients, were soon demonstrated to be prone to very early calcification, which led to progressive and severe valvar stenosis. Our own experience confirms this accelerated rate of biodegradation. From 1976 to 1980, glutaraldehyde-preserved porcine bioprostheses were implanted, in the mitral position only, in all our patients. Only 19% of those under 20 years of age were alive with their original prosthesis after a period of seven years. The rate of degeneration in these patients was 22.4% per patient-year, when compared to a structural failure of 4.0% per patient-year in patients over 20 years.[4] The generalized concept that failure of bioprostheses is a slow, relatively benign process appears fallacious. Many of our patients died in hospital while waiting for surgery scheduled for the next few days. Furthermore, recent reports appear to indicate that these valves fail after a mean period of 10–12 years in older patients.[5]

Mechanical prostheses are, thus, the only alternative device for replacement of diseased valves in children.* Prosthetic thrombosis and systemic thromboembolism, however, remain a significant complication and the main causes of failure of these prostheses. When the intensity of anticoagulation is increased, the incidence of hemorrhagic complications increases as significantly as the thromboembolic phenomena decrease.

It has been suggested that mechanical prostheses are safe with low-dose anticoagulation or no anticoagulation at all.[6] Verrier, et al.[7] found that "children with mechanical aortic valves in normal sinus rhythm can be safely treated with aspirin (or aspirin with dipyridamole) with little risk of thromboembolic events, valve thrombosis, or valve failure." On the other hand, the results of Ribeiro et al.[8] "indicate that anti-

platelet drugs alone are associated with a very low risk of embolism but are insufficient to prevent thrombosis of St. Jude medical aortic valves, even when the patients have sinus rhythm."

Our series appears to confirm a significantly lower incidence of serious systemic thromboembolism in children (1.6% per patient-year) when compared with that observed in older patients (3.3% per patient-year).[9] However, the incidence of prosthetic valvar thrombosis was similar in the two groups of patients. These incidences in an anticoagulated, albeit doubtfully compliant, population group strongly suggest the need for adequate anticoagulation of all patients with mechanical prostheses, irrespective of their age. A similar conclusion was derived by Robbins et al.[10] In their series, seven of the 11 patients who did not receive anticoagulation experienced major thromboembolic events. Many of the reports suggesting a lower incidence of thromboembolic and thrombotic complications in unanticoagulated children were based on relatively short periods of follow-up. Experience clearly teaches cautiousness, especially in the interpretation of early data regarding replacement of diseased valves. Reoperation was required in 22 patients (3.8% per patient-year). Nevertheless, 84% of the patients were free from reoperation at five years, a considerable improvement over the figures obtained in the previously mentioned series using bioprosthesis as the substitutes for diseased valves performed in the same population group.[1] Even the actuarial global survival rate of 77% was considerably better. Furthermore, most of the late deaths were unrelated to the prosthetic valve.

The evidence uncovered by this study appears to vindicate our recent recommendation that mechanical prostheses having the pattern of the newer generation of tilting discs (Medtronic-Hall) or bileaflet (St. Jude) be used for replacement of diseased valves in children in whom bioprostheses demonstrate intolerably high rates of structural failure. The incidence of thromboembolic

---

* *Editor's note:* Aortic homografts could also be used: see chapter 3.9 in Section III.

episodes, however, remains of concern and the use of adequate anticoagulation is strongly recommended.

References

1. Antunes MJ. Bioprosthetic valve replacement in children: Long-term follow-up with 135 isolated mitral valve implantations. Eur Heart J 1984;5:913–8.
2. Silver MM, Pollack J, Silver MD, et al. Calcification in porcine xenograft valves in children. Am J Cardiol 1980;45:685–9.
3. Geha AS, Laks H, Stansel HC Jr, et al. Late failure of porcine valve heterografts in children. J Thorac Cardiovasc Surg 1979;78:351–64.
4. Antunes MJ, Santos LP. Performance of glutaraldehyde-preserved porcine bioprostheses as a mitral valve substitute in a young population group. Ann Thorac Surg 1984;37:387–92.
5. Foster AH, Greenberg GJ, Underhill DJ, et al. Intrinsic failure of Hancock mitral bioprostheses: 10 to 15 year experience. Ann Thorac Surg 1987;44:568–77.
6. Weinstein GS, Mavroudis C, Ebert PE. Preliminary experience with aspirin for anticoagulation in children with prosthetic cardiac valves. Ann Thorac Surg 1982;33:549–53.
7. Verrier ED, Tranbaugh RF, Soifer SJ, et al. Aspirin anticoagulation in children with mechanical aortic valves. J Thorac Cardiovasc Surg 1986;92:1013–20.
8. Ribeiro PA, Zaibag MA, Idris M. Antiplatelet drugs and the incidence of thromboembolic complications of the St. Jude medical aortic prosthesis in patients with rheumatic heart disease. J Thorac Cardiovasc Surg 1986;91;92–8.
9. Antunes MJ, Wessels A, Sadowski RG, et al. Medtronic-Hall valve replacement in a third world population group. A review of the performance of 1000 prostheses. J Thorac Cardiovasc Surg 1989;95:980–93.
10. Robbins RC, Bowman FO, Malm JR. Cardiac valve replacement in children: A twenty-year series. Ann Thorac Surg 1988:45:56–61.

Aortic Valvar Surgery in the Young

M. R. Al Fagih, A. Ashmeg, S. Al Kasab, Y. Al Faraidi,
and W. Sawyer

Introduction

Between 1980 and 1987, 103 surgical procedures on the aortic valve were performed at the Riyadh Cardiac Centre in 102 symptomatic patients, aged up to 18 years at the time of surgery. Seven patients were below 1 year old, 29 were 2–12 years old, and 66 were 13–18 years old. The youngest patient was 1 month old. The lesions were rheumatic in 76% of cases and congenital in 24%. Incompetent valves accounted for 70% of the procedures, stenotic lesions for 18%, and valves that were both incompetent and stenotic made up the remainder. One patient had endocarditis at the time of surgery. The results of their procedures form the basis of this article.

Surgical Procedures

Surgery was confined to the aortic valve in 72% of the population. Another valve (mitral or pulmonary) needed attention in 21%, and three valves were involved in 6%. Replacement of the valve was by far the most common procedure. Of the 70 valves inserted, 27 were bioprosthetic (Carpentier, Edwards, or Hancock), and 43 were mechanical (St. Jude or Duromedics). The aor-

tic root was enlarged when necessary in some cases of valvar replacement. The techniques used included gusset enlargement, which in some cases was extended into the roof of the left atrium, and aortoventriculoplasty (Konno procedure). There was no related morbidity or mortality with these procedures.

Sixteen incompetent aortic valves were repaired. In nine of these, a new technique was used. The three native cusps were extended with specially shaped pieces of bovine pericardium treated with glutaraldehyde.[1] This technique retains the hinge mechanism of the native leaflets and restores their coaption, resulting in valvar competence without the introduction of large amounts of foreign tissue or a rigid ring (Figs. 1 and 2). Following repair with this technique, there was no gradient across the valve, in contrast to the gradients that have been reported after insertion of porcine or mechanical valves.[2,3] On postoperative cross-sectional echocardiography, the left ventricular end systolic dimension decreased from a mean ($\pm$SD) of 4.1 $\pm$ 1 to 3.4 $\pm$ 0.6 cm, while the end diastolic dimension decreased from 6.2 $\pm$ 1.4 to 4.8 $\pm$ 0.8 cm. These improvements were both statistically significant. Anticoagulation is not required. The remaining seven repairs of the

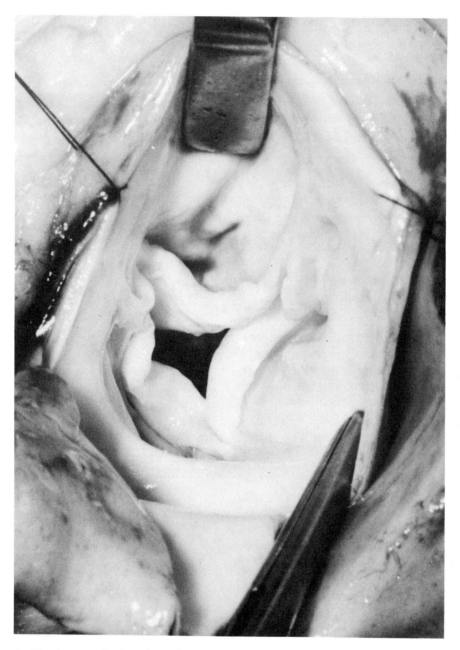

Figure 1. The incompetent aoritc valve, showing thickened and retracted leaflets which fail to coapt.

aortic valve involved suspension of the leaflets at the commissures.

Fifteen valvotomies were performed. In one other case the aortic valve was simply dilated. One valve was completely replaced using bovine pericardium to recreate the leaflets. Seven of the procedures were reoperations (Table 1).

Of the 41 patients who received a mechanical valve and survived the periopera-

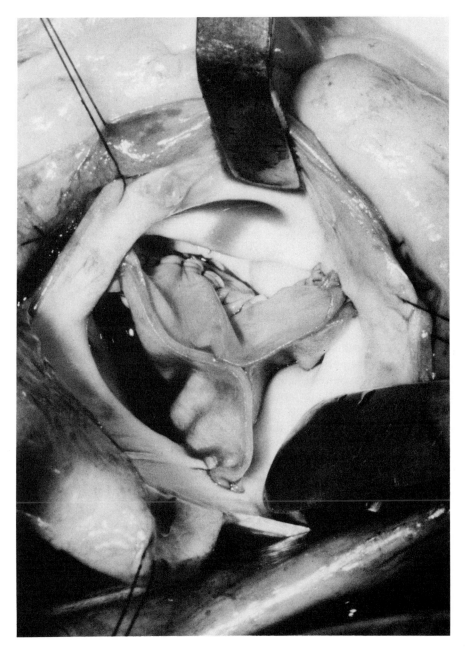

Figure 2. The same valve after extension of the leaflets with bovine pericardium. Note the restored coaption.

tive period, 26 (63%) were anticoagulated with warfarin from the time of surgery. No difficulties were experienced in the management of these patients, despite fears of noncompliance and the increased risk of trauma. Antiplatelet therapy by means of aspirin with persantin was used in 12 patients (32%). On the basis of our previous observations,[4] five of this latter group were subsequently changed to anticoagulation by

Table 1

Reoperation

Original procedure	n	Years after first operation	Cause
Valvotomy	1	9	Restenosis
Mechanical valve	1	3	Thrombosis
Bioprosthesis	5	3, 3, 5, 5, 7	Degeneration

means of warfarin where local provision for control was adequate. One patient took aspirin alone. In this case, unfortunately, the mechanical valve thrombosed and was replaced (Fig. 3).

Results

There were nine deaths in the series of 103 procedures. All were perioperative, and three occurred in infants below the age of 3 months. A further seven patients were lost to follow-up, giving a follow-up rate of 92%. The mean period of follow-up for the remaining 86 patients was 25 months, with a range of 2–92 months. When last seen at follow-up, the majority of patients were asymptomatic; only four were short of breath on severe exertion. One patient has undergone a normal pregnancy and delivery, and another has become pregnant.

Apart from the previously mentioned thrombosis in a mechanical valve in the patient who was taking aspirin alone, no other thromboembolic phenomena have occurred. No patient developed endocarditis.

Discussion

For patients up to 18 years of age, repair of incompetent aortic valves is preferable, whenever possible, to replacement. The implantation of bioprosthetic valves should be avoided. Our experience confirms that they degenerate quickly in the young subject. Mechanical valves with anticoagulation

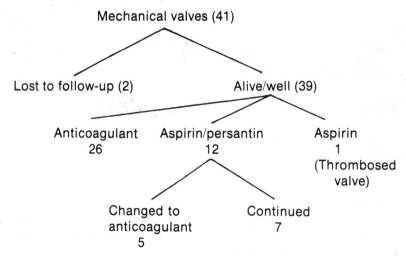

Figure 3. Progress of patients in whom mechanical valves were inserted.

give satisfactory long-term results. Provided that the patient is within reach of a center with the appropriate facilities, careful management of anticoagulation in this age group is possible with few problems, and it should be preferred to antiplatelet therapy. Aortic root enlargement should be performed if necessary, providing better hemodynamics with low risk.

References

1. Al Fagih MR, Al Kasab SM, Ashmeg A. Aortic valve repair using bovine pericardium for cusp extension. J Thorac Cardiovasc Surg 1988; 96:760–64.

2. Reis RL, Hancock WD, Yarbrough JW, et al. The flexible stent; a new concept in the fabrication of tissue heart valve prostheses. J Thorac Cardiovasc Surg 1971;62:683–89.

3. Bjork VO, Henze A, Holmgren A, et al: Evaluation of the 21 mm Bjork-Shiley tilting disc valve in patients with narrow aortic roots. Scand J Thorac Cardiovasc Surg 1973;7:203–213.

4. Ribeiro PA, Al Zaibag M, Idris M, et al. Antiplatelet drugs and the incidence of thromboembolic complications in the St. Jude medical aortic prosthesis in patients with rheumatic heart disease. J Thorac Cardiovasc Surg 1986;91:92–8.

Multivalvar Surgery in Children with Rheumatic Heart Disease

C. A. Moraes, J. V. Rodrigues, C. L. Santos, and I. Cavalcanti

Introduction

Multivalvar surgery in children is a procedure routinely performed in cardiothoracic centers of developing countries where rheumatic heart disease continues to be a challenging problem. Young people from the lower strata of the population often have an accelerated and severe form of disease that produces early valvar damage. Although the majority of the young subjects present with mitral stenosis or incompetence, it is not uncommon to see children with marked disability due to multivalvar lesions. In this article, we describe our experience with 60 patients below the age of 17 years with multiple valvar disease of rheumatic origin.

Patients and Methods

During the past 20 years (1967–1987), 1,474 patients underwent open-heart operations for rheumatic valvar disease at the Medical School of the Federal University of Pernambuco and at the Real Hospital Portugues, Recife, Brazil. Two hundred twenty-seven (15.4%) were children under the age of 17 years. Among these 227 patients, 60 (26.6%) had multiple valvar disease, and

they form the basis for this article. There were 35 boys and 25 girls, ranging in age from 7 to 17 years with a mean of 15 ± 2.3 years. None had undergone any previous operation. Fifty-two (86.6%) had a history of rheumatic fever or exhibited active carditis at the time of admission. Most patients were in poor general condition with a poor nutritional status, their weights ranging from 14 to 48 kg (average 20 ± 7.5 kg). All the children were seriously disabled and, as classified following the criteria of the New York Heart Association, 38 (63.3%) were in functional class IV and 22 (36.7%) were in class III.

Forty-two (70%) patients had mitral and aortic lesions, 15 (25%) had mitral and tricuspid valvar disease, and three (5%) had triple valvar disease. Of the 123 diseased valves, 30 (24.3%) were preserved and 93 (75.5%) were replaced. The procedures performed in this series included replacement of the aortic valve in 45 patients, mitral valve in 42, tricuspid valve in 46, mitral commissurotomy in 14; mitral annuloplasty in 4; and tricuspid annuloplasty in 12.

The type of prosthesis implanted varied over the years, reflecting improvements in the design of prostheses and changes in our policy. Sixty-four bioprosthetic and 29 mechanical valves were implanted. The tissue valves were constructed of fascia lata in one case, porcine heterografts in two, dura mater in 33, and of bovine pericardium in 28. The mechanical prosthesis implanted were of the Starr-Edwards type in 27 and Medtronic-Hall in two. Long-term therapy with warfarin sodium was prescribed for the recipients of mechanical valves.

Results

The operative mortality (up to one month after operation) was 20% (12/60). It was 19% (8/42) in the group undergoing mitro-aortic surgery, 20% (3/15) in those having surgery of the mitral and tricuspid valves, and 33.3% (1/3) in the patients with triple valvar disease. The causes of early deaths included low cardiac output in eight, arrhythmias in two, neurologic lesions in one, and sudden death in another.

The total follow-up for the 48 surviving patients was 1,569 patient-months (mean 27 months). Four (6.6%) patients were lost to follow-up. Fourteen (23.3%) children had clinical evidence of rheumatic reactivity between six months and two years after the operation. Prophylactic antibiotic therapy was always prescribed but, due to a low social and economic standing, many patients were not compliant. Reoperation for failure of tissue valves was needed in eight (13.3%) patients. Thromboembolic episodes occurred in four patients with mechanical valves (6.6%). Finally, three (5%) children with tissue valves developed endocarditis.

Late mortality was 26.6% (16/60), resulting in an overall mortality of 46.6% (28/60). The causes of the late deaths were congestive heart failure due to rheumatic reactivity in six, reoperation in four, endocarditis in three, and thromboembolism in the remaining three.

Twenty-eight (46.6%) patients are alive at present. All of them are in functional class I or II as judged by the criteria of the New York Heart Association. Five-year actuarial survival was 32% (Fig. 1).

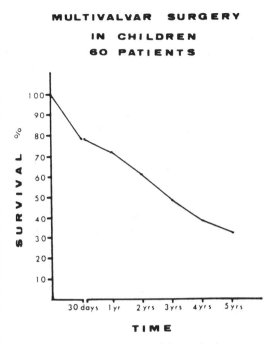

Figure 1. Five-year actuarial survival curve.

Discussion

It is well known that in many areas of the Third World rheumatic heart disease affects poor young people in a much more severe form than in developed regions. In Recife, the largest city of northeastern Brazil, 15.4% of all patients requiring surgery for rheumatic valvar disease in the last 20 years were children under 17 years of age. The majority presented with isolated mitral stenosis or incompetence, but 60 children had multivalvar disease. This subgroup of patients represents the most advanced and severe form of rheumatic heart disease. All of them were seriously disabled and in poor general condition prior to surgery, showing, at operation, extensive valvar deformities. It is not surprising that surgical treatment in this series resulted in an operative mortality of 20%. Similar figures have been reported by others.[2-4] Low cardiac output was the leading cause of early death and reflects the severity of myocardial impairment.

Selection of the ideal surgical procedure for children with multivalvar lesions poses a dilemma. Although reconstruction, especially of the mitral and tricuspid valves, would seem to be the ideal surgical procedure, the severe deformities frequently seen precluded such reparative operations in many patients of this series. The choice of a valvar substitute for children is another problem. Despite the generally unsatisfactory results using tissue valves in the pediatric age range,[5-7] we favored use of bioprostheses because, in most patients, long-term control of anticoagulation was not considered possible. We have used mechanical valves only in patients living near a medical center. Even so, four of 29 children who underwent implantation of a mechanical prosthesis had thromboembolic complications.

Follow-up for the 48 surviving patients (1,569 patient-months with a mean of 27 months), revealed unsatisfactory results due to calcification (13.3%) and endocarditis (5%) in children with tissue valves and thromboembolism (6.6%) in patients with mechanical prostheses. Moreover, there was a high incidence (29.1%) of recurrence of rheumatic endocarditis. This latter finding is discordant with reports from Israel[4] and India.[6] Its occurrence in the late postoperative period suggests that surgery itself cannot be responsible for this complication. Possibly, it is due to discontinuation by the patients of their recommended penicillin prophylaxis. As the result of these various complications, there was a late mortality of 26.6%. The calculated five-year actuarial survival was only 32%.

In conclusion, all problems experienced with multivalvar replacement in older patients are also experienced in children. But, in addition, this latter group present their own problems related, for example, to calcific stenosis of tissue valves and difficulties with long-term anticoagulation. Those problems are more pronounced in developing countries where, in our experience, there is also a significant incidence of rheumatic reactivity. It is obvious, therefore, that surgery for multivalvar rheumatic heart disease in children is essentially a palliative procedure.

References

1. Moraes CR, Arruda M, Lagreca JR, et al. Mitral valve surgery in children. Vasc Surg 1978; 12:176–84.
2. Mathews RA, Park SC, Neches WH, et al. Valve replacement in children and adolescents. J Thorac Cardiovasc Surg 1977;73:872–6.
3. Gardner TJ, Roland JMA, Neill CA, Donahoo JS. Valve replacement in children. A fifteen-year perpsective. J Thorac Cardiovasc Surg 1982;83:178–85.
4. Vidne B, Levy MJ. Heart valve replacement in children. Thorax 1970;25:57–61.
5. Wada J, Yokoyama M, Hashimoto A, et al. Long-term follow-up of artificial valves in patients under 15 years old. Ann Thorac Surg 1980;29:519–21.
6. John S, Bashi VV, Jairaj PS, et al. Mitral valve replacement in the young patient with rheumatic heart disease. Early and late results in 118 subjects. J Thorac Cardiovasc Surg 1984;88:217–24.
7. Robbins RC, Bowman FO Jr, Malm JR. Cardiac valve replacement in children: A twenty-year series. Ann Thorac Surg 1988;45:56–61.

Valvar Replacement in Children

A. Pellegrini, E. Quaini, P. Austoni, T. Colombo, E. Vitali, and
F. Donatelli

Introduction

In this article, we review our experience with replacement of valves in children in an attempt to assess more precisely the difficulties occurring in this special group of patients considering the potential problems related to expected somatic growth, the need for long-term anticoagulation, and the choice for valvar substitutes.

Patients and Methods

From January 1970 to December 1987, 72 patients younger than 15 years of age underwent valvar replacement. Forty-two were boys and 30 girls. Their ages ranged from 1 to 15 years, with a mean of 11.3 ± 3.8 years. Evidence of impaired growth (less than 10th weight percentile) was present in 59.7% of the cases.

All patients had advanced stages of heart disease. Only 16 were in the classes I or II of the New York Heart Association; 21 were in class III; 13 in IV; and 8 in V.

Chest Roengtenogram showed marked cardiomegaly in the majority of patients. The cardiothoracic ratio ranged from 0.46 to 0.80, with a mean of 0.61 ± 0.08.

The most common etiological factor was congenital heart disease which was present in 35 patients. A history suggestive of rheumatic fever was elicited in 30 patients. In seven cases, valvar disease was due to active endocarditis. Endocarditic lesions were present in a further two patients, with congenital valvar disease in one case and with rheumatic valve disease in the other. The intrinsic valvar lesions causing replacement of the aortic valve in 25 patients, of the left atrioventricular valve in 37, and of both the mitral and aortic valves in 10 are shown in Table 1.

Other intracardiac congenital abnormalities complicated the valvar disease in 36 patients, specifically an intracardiac shunt in 12 cases; a mitral web in three cases; various types of atrioventricular septal defect in seven cases; simple or complex types of subaortic obstruction in three cases; congenitally corrected transposition together with a ventricular septal defect in one case; double-inlet right ventricle with two atrioventricular valves, a rudimentary left ventricle with concordant ventriculo-arterial connection in one case; a common arterial trunk in one case; acute aortic dissection in one case; supravalvar aortic stenosis in two cases; a sinus of Valsalva aneurysm in one case; aortic coarctation in one case; cardiomyopathy in one case; and ventricular

Table 1

Type of Lesion

Aortic valve	25
AS	6
AR	14
AR/AS	5
Left A-V valve	37
MS	1
MR	31
MR/MS	5
Mitral and aortic valves	10
MR + AR	6
MR + AR/AS	2
MR/MS + AR	2

AS = aortic stenosis; AR = aortic regurgitation; MS = mitral stenosis; MR = mitral regurgitation.

preexcitation of the Wolff-Parkinson-White in two cases.

Fifteen patients had undergone one or two previous cardiac operations. Most of them were conservative procedures aiming at the repair of the diseased valve.

The indication for valvar replacement was elective in 52 patients, urgent in five, and emergency in 15. Urgent or emergency indications were due to the presence of a low cardiac output syndrome, either controlled or not controlled with inotropic and vasodilator drugs at the maximum level of the therapeutic range.

The final decision for replacement versus valvar repair was made at the time of the operation. Operation was performed with cardiopulmonary bypass and moderate hypothermia, using potassium cardioplegia since 1977.

Mechanical prostheses were used in 73 cases and bioprostheses in nine. The ratio between the effective orificial area of the prostheses used and the anticipated valvar area according to body surface was calculated according to the formula of Lev. This ratio was over one in 62 cases (86.1%). Except for one case, it has always been possible to implant a prosthesis of 25 mm or greater diameter in mitral position and, except for two cases, of 19 mm or greater in aortic position.

Associated intracardiac procedures were performed in 17 patients (Table 2). Hospital and late mortality was analyzed using stepwise multiple logistic regression analysis in attempt to identify incremental risk factors.[1]

Results

There were 13 hospital deaths, giving a hospital mortality rate of 18.05%. The causes of hospital deaths were the impossibility to wean the patient from cardiopulmonary bypass in six cases, hemorrhage and myocardial infarction in one case each, low cardiac output in three cases, and an early periprosthetic leak in two cases.

Stepwise multiple regression analysis was carried out among 13 pre- and intraoperative variables. The variables considered were: age, sex, body surface area, etiology, site of prosthesis, associated anomalies, previous cardiac operation, class within the criteria of the New York Heart Association, cardiothoracic ratio, time of cardiopulmonary bypass, time of aortic cross-clamping, associated cardiac procedures,

Table 2

Simultaneous Cardiac Procedures in 27 Patients

Closure of ventricular septal defect	7
Excision of subaortic fibrous shelf	2
Closure of atrial septal defect	1
Complete correction of atrioventricular septal defect	2
Mitral commissurotomy	1
Mitral annuloplasty	1
Aortic commissurotomy	1
De Vega repair of tricuspid valve	5
Bentall procedure	1
Patch enlargement of ascending aorta	1
Enlargement of aortic root	2
Correction of common arterial trunk	1
Atrioventricular deconnection	1
Implantation of pacemaker	1

Table 3

Hospital Mortality: Incremental Risk Factors

Multivariate Analysis

	Logistic coefficient (CL)	p value
NYHA	0.194 (0.155–0.234)	0.0001
CPB time	0.005 (0.003–0.006)	0.0015
Age	−0.047 (−0.068/−0.027)	0.0172
BSA	0.432 (0.194–0.671)	0.0629
Intercept 0.348		

NYHA = New York Heart Association; CBP = cardiopulmonary bypass; BSA = body surface area.

and the year of operation. This analysis shows that the most powerful statistical predictor for hospital death is preoperative categorization within the criteria of the New York Heart Association followed by the time of cardiopulmonary bypass and age (Table 3).

Each of the 59 hospital survivors has been followed-up for periods ranging from 6 to 204 months with a mean follow-up of 72.6 months. All the patients with mechanical prostheses have been managed chronically with warfarin. Fatal or nonfatal valve-related or cardiac complications occurred in 14 cases. Reoperation was necessary in seven cases. Embolism occurred in one case and, in the group of patients with mechanical prostheses inserted at the site of the mitral valve, endocarditis in one case, progressive heart failure in three cases, and arrythmias in two cases.

Three re-replacements were performed because of degeneration of bioprostheses in three cases. These were performed 36, 15, and 12 months after the first implant, respectively. Re-replacement in four patients (three with mechanical valves and one with a bioprosthesis) was performed because of a periprosthetic leak. An orthotopic heart transplant was carried out in one patient for cardiomyopathy developing 11 years after replacement of the aortic valve.

There were nine late deaths; they were due to reoperation in two cases, sudden death in four cases, progressive heart failure in one case, and acute endocarditis in the remaining case. Stepwise multiple logistic regression analysis was performed for late deaths or eight pre- and intraoperative variables (etiology, associated anomalies, New York Heart Association class, previous cardiac operation, cardiothoracic ratio, associated intracardiac procedure, type and site of implantation of prosthesis). The only sta-

Table 4

Late Mortality: Incremental Risk Factors

Multivariate Analysis

	Logistic coefficient (CL)	p value
Prosthesis	0.323 (0.177–0.468)	0.0243
Associated procedure	0.157 (0.057–0.256)	0.1057
Intercept	0.582	

tistically significant variable is the use of bioprostheses (Table 4). Among the 50 late survivors, 49 are in New York Heart Association class I, and one is in class III.

Discussion

Early results of valve replacement are apparently worse[2-5] in pediatric patients when compared with those obtained in adult cases. The data are confirmed by our computerized and monthly revised analysis regarding the whole group of valvar replacements performed in recent years at our institution, which now includes more than 2,900 patients. The apparent difference between these observations are, no doubt, related to the high incidence of severely compromised preoperative clinical conditions in our group of pediatric patients. Our data confirm that the categorization within the classes of the New York Heart Association is the most powerful statistical variable in determining hospital mortality.[6] The influence of cardiopulmonary bypass time is no doubt overestimated and reflects the unsuccessful attempts at weaning patients from cardiopulmonary bypass. Late mortality is influenced by the use of bioprosthesis. This is influenced by the hospital mortality at time of re-replacement. It is noteworthy to observe that all three patients reoperated because of degeneration of a bioprosthesis presented at reoperation in functional class

V. This observation indicates that mechanical prostheses are the valvar substitutes of choice in pediatric patients.[7] No patients outgrew their prostheses.

Our experience has also confirmed the importance of anticoagulant therapy in pediatric patients. Only one embolism but no hemorrhagic complications occurred and we did not encounter any particular problem in managing anticoagulation by means of oral anti-vitamin K drugs.

References

1. Kirklin JW, Barratt-Boyes BG. Cardiac Surgery. New York, John Wiley & Sons, 1986, pp 177–204, 1493–1524.
2. Ben-Ismail M, Kafsi N, Ayari M. Evolution a long terme des heterogreffes en position mitrale. Arch Mal Coeur 1984;77:180–8.
3. Antunes MJ. Bioprosthetic valve replacement in children: Long-term follow-up of 135 isolated mitral valve implantations. Eur Heart J 1984;5:913–8.
4. El Makhlouf A, Friedli B, Oberhansli I, et al. Prosthetic heart valve replacement in children. Results and follow-up of 273 patients. J Thorac Cardiovasc Surg 1987;93:80–5.
5. Spevak PJ, Freed MD, Castaneda AR, et al. Valve replacement in children less than 5 years of age. J Am Coll Cardiol 1986;8:901–8.
6. Miller DC, Oyer PE, Stinson EB, et al. Ten to fifteen year reassessment of the performance characteristics of the Starr-Edwards model 6120 mitral valve prosthesis. J Thorac Cardiovasc Surg 1983;85:1–20.
7. Quaini E, Colombo T, Donatelli F, et al. Left a-v valve replacement in patients under fifteen years of age. J Cardiovasc Surg 1985; 26(Suppl):9–10.

Late Postoperative Functional Status of Patients with Rheumatic Heart Disease

C. Vongprateep, P. Sakornpant, and S. Utapisarnsuradi

Introduction

Rheumatic fever and rheumatic heart disease are still a major health problem in many parts of the world, particularly in developing countries. The disease usually occurs in children. In our series, extending over 15 years of follow-up, about half the patients seen at the Children's Hospital, Bangkok, were left with permanent cardiac damage. Management is usually done by medical means except in some rare cases where life-threatening carditis cannot be controlled or severe valvar lesions develop, causing severe hemodynamic compromise. In those circumstances, cardiac surgery may be considered. Valvotomy, repair, and replacement are the common forms of surgical therapy that are mostly done in adults. Many physicians, along with the parents of children and adolescents, are reluctant to contemplate surgery in view of the potential operative risk, the fact that it is rarely curative, and because of uncertainty regarding the long-term result.

In this article, we evaluate the long-term result of surgical management for rheumatic heart disease in children and adolescents performed in our institute.

Material and Methods

Statistical analysis carried out in Thailand, over a period of 50 years (1933–1983), in five hospital centers showed no change in the admission rate for rheumatic heart disease.[1] It is the commonest cause (35%) among all admittances for heart disease. Review of those cases that underwent cardiac surgery at the Heart Centre for Children and the Rajvitee Hospital, Bangkok, Thailand, during 1970–1987, disclosed 91 cases under the age of 18 years that were available for analysis. There were 46 males and 45 females. The mitral valve was by far the most common valve involved. Valvotomy and valve replacement were the forms of surgical treatment performed. Follow-up by means of clinical findings, serial electrocardiogram, chest x-rays, and blood tests were done routinely in every patient. Cardiac catheterization and cross-sectional echocardiography were performed in some.

Results

Mitral Valvotomy

A total of 37 cases underwent valvotomy. There were 20 males and 17 females, whose ages ranged from 13 to 18 years with a mean age of 15.9 years. The period of follow-up ranged between 1 month and 12 years. Ten cases were lost to follow-up in this period (27%). There was only one late death. This occurred after 10 years because of congestive heart failure in a patient having replacement of the mitral and tricuspid valves. There was no incidence of embolism. Six cases showed some evidence of valvar calcification. At catheterization, 20 cases had evidence of pulmonary hypertension, and six cases showed evidence of additional valvar lesions involving the aortic and tricuspid valves. Mitral regurgitation was found in nine cases prior to surgery and 15 cases after surgery. All patients were improved clinically with a decrease in heart size in their roentgenograms (Fig. 1) and improvement in the electrocardiogram. Before surgery, 14 cases were in functional class II of the New York Heart Association, 19 were in class III, and 4 were in class IV. After surgery, none were in classes III or IV, 16 cases were in class I, and 12 in class II.

Valve Replacement

Valvar replacement was carried-out in 54 patients (26 males and 28 females). Their ages ranged from 8 to 18 years with a mean of 14.2 years. There were 10 early deaths (18.5%) and four late deaths (7.4%). Of the latter, one was due to cerebral embolism and one to myocardial dysfunction. Infection was the cause of the two remaining deaths. Follow-up ranged from 1 to 14 years, and six cases (13.6%) were lost to follow-up over this period. Only one case was in functional class III prior to surgery, all the rest being in class IV. Postoperatively, 11 cases were

in class I, 17 cases were in class II, and four were in class III. There was only one case in class IV. Eight cases had clinical evidence of thromboembolism (18.2%) despite anticoagulant therapy and one of these died. Six had episodes of atrial fibrillation. The survival rate at one year was 72%, at five years was 58% and at 10 years was 50%.

Those who had cross-sectional echocardiography performed showed a good siting and function of the mechanical valve, with 83.8% of the cases showing evidence of good myocardial function.

Discussion

Open-heart commissurotomy is the technique used in most centers for treatment of rheumatic mitral stenosis, but closed commissurotomy continues to be used in some developing countries.[2,3] The early and long-term results in these centers are comparable to our own. Repair has been used successfully for selected cases of mitral regurgitation or mixed stenosis and regurgitation. In our cases, we found that mitral commissurotomy had many advantages. It is less expensive, more simple, carries a very low mortality, and requires no anticoagulation with a low incidence of embolism. Its disadvantages are a high incidence of residual pulmonary hypertension (almost 50%) and residual stenosis (67%). Six cases developed mitral regurgitation following surgery (16.2%).

There was a significant improvement of functional class after surgery in all our patients. This experience is also similar to previous reports. In the majority of our surgical cases, with severely malformed and calcified valves and serious damage of the subvalvar apparatus, replacement of the valve was necessary. The mortality rate (both early and late) was much higher in this group. Another disadvantage is that those patients needed long-term anticoagulant therapy

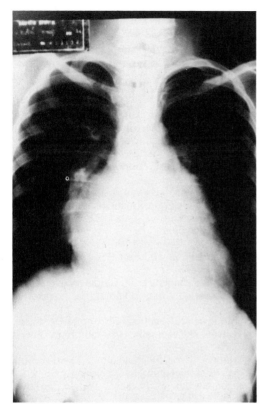 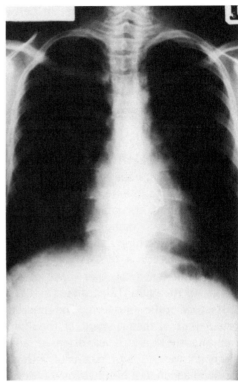

Figure 1a   **Figure 1b**

Figures 1a and 1b. Chest x-rays before (left) and after (right) mitral valve replacement.

and, in spite of that, there was a high incidence of thromboembolism, as also reported by others,[4-6] and atrial fibrillation. The cardiac status of the group of patients requiring valve replacement, nonetheless, was much worse prior to the procedure. All were in functional class IV except one who was in class III. There was a significant improvement in functional class in all of the survivors except five cases who were still in functional classes III and IV. These five patients had long-standing disease with severe heart failure and poor myocardial function preoperatively along with multiple recurrences of rheumatic activity.

We found that the surgical risk and late postoperative functional status depended upon the severity of the cardiac lesion, a late timing of surgery and poor myocardial func-

tion at the time of operation. As a whole, patients, albeit not cured, were much improved clinically. They still required close medical attention, including careful institution of a program of secondary prophylaxis to prevent the recurrence of rheumatic fever. Surgery helped to improve the functional status dramatically and the young girls who experienced child-bearing had no problems. Most of the survivors could resume their normal activities and jobs.

In conclusion, surgery for rheumatic heart disease in children and adolescents is expensive and, in many countries, is available only in highly specialized medical centers. It has proved capable of prolonging survival, improving the quality of life, and has permitted our patients to resume socially and economically productive activities, including child-bearing in women. It must be considered essential, therefore, in severe cases with pronounced disability that might result in death. Treatment by means of surgery should not be delayed until severe pulmonary vascular changes and myocardial damage have occurred. These, indeed, are the major factors responsible for a poor late functional result.

The problems of residual pulmonary hypertension, residual stenosis and/or regurgitation after commissurotomy, the relatively high mortality rate, the need for lonterm or lifetime anticoagulant therapy with a high incidence of embolism and, perhaps, a question concerning the durability of an artificial valve for a lifetime after valvar replacement[7] taken together make cardiac surgery for rheumatic heart disease still unsatisfactory in the long term. The most important part of management of rheumatic fever and rheumatic heart disease, therefore, is its prevention by means of both primary and secondary prophylaxis.

References

1. Proceeding's, Workshop on the Community Control and Prevention of Rheumatic and Rheumatic Heart Disease in Thailand. Department of Medical service. Ministry of Health, Thailand, 1983.
2. John S, Bashi VV, Jairaj PS, et al. Surgery for rheumatic valvular disease in the young subject in: Pediatric Cardiology. Proceeding of the Second World Congress of Pediatric Cardiology. New York, Springer-Verlag, 1986, pp 1025-9.
3. John S, Krishnaswami S, Jairaj PS, et al. The profile and surgical management of mitral stenosis in young patients. J Thorac Cardiovasc Surg 1975;69:631-8.
4. Freed MD, Bernhard WF. Prosthetic valve replacement in children. Prog Cardiovasc Dis 1975;17:475-87.
5. Sade RM, Ballenger JF. Cardiac valve replacement in children. J Thorac Cardiovasc Surg 1979;78:123-7.
6. Bloodwell RD, Hallman GL, Cooley DA. Cardiac valve replacement in children. Surgery 1968:63:77-89.
7. John S, Jairaj PS, Ravikumar E, et al. Mitral valve replacement in the young patient with rheumatic heart disease. J Thorac Cardiovasc Surg 1983;86:209-16.

V

Transplantation

5.1

Introduction

G. Crupi and R. H. Anderson

Transplantation of the heart, or the heart together with the lungs, is now a well-accepted procedure in adults and is performed with increasing frequency in multiple centers. The indications for transplantation in infants and children are less well established, and most procedures are performed in a relatively small number of centers.

Transplantation of the heart in neonates is now proved possible and successful, but the greatest experience in these very young patients has been performed for the hypoplastic left heart syndrome by the team of Bailey working at Loma Linda.[1] The articles of this section review the experiences with heart and heart-lung transplantation in children and adolescents, performed because of pulmonary vascular disease, cardiomyopathy, or else because of congenital cardiac malformations. Musumeci discusses the patients from the extensive experience of Yacoub who underwent transplantation because of the existence of congenital cardiac lesions. There were 11 patients undergoing heart transplantation, ranging in age from 9 days to 28 years. Heart-lung transplantation was performed in 53 patients, all with Eisenmenger's reaction, and they ranged in age from 10 weeks to 52 years. The experience reported by Le Bidois and

his colleagues from Paris is confined to infants and children. Sixteen patients underwent operation, 13 for transplantation of the heart and 3 for both heart and lungs. Siclari and his colleagues report their experience with 10 patients below the age of 18, all having transplantation of the heart alone. None underwent operations because of congenital lesions. All had cardiomyopathy, one together with endocardial fibroelastosis. The combined results of these series underline the feasibility of performing these procedures even in the pediatric age group. The likely indications are noncorrectable congenital lesions. It remains to be seen if the transplantation in the neonatal period will supplant use of the Norwood procedure for the surgical treatment of hypoplastic left heart syndrome. Problems with immunosuppression and the inducement of neoplastic disease will probably need to be overcome before the procedure becomes widely accepted.

Reference

1. Bailey LL, Nehlsen-Cannarella SL, Doroshow RW, et al. Cardiac allotransplantation in newborns as therapy for hypoplastic left heart syndrome. N Engl J Med 1986;315:949–51.

Heart and Heart-Lung Transplantation for Congenital Heart Disease

F. Musumeci, A. Khaghani, N. Banner, S. Aranki,
R. Radley-Smith, and M. Yacoub

Introduction

Cardiac transplantation has been shown to be an effective treatment for patients with end-stage myocardial disease. Its role in the management of those patients with congenital cardiac anomalies who are not amenable to conventional surgery, however, has not been established. In this article, we review our experience in transplantation for congenital heart defects and attempt to define specific problems related to those patients.

Patients and Methods

Between October 1980 and April 1988, a total of 717 patients underwent transplantation at Harefield Hospital. From September 1982, postoperative immunosuppression consisted of cyclosporine and azathioprine with minimal or no oral steroids.

Heart Transplantation

Out of 551 patients who underwent cardiac transplantation during the study period,

11 (2%) had a congenital heart defect. Their ages (Fig. 1) ranged from 9 days to 28 years (mean 13 years). The 3 younger patients had the hypoplastic left heart syndrome, while uncorrected and complex congenital heart defects with poor ventricular function were present in the other 8. There were 7 hospital deaths (63.7%). The causes of death were right heart failure in three patients, failure of multiple organs in 3, and failure of the donor heart in 1.

In contrast to our experience with acquired heart disease, for recipients with congenital heart defects a moderate but potentially reversible elevation of pulmonary vascular resistance (> 4 Wood units) had an adverse effect on early survival. The four survivors in this series included two patients who had pulmonary vascular resistance less than 4 Wood units. In two further patients, "conditioned" hearts from live donors (heart-lung recipients with primary pulmonary hypertension) were successfully used to avoid the risk of peri- and postoperative right ventricular failure. All the four survivors are asymptomatic 2 to 34 months postoperatively (Fig. 2).

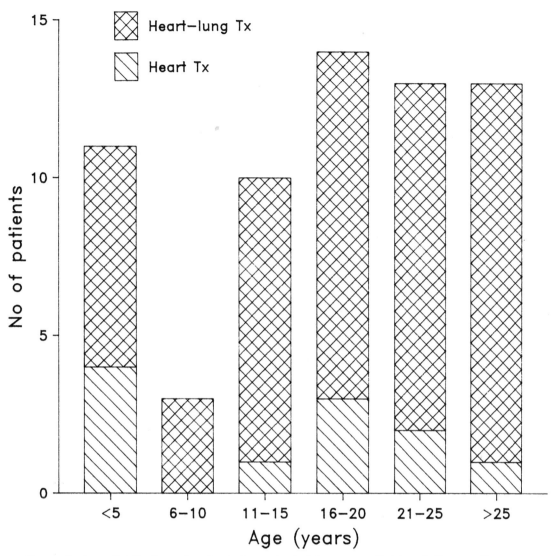

Figure 1. Age distribution of patients transplanted for congenital heart disease. Tx, transplantation.

Combined Heart-Lung Transplantation

In patients with irreversible pulmonary vascular disease (Eisenmenger's syndrome), heart-lung transplantation remains the only surgical option. Fifty-three of the 166 patients (32%) who underwent heart-lung transplantation at Harefield Hospital had Eisenmenger's syndrome. The anomalies present are listed in Table 1. Their ages (Fig. 1) ranged between 10 weeks and 52 years (mean 19.4 years).

The hospital mortality was 33.8% (18/53). The causes of death were bleeding in 5 patients; failure of multiple organs in 5, infection due to *Pseudomonas aeruginosa,* cytomegalovirus, and *Mycoplasma pneumoniae,* respectively, in 3; rejection in 2; failure of donor organs in 2; and tracheal hemorrhage in the remaining patient. The surgical outcome was significantly affected by previous thoracotomy. Nine of the 34 (23%) patients who had no previous surgery and one of the six (16.6%) patients who had had pre-

Heart Transplantation

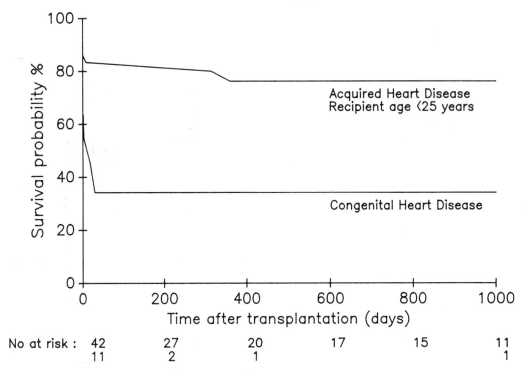

No at risk :   42   27   20   17   15   11
                11   2   1   1

Heart–Lung Transplantation

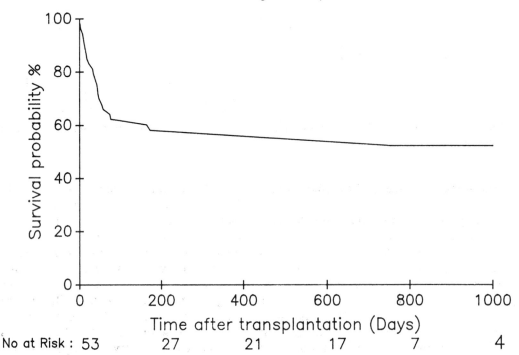

No at Risk : 53   27   21   17   7   4

Table 1

Preoperative Diagnosis in Patients Who
Had Heart-Lung Transplantation

Diagnosis	Patients (n)
Atrial septal defect	2
Totally anomalous pulmonary venous connection	1
Complete transposition	4[a]
Complete AV septal defect	3
Ventricular septal defect	15
Double inlet ventricle	9[a]
Congenitally corrected transposition	3
Double outlet right ventricle	2
Tricuspid atresia	2[a]
Common arterial trunk	5
Aorto-pulmonary window	1
Persistent patency of arterial duct	5
Pulmonary atresia & intact ventricular septum	1[a]

[a] Patients who had a systemic-pulmonary shunt.
AV, atrioventricular.

vious sternotomy died, while there were eight deaths among the 13 patients who had had previous lateral thoracotomies (61.5%) (p < 0.05). Univariate analysis showed no correlation between hospital mortality and age at operation, length of the bypass, or time of graft ischemia.

The mean follow-up for the 35 patients who survived heart and lung transplantation (Fig. 2) was 19.9 months (4–39 months). One patient died 5½ months after surgery following chronic lung infection due to *Staphylococcus aureus*. Nine other survivors

(25.6%) manifested evidence of impaired lung function 6 to 18 months postoperatively, characterized by increasing airway obstruction with a fall in tests of respiratory function suggestive of obliterative bronchiolitis. This has been the cause of death of one patient 25 months postoperatively. A second patient underwent successful retransplantation 12 months after the first procedure. Obliterative bronchiolitis developed in the retransplanted lungs and she died 5 months postoperatively. A further patient is waiting for retransplantation 19 months after the first procedure.

Annual cardiac catheterization and angiography has shown intracardiac pressure within normal ranges, normal ventricular function, and no evidence of coronary atherosclerosis.

Conclusion

The use of cyclosporine and azathioprine with no routine steroids has enabled us to transplant infants and children. In patients with congenital heart defects, cardiac transplantation has produced good results only in the absence of any degree of increased pulmonary vascular resistance. "Conditioned" hearts from live donors can be used for patients with a potentially reversible increase in pulmonary vascular resistance. Heart-lung transplantation is effective for treatment of Eisenmenger's syndrome. Concern remains, however, over the risk of obliterative bronchiolitis developing late after transplantation.

←——————————————————————————

Figure 2. *Top panel:* Actuarial patient survival following heart transplantation for congenital heart disease compared to survival for patients transplanted for acquired heart disease (age < 25 years). *Bottom panel:* Actuarial patient survival following heart-lung transplantation for Eisenmenger's syndrome.

Heart and Heart-Lung Transplantation in Infants and Children
A Study of Sixteen Cases

J. Le Bidois, P. Vouhé, J. Kachaner, J. Y. Neveux, D. Sidi, G. Touati, and S. Guarnera

Transplantation of the heart or the heart and lungs in children was started only a few years ago[1,2] when the use of cyclosporine was seen dramatically to improve the long-term results.[3] More recently, transplantation has even been performed in neonates with encouraging results subsequent to the introduction of newer immunosuppressive regimens.[4] We started our transplantation program in January 1987 and report here our first experiences with transplantation of 13 hearts and 3 heart-lung preparations.

Patients and Methods

Heart Transplantation Alone

Up to June 1988, 13 children (8 boys and 5 girls) underwent heart transplantation. All were in severe and intractable congestive heart failure, and there was no other surgical alternative. Among them, 4 were 2 to 26 weeks old and had various forms of left ventricular obstruction with ventricular hypoplasia and fibrosis. The other 9 patients (5 between 6 and 36 months, and 4 between 5 and 15 years) had either idiopathic cardiomyopathies (5 cases) or complex cardiac malformations (4 cases).

Compatibility between donor and recipient was always respected with regard to blood grouping according to the rules usually followed for transfusion. Heart size was within 25% of the expected heart size (for the body surface area of the recipient) in all but one patient. In this case, the heart of the donor was more than half again greater than the ideal recipient heart size. Each donor had been in a good hemodynamic condition prior to the harvesting. Only one patient underwent a prolonged cardiac resuscitation. He was, nevertheless, accepted for transplantation in view of a complete recovery and normal left ventricular function. The duration of cold ischemia was between 50 and 270 minutes (mean 125 ± 35 minutes). One of the hearts was obtained from a recipient of heart-lung transplantation.

178

The transplantation was performed according to the technique described by Lower and Shumway.[5] Vascular sutures were accomplished without difficulty in two patients with discordant ventriculo-arterial connection. In two of the neonates, it was also necessary to repair a narrowed aortic isthmus at the time of the transplantation according to the technique of Bailey and his colleagues.[6]

The immediate postoperative immunosuppression included rabbit antithymocyte globulin (5 mg/kg/day), methylprednisolone (100 mg/m²/day), and cyclosporine starting intravenously (2 mg/kg/day) with increasing doses. By the 5th day, the rabbit globulin was discontinued, methylprednisolone decreased, and cyclosporine given orally in order to ensure residual plasma levels of 100 to 150 ng/ml. Azathioprine was then started orally (2 mg/kg/24 h). Cyclosporine and azathioprine were the only immunosuppressive drugs by the 10th postoperative day. Endomyocardial biopsies were not performed as a routine procedure. As soon as rejection was suspected on the basis of the noninvasive criteria suggested by Bailey et al.,[4] however, endomyocardial biopsies were performed even in neonates through a femoral vein approach with a 6 French bioptome. Histologic criteria of rejection as described by Billingham[7] were used to quantify the degree of acute rejection. Mild to moderately acute rejection was treated by methylprednisolone (1 g/1.73 m²/day) given for 3 days with a control biopsy 1 week later. Severe acute rejection required additional treatment with rabbit antithymocyte globulin or other antiglobulin treatment.

The patients were followed up in our outpatient clinic and were seen twice a week over the first postoperative month and once a month after the first 6 months. Endomyocardial biopsies and kidney biopsies were systematically performed 6 to 12 months after the transplantation.

Four infants died in the immediate postoperative period (31%). Death was due, in two cases, to transplantation of inadequate donor heart (the case with prolonged cardiac resuscitation and the case in which the donor heart was too big). One patient died from persistent postcapillary pulmonary hypertension with acute right ventricular failure, while the other had a fulminant pulmonary infection caused by *Pseudomonas aeruginosa*.

There was no late death but, among the nine early survivors, one (a neonate) is in severe heart failure 3 weeks postoperatively with a persistent hypokinetic left ventricle but no histologic signs of rejection. No improvement has occurred, nonetheless, following institution of antirejection therapy. He is, therefore, a candidate for retransplantation. Another is still in the early postoperative period.

The other seven patients were discharged 3 to 12 weeks postoperatively and have been followed up for 11 ± 4 months (7 to 17 months). Only one has had two episodes of moderately acute rejection in the first postoperative month which responded well to treatment.

All survivors are in excellent clinical condition and are being treated with cyclosporine and azathioprine alone. The heart was judged normal on clinical, electrocardiographic, x-ray, and echocardiographic evaluation, while histology was normal in the three endomyocardial biopsies obtained thus far 1 year postoperatively. No patient showed systemic hypertension or alteration of kidney functions, but three of the six patients who have undergone histological control showed some tubular and interstitial lesions.

Heart-Lung Transplantation

During the same period, three children (9, 10, and 11 years old) with severe primary or secondary pulmonary hypertension (two cases) or pulmonary disease (one case) underwent heart and lung transplantation. For this purpose we require a strict similarity between the size of the donor and the recipient. Steroids were avoided so as to permit adequate healing of the tracheal sutures. The early postoperative course was much more difficult than for heart transplantation alone. Early complications have been common: such as hemorrhage; bacterial, viral, and mycotic pulmonary infections; and lung rejection. One patient had a severe tracheal stenosis that required complex therapy. Nevertheless, all our three patients are alive and doing well 1, 4, and 6 months postoperatively.

Conclusions

Despite the many remaining long-term uncertainties, heart and heart-lung transplantation are, in some infants and children, a reasonable therapeutic option when there are no suitable alternatives. The early mortality is still high but should be improved by better assessment of pulmonary hypertension in the recipient and a more strict policy of graft selection. Our protocol of treatment in the postoperative period and follow-up seems light enough to allow a good quality of life with a very low incidence of rejection.

References

1. Pennington DG, Sarafian J, Swartz M. Heart transplantation in children. Heart Transplant 1985;4:441–5.
2. Griffith BP, Hardesty RL, Trento A, et al. Heart-lung transplantation: Lessons learned and future hopes. Ann Thorac Surg 1987;43:6–16.
3. Cabrol C, Grandjbakhch I, Pavie A, et al. Cardiac transplantation in France. Current problems. Transplant Proc 1987;19(suppl 5):12–15.
4. Bailey LL, Nehlsen-Canarella SL, Doroshow RW, et al. Cardiac allotransplantation in newborns as therapy for hypoplastic left heart syndrome. N Engl J Med 1986;315:949–51.
5. Lower RR, Shumway NE. Studies on orthotopic homotransplantation of the canine heart. Surg Forum 1960;2:18–20.
6. Bailey LL, Conception W, Shattuck H, Lou H. Method of heart transplantation for treatment of hypoplastic left heart syndrome. J Thorac Cardiovasc Surg 1986;92:1–5.
7. Billingham ME. Cardiac transplant atherosclerosis. Transplant Proc 1987;19:19–25.

Results of Orthotopic Heart Transplantation in Children and Young Adults

F. Siclari, A. Haverich, G. Herrmann, G. Ziemer, C. Kallfelz, and H. G. Borst

Introduction

Since the introduction of cyclosporin A, heart transplantation has gained increasing acceptance. This new therapeutic option, however, has been employed predominantly in adults. This discrepancy is explained not only by the paucity of suitable donors but also on the basis of questionable tolerance of immunosuppression; the unknown nature of its influence on growth; the limited vascular access; and the psychological impact of the procedure and its sequels, just to name some of the problems.[1] As a result, experience worldwide with heart transplantation in children is still limited.[2] An analysis of our patients represents the basis of the experience described in this article.

Patients and Methods

At our institution, from July 1983 to May 1987, 232 orthotopic heart transplantations have been performed in 222 patients aged 9 to 59 years (43.2 mean). Ten patients were under 18 years. In this group, there were nine males and one female. The ages ranged from 9 to 17 years with a mean of 13.9 years. All patients but one were affected by dilatative cardiomyopathy, which was familial in two and idiopathic in the others. The remaining patient had endocardial fibroelastosis. All patients were in New York Heart Association class IV, with seven of them requiring intravenous inotropic and diuretic treatment. There was one early death (10%). This 15-year-old boy had end-stage biventricular failure with renal and hepatic insufficiency. On the day of surgery, he had a low grade fever and a slight increase in his white cell count. A chest roentgenogram showed a localized pneumonia. He died 14 days after the operation from a gram-negative sepsis. All the survivors, to date, are alive and well. Follow-up is complete, with a range from 10 to 38 months and a mean of 23.4 months.

Immunosuppression

The immunosuppressive regimen was essentially the same for children and adults

Table 1

Heart Transplantation in Children: Immunosuppressive
Regimen

	Day				
Early	*0–4*	*8*	*14*	*21*	*28*
Azathioprine (mg/kg)	2.0	1.5	1.4	1.5	1.6
Prednisone (mg/kg)	0.5	0.5	0.5	0.4	0.3
Cyclosporin A (mg/kg)	5.0	8.0	8.0	7.5	7.5
ATG (mg/kg)	1.5	—	—	—	—

	Months		
Late	*3*	*6*	*12*
Azathioprine (mg/kg)	1.4	1.4	1.0
Prednisone (mg/kg)	0.25	0.25	0.13
Cyclosporin A (mg/kg)	7.0	5.25	5.0

ATG, antithymocyte globulin.

and was based on a quadruple combination including cyclosporin A, azathioprine, prednisone, and rabbit antithymocyte globulin (Table 1). Due to the possibility of inducing malignancies, we did not give rabbit antithymocyte globulin to our last three patients. Treatment of rejection was based primarily on routine endomyocardial biopsy performed under local anesthesia. Noninvasive diagnosis of rejection by means of cytoimmunologic monitoring and/or echocardiography has also been carried out, but treatment was given only on the basis of the result of biopsies. In terms of incidence, we have found no difference in rejection between adults and children (3.1 vs. 2.8 episodes in the first 3 months, respectively). This has also been true for the second and third trimesters (1.6 vs. 2.0 and 2.0 vs. 1.8). Renal function was impaired preoperatively in all patients because of low cardiac output. Following transplantation, however, we observed a dramatic improvement in renal function with the levels of serum creatinine decreasing to the normal range. One year postoperatively, creatinine levels stabilized at a high-normal level (100 mol/L) when whole blood levels of cyclosporin A were kept at 500 to 600 ng/ml (Fig. 1).

Complications

Two children developed infection with the cytomegalovirus (pneumonia in one case and generalized in the other), which was successfully treated with cytomegalovirus-hyperimmuneglobulin and antibiotic therapy. One child developed cutaneous herpes simplex, which was successfully treated with acyclovir. The only bacterial infection occurred in the patient who had a pulmonary infiltration preoperatively. This caused septicemia and, eventually, the death of the patient 14 days after the transplantation. On two occasions, in two different patients, severe rejection occurred after treatment of milder episodes of rejection with steroids. In both cases, intravenous rabbit antithymocyte globulin was administered for 3–4 days and led to prompt remission. One patient, early after the operation, developed several episodes of atrial flutter with transient cardiac failure which was treated by means of oral verapamil and, later, cardioversion. All the survivors had a normal postoperative weight gain (Table 2). Cardiac catheterization has been performed in six of the patients 12 months postopera-

HEART TRANSPLANTATION IN CHILDREN
Creatinine levels after transplantation

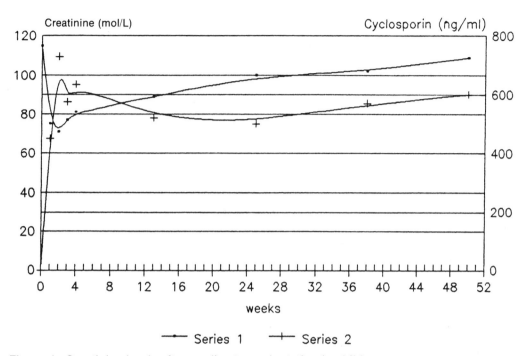

Figure 1. Creatinine levels after cardiac transplantation in children.

tively to assess myocardial function and coronary arterial morphology. No abnormalities of the arterial tree were found, and indices of both right and left ventricular function were normal. Since coronary arterial lesions have been described early after heart transplantation, even in young patients, we have planned a program of yearly angiography.

All children returned to school, and five of them are also active in sports (Table 3).

Discussion

One of the major concerns following heart transplantation in children is the impact of immunosuppression on the growing child and its side effects.[3,4] Among the various side effects of cyclosporin A, nephrotoxicity is the most serious, since damage to tubular cells is well known. Although the renal impairment is fully reversible after acute administration of the drug, very little is known following chronic administration. Atrophic tubular injury, as well as interstitial fibrosis, have been shown to occur chronically, suggesting irreversibility of the process.[5]

Glomerular alterations may also take place secondarily as suggested by the observed increase in creatinine levels. Learning from this experience, we titrate the dosages of cyclosporin A so as to achieve drug levels in the whole blood of 300 ng/ml. If irreversibility of the renal changes is confirmed, we will need to search for an alternative chronic immunosuppressive regimen without cyclosporin A. Steroids also have major drawbacks when administered chronically. Although they are very useful in the treatment of acute rejection, their role as the

Table 2

Heart Transplantation in Children: Postoperative Growth

Patient no.	Follow-up (months)	Height (cm)		Weight (kg)	
		pre	post	pre	post
1	22	153	158	29.7	50.4
2	21	184	188	65.5	72.5
3	17	165	170	44.0	56.4
4	8	178	181	61.0	76.8
5	4	166	168	47.0	56.0

main immunosuppressive agent has been questioned recently.[6] Thus far, in our patients, we have had no problems. On the basis of this experience, we believe that steroids still have a place in the early immunosuppressive therapy. With our regime, we have experienced only two episodes of acute rejection and two instances of viral infection, suggesting that our immunosuppressive approach is satisfactory. How the approach will require adjustment in long-term survivors will depend on if and when tolerance occurs and on how the present regime is tolerated by the patients. All of our survivors have resumed the activities appropriate to their age, while some have even participated in sports, as reported by others.[7,8] Thus, there is increasing evidence that heart transplantation in children is not only life-saving but also allows the survivors to return to their normal and enjoyable activities.

References

1. Allen DH. Is cardiac transplantation in children an experimental procedure? Am J Dis Child 1986;140:1105–06.
2. Pennington DG, Sarafian J, Swartz M. Heart transplantation in children. J Heart Trans 1985;IV;441–445.
3. Hanto DW, Sakamoto K, Purtilo TD. The Epstein virus in the pathogenesis of post transplant lymphoproliferative disorders. Surgery 1981;90:204–213.
4. Dummer JS, Bound LM, Sing G. Epstein-Barr virus induced lymphona in a cardiac transplant recipient. Am J Med 1984;77:179–184.
5. Meyers BD, Ross J, Newton L, et al. Cyclosporin associated chronic nephropathy. N Engl J Med 1984;311:699–705.
6. Katz MR, Barnhart GR, Szenpetery S, et al. Are stroids essential for successful maintenance of immunosuppression in heart transplantation? J Heart Trans 1987;6:293–297.
7. Dunn JM, Cavarocchi NC, Balsara RK, et al. Pediatric heart transplantation at St. Christopher Hospital for children. J Heart Trans 1987;6:344–342.
8. Fricker FJ, Griffith BP, Hardesty Rl, et al. Experience with heart transplantations in children. Pediatrics 1987;79:138–146.

Table 3

Heart Transplantation in Children: Current Functional Status

Functional class	Patient capabilities	No.
I	Attends school, participates in sport, works	5
II	Attends school, no sports	5
III	Unable to attend school	0
IV	Bedridden	0

VI

Cardiopulmonary Bypass and Myocardial Protection

Introduction

G. D. Buckberg, P. L. Julia, D. S. Steed, E. Rosenkranz,
H. Becker, and E. F. Kofsky

Intraoperative myocardial damage is the most perplexing complication of pediatric cardiac surgery, as impaired postoperative cardiac performance remains the principal cause of death after technically successful cardiac repair.[1] Surgical correction of complex congenital heart defects requires several special considerations, including the adequate perfusion of immature hearts during extracorporeal circulation, the frequent need for deep hypothermia and circulatory arrest, and the high incidence of emergency procedures in hearts depleted of energy due to preoperative stress. In the introductory article to this section, we will review our data on these issues in an effort to help clarify the pathophysiology of intraoperative damage during pediatric cardiac surgery and allow for formulation of strategies for safer operations. These will then be amplified in the succeeding articles.

Myocardial Perfusion

The subendocardial muscle of the working right ventricle receives its blood supply only during diastole, and a similar pattern of flow exists when the working ventricle is hypertrophied by generation of systemic pressure. Our previous studies in adult hearts show that potential diastolic subendocardial perfusion becomes reduced by 24% during normothermic total vented bypass. It is lowered by an additional 18% (42% of control) when myocardial temperature is reduced to 28°C. We presume that the relative inability to maintain constant subendocardial perfusion during vented bypass, especially with hypothermia, is caused by distortion of coronary vessels produced by an altered ventricular geometry, whereby the ratio of lumen to wall thickness falls with ventricular decompression. Muscular diastolic relaxation is then less complete with hypothermia.

The critical nature of altering the ventricular/wall ratio on myocardial perfusion becomes magnified in puppy hearts (3–5 kg body weight) where we measured nutritive flow by radioactive microspheres. Hypothermic (28°C) vented bypass raised subendocardial vascular resistance 200% in puppy hearts as opposed to only 80% in adult hearts ($p < 0.05$). These observations were made in normal hearts, where perfusion pressure was kept at 80 mmHg. We expect these findings would be more pronounced if ventricular hypertrophy were present and/or if perfusion pressure were lowered. These data suggest that it may be difficult to maintain adequate myocardial perfusion in hypertrophied infant hearts unless the perfusion pressure is kept at high levels; that increased vascular resistance may impede cardioplegic delivery; that the capacity to ensure postischemic reactive hyperemic flow to provide added oxygen to enhance metabolic recovery after ischemia may be impaired; and that it is imperative to develop effective strategies for cardioplegic delivery to optimize myocardial protection during pediatric cardiac surgery and thus minimize global ischemia during aortic clamping.

Profound Hypothermia in Circulatory Arrest

Repair of complex congenital lesions in small hearts requires a flaccid empty heart devoid of bronchial flow and cannulas. These technical considerations often make it necessary to use profound hypothermia and circulatory arrest. Our experimental studies have compared the three different strategies for maintenance of pH which can be used during clinical cooling and rewarming. Puppy hearts were subjected to 1 hour of circulatory arrest with the "ideal" blood cardioplegic solution (allowing 4 hours of safe aortic clamping in adult hearts).[2]

These strategies were followed first to keep pH and pCO_2 "normal" at 7.4 and 40 mmHg at all temperatures as occurs in hibernating warm-blooded (euthermic) mammals. This is the "constant pH strategy" or $\Delta pH/°C = 0.00$. The second is to match the changes in acidity or alkalinity seen in cold-blooded (ectothermic) mammals that raise pH and reduce pCO_2 as temperature falls to maintain a constant net charge on proteins.[3] This is the so-called stat or neutral strategy ($\Delta pH/°C = 0.017$). The third is to raise the pH to the most alkaline range of ectotherms—the so-called alkaline strategy ($\Delta pH/°C = 0.33$).

Our initial studies[4] compared the alkaline and constant pH strategies at 28°C and showed that the alkaline strategy allowed

better myocardial performance, more effective oxidative and lactate metabolism, and more subendocardial perfusion than was possible at pH 7.40. These findings explain the clinical observations of reduced cardiac output, acidosis, and ventricular fibrillation that occur during surface cooling at 28°C when pH is kept "normal".

Our subsequent studies compared the "stat" (neutral) to the alkaline strategy during surface and perfusion hypothermia and circulatory arrest.[5,6] Reduction of pCO_2 to 10 mmHg while following the alkaline strategy during surface cooling ensured better cerebral blood flow (brain stem, cerebrum, cerebellum) than keeping pH at 40 mmHg (25% vs. 75% reduced flow, $p < 0.05$),[6] and keeping the pH meter reading at 7.4 (α stat). The neutral pH (α stat) policy failed to avoid profound depression in coronary or cerebral blood flow, or ventricular fibrillation, as temperature was lowered below 24°C during surface cooling, or repeated defibrillations during rewarming after perfusion hypothermia. Conversely, the alkaline strategy provided the best results, with excellent maintenance of cardiac output and organ perfusion during surface cooling to 22°C. It prevented lactate acidosis, allowed spontaneous return of sinus rhythm after unclamping, and assured complete recovery of cardiac performance after discontinuation of bypass (vs. 50% and 65% depression after perfusion and surface cooling using the neutral pH (α stat) strategy.[5,6]

These findings suggest that failure of cardiac recovery after the clinical counterpart of this experiment may be avoided by adjusting pH more appropriately before and after circulatory arrest. We suspect that the alkaline strategy delays build-up of acid metabolites when extracorporeal circulation is stopped and produces an effect similar to that of hyperventilation before breath-holding, which increases tolerance to a given period of hypoxia.

These findings suggest that constraining pH to 7.4 (corrected or uncorrected) during hypothermia causes a degree of myocardial damage and "limitation" of myocardial protection. This is avoidable by adjustment of the pH during cooling and rewarming and must be sought in humans, as our findings may have major implications in the routine management of hypothermia during all cardiac operations.

Energy Depletion

The normal newborn heart is more tolerant to hypoxia than the adult heart because of its higher glycogen content and better production of anaerobic energy.[7] Our recent studies have documented the increased tolerance of immature hearts (3–5 kg puppies) to 45 minutes of normothermic global ischemia, a period which produces profound damage to adult hearts. All puppies survived, and left ventricular function returned to 80% of normal. In contrast, 3 of 10 adult dogs died of low output syndrome, and the index of stroke work returned to only 80% of control in survivors (Fig. 1). These findings suggest that more severe is-

chemic models must be sought to test strategies for myocardial protection in infant hearts.

Our metabolic studies show that infant hearts produce more lactate (99 vs. 42 μmol/L) than adult hearts but have comparable levels of glycogen before and during ischemia. The findings suggest that anaerobic glycolysis alone was not responsible for reduced susceptibility to damage. Analysis of tissue amino acids showed that puppy hearts contained more preischemic glutamate (23 vs. 14 μmol, $p < 0.05$), utilized (Figs. 2a and b) more glutamate during ischemia (15 vs. 9 μmol), and demonstrated evidence of substrate level phosphorylation. Production of alanine (19 vs. 6 μmol) and accumulation of succinate (19 vs. 8 μmol) were higher. These observations suggest that amino acid metabolism provides an important source of anaerobic energy to increase the resistance of neonatal hearts to ischemia. They may have implications in the design of cardioprotective solutions for neonatal hearts. Conceivably, depletion of amino acids could be replenished by preoperative intravenous infusions as these in-

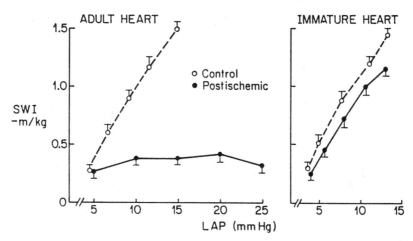

Figure 1. Left ventricular (LV) performance before and after 45 minutes of 37°C global ischemia in adult and immature hearts. See text for description. SWI, stroke work index.

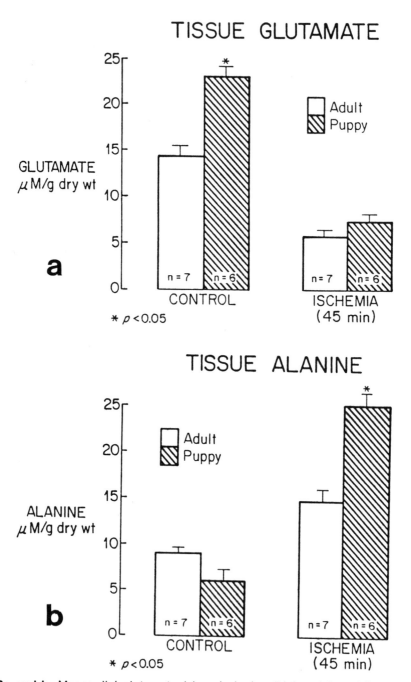

Figures 2a and b. Myocardial glutamate (a) and alanine (b) in adult and immature hearts before and after 45 minutes of 37°C global ischemia. See text for description.

fants are transported to the catheterization laboratory and operating room for diagnosis and correction of congenital defects.

Infants with severe cyanosis and frequent bouts of cardiopulmonary arrest are particularly vulnerable to intraoperative damage, and the aforementioned defense mechanisms may be unavailable to them.

Blood cardioplegia may be particularly well-suited for use in infant hearts, because it prevents further energy loss when it is administered cold during aortic clamping. It also avoids reperfusion damage when it is given as a warm reperfusate before unclamping.[8] Induction of blood cardioplegia in energy-depleted hearts is, in reality, the first phase of reperfusion so that the warm induction of blood cardioplegia may be used as a method of "active resuscitation".

Our previous studies document that adult hearts subjected to 2 hours of normothermic global ischemia can undergo an additional 2 hours of aortic clamping with multidose cold blood cardioplegia. There is then 90% recovery of left ventricular stroke work index if cardioplegia is induced with warm substrate energy aspartate/glutamate blood cardioplegia.[9] Conversely, cold cardioplegia without amino acid supplementation resulted in only 33% of recovery of left ventricular performance after unclamping. We have employed these principles of supplementation of amino acids using warm induction and warm reperfusion in adults with cardiogenic shock at high risk, and have observed substantially improved results over our previous techniques of cold blood cardioplegia alone.[10]

These findings suggest that the principles of supplementation of amino acids and warm cardioplegic induction may be beneficial also to energy-depleted hearts during pediatric cardiac surgery. It is hoped that better understanding of the principles of myocardial protection described herein, which are applicable directly to pediatric cardiac surgical patients, will improve surgical results and define the role of surgical intervention in the natural history of congenital heart disease.

References

1. Kirklin JK, Blackstone EH, Kirklin JW, et al. Intracardiac surgery in infants under 3 months: Predictors of postoperative in-hospital cardiac death. Am J Cardiol 1981; 48:507–12.
2. Robertson JM, Vinten-Johansen J, Buckberg GS, et al. Prolonged safe aortic clamping (4 hours) with cold glutamate enriched blood cardioplegia. Circulation 1981;64(suppl 4):147(abstr).
3. Rahn H, Reeves RB, Howell BJ. Hydrogen ion regulation, temperature, and evolution. Am Rev Respir Dis 1975;112:165–72.
4. McConnell DH, White F, Nelson RL, et al. Importance of alkalosis in maintenance of "ideal" blood pH during hypothermia. Surg Forum 1975;26:263–5.
5. Buckberg GD, Becker H, Vinten-Johansen J, et al. Myocardial function resulting from varying acid-base management during and following deep surface and perfusion hypothermia and circulatory arrest. In: Rahn H, Prakash O (eds), Acid-Base Regulation and Body Temperature. Boston, Martinus Nijhoff, 1985, pp 135–60.
6. Becker H, Vinten-Johansen J, Buckberg GD, et al. Myocardial damage caused by keeping pH 7.40 during systemic deep hypothermia. J Thorac Cardiovasc Surg 1981;82:810–20.
7. Jarmakani JM, Nagatomo T, Nakazama M, Langer GA. Effect of hypoxia on mechanical function in the neonatal mammalian heart. Am J Physiol 1978;235:469–74.
8. Buckberg GD. Strategies and logic of cardioplegic delivery to prevent, avoid, and reverse ischemic and reperfusion damage. J Thorac Cardiovasc Surg 1987;93:127–39.
9. Rosenkranz ER, Okamoto F, Buckberg GD, et al. Safety of prolonged aortic clamping with blood cardioplegia. III. Aspartate enrichment of glutamate blood cardioplegia in energy depleted hearts after ischemic and reperfusion injury. J Thorac Cardiovasc Surg 1986; 1,3:428–35.
10. Rosenkranz ER, Buckberg GD, Mulder DG, Laks H. Warm induction of cardioplegia with glutamate-enriched blood in coronary patients with cardiogenic shock who are dependent on inotropic drugs and intra-aortic balloon support: Initial experience and operative strategy. J Thorac Cardiovasc Surg 1983;86:507–18.

Perfusion Primes, Flow Rates, and Perfusion Pressures for Cardiopulmonary Bypass in Pediatric Practice

J. J. Amato, J. V. Cotroneo, R. J. Galdieri, E. Heldmann, F. E. Stark, J. Bushong, and C. Lepeniotis

Introduction

It is well recognized that pediatric perfusion techniques differ from adult methods in all considerations. The historical full blood prime has been minimized in the past because hemodilution was not only recognized as beneficial by decreasing viscosity, vasoconstriction, and pulmonary and coagulation complications, but was also known to increase tissue perfusion, blood flow, and renal function. While the major objection to the use of blood had come from Jehovah's Witnesses, the generalized fear of infectious contamination of blood, especially with the human immunodeficiency virus, is a reality.[1] Although blood samples can be screened for some viruses (Table 1), there is now more cause for consideration of "the bloodless prime." While presently accepted in adults, limiting the use of blood in the prime for children was reported by Scott and Subramanian[2] in 1979. In 1981[3] and 1984,[4] a total bloodless prime was used. Preoperative considerations were normal or elevated hemoglobin, a median weight of 10 kg (range 4.7 to 19.3), and minimal preoperative laboratory blood work.

Intraoperative techniques included meticulous placement of lines with minimal blood loss, reduced time of cardiopulmonary bypass by surface cooling, moderate hypothermia with reduced bypass or deep hypothermia with circulatory arrest to reduce trauma to the red blood cells, reduction of prime by decreasing tubing length and diameter, no filtration and the use of a device for saving red-cells. Postoperative considerations were reduction of postoperative laboratory tests and early iron therapy. Necessary transfusions were given only if the hematocrit dropped below 13 on cardiopulmonary bypass, 20 postoperatively, or if acidosis occurred. While this methodology can be used in many cases, most of the children reported weighed above 8 kg with few children in the categories of lower weight.

Table 1

Blood Bank Test for Organisms Transmitted by Transfusion of Blood and Blood Products

Tests	Organisms
+	Hepatitis B virus
+	Hepatitis, non-A, non-B virus(es)
0	Hepatitis delta virus
+	Cytomegalovirus
0	Epstein-Barr virus
+	Syphilis spirochete (*Treponema pallidum*)
0	Colorado tick fever virus
0	Malaria parasite (Plasmodium)
0	*Trypanosoma cruzi* (Chagas' disease)
0	*Rickettsia rickettsii* (Rocky Mountain Spotted Fever)
0	Babesia
+	Human immunodeficiency virus

Clinical Experience

Since most of the patients undergoing operation at the Children's Hospital of New Jersey are neonates and children weighing less than 10 kg, our technique of necessity reflects the minimal use of blood. In 1987, 39% of our patients were below 10 kg, while, from January to June of 1988, 57% were below 10 kg, reflecting more complex surgery being performed earlier. The alternative to the bloodless prime is the use of directed blood donations. Concerned parents have forced the concept of donation by relatives and friends. We use a lactated Ringer's solution supplemented with albumin and packed red blood cells which are heparinized, recalcified, and buffered. Relative concentrations of each are based on the calculation of the hematocrit, blood volume, and circulating volume on bypass. We utilize a total prime of 800 cc in an infant weighing 10 kg or less, with the addition of up to 200 cc of volume as size approaches 20 kg. We prefer to use arterial filters and also maintain the hematocrit at 20 to 25 with heavy

reliance on the use of hemofiltration and cell saving at the end of bypass. The hematocrit is restored postoperatively to 30 to 35 and even higher in the neonate. We have not used low molecular weight dextran but have used Hetastarch in certain cases. The newer fluorocarbons are used experimentally in the United States, and we understand that denatured gelatins are currently being used primarily in Europe.

Flow rates in children are predicated on the degree of hypothermia used. According to Kirklin and Barratt-Boyes[5] perfusion is related to the oxygen consumption and, accordingly, with each 10°C decrease in temperature the oxygen consumption is decreased approximately by 50%. We calculate the estimated flow rates utilizing a range of 1.8 to 2.4 L/min/m^2 for normothermic perfusion. In the case of neonates, we correlate this measurement with the calculation of 100 ml/kg/min. Below 22°C we will perfuse at 0.5 liters/min/m^2 for a period of 45 minutes. The sizes of cannulas are standard, and use of two venous cannulas is normal practice with us. Presently, we utilize the DLP straight plastic arterial cannula or the curved Argyle catheter. For venous cannulation, the U.S.C.I. lighthouse tip or the Pacifico curved metal-tipped cannulas are used.

The total adequacy of perfusion is monitored by pH, venous pO$_2$, blood pressure, urine output, and so on. While circulatory arrest is not within the scope of this article, we firmly adhere to the concept taught by Kirklin that the most powerful weapon for myocardial protection in the young child is deep hypothermia. So, the younger the patient, the less the added protection from cardioplegia. We have been experimenting with a pediatric cooling device which we designed in 1983 and are currently testing (Fig. 1). The use of this device placed around the myocardium maintains a mean myocardial temperature from 7 to 12°C between cardioplegic dosages, thus further protecting the myocardium. While these results are prelim-

TOPICAL COOLING DEVICE
SIZE COMPARISON
(Actual Size)

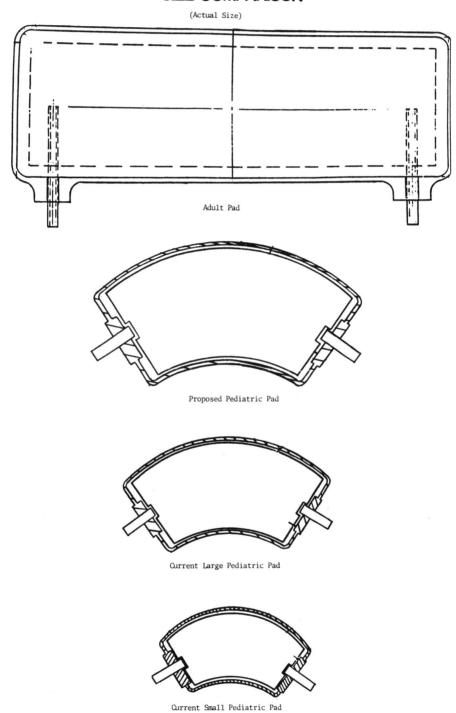

Adult Pad

Proposed Pediatric Pad

Current Large Pediatric Pad

Current Small Pediatric Pad

Figure 1. The Amato/Cobe topical cooling device currently being tested for children.

inary, we are encouraged in its use even in the newborn cardiac patient.

Perfusion pressures are usually measured during cardiopulmonary bypass with one long arterial line passed centrally either through the radial artery or the posterior tibial artery. While the use of the femoral artery has been advocated,[6] we would caution its use because of potential complications such as thrombosis or hematomas, which can create an environment of litigation among the other obvious problems of femoral exploration and re-establishment of flow. Central venous pressure is usually measured by two centrally placed venous catheters. It is currently our policy to attempt to introduce one or two long venous catheters into the left atrium to record left-sided pressures. These catheters are passed through either an existing patent oval foramen or a small stab in the atrial septum.

The arterial pressure is maintained at between 40 to 50 mmHg and, even at the inception of perfusion, should not drop lower than 30 mmHg. We take care to verify that any arterio-venous shunts, whether artificially placed (central or Blalock-Taussig shunts) or naturally occurring (a patent arterial duct), are occluded before bypass. If high venous pressures are recorded, one must verify that the lower venous cannula is not in some way occluded, or compressed in the leg, or that the catheter in the arm is not stretched with the opening of the chest by the retractor. When doubtful, the inadequacy of perfusion can be judged by suffusion of the head or development of acidosis while on bypass. At the conclusion of bypass, the suture at the site of arterial cannulation is always reinforced with a full thickness suture to prevent the occurrence of an aortic aneurysm. Currently, we attempt to perform the majority of our cases with low flow cardiopulmonary bypass but will not hesitate to convert to circulatory arrest for periods of 30 to 60 minutes whenever the anatomy requires a clear surgical field. Whatever the methods used by the surgeon, meticulous attention to each step is important for the proper conduct of perfusion in the child.

References

1. Baldwin S, Stagno S, Whitley R. Transfusion-associated viral infections. Curr Probl Pediatr 1987;17:395–443.
2. Scott CW, Subramanian S. Limited prime pediatric perfusion. J Extra-corporeal Technol 1980;12:26–8.
3. Levinsky L, Srinivasan V, Choh JH, et al. Intracardiac surgery in children of Jehovah's Witnesses. Johns Hopkins Med J 1981; 148:196–8.
4. Kawaguchi A, Bergsland J, Subramanian S. Total bloodless open heart surgery in the pediatric age group. Circulation 1984;70(suppl 1):30–7.
5. Kirklin JW, Barratt-Boyes BG. Hypothermia and total circulatory arrest. In: Cardiac Surgery. New York, John Wiley & Sons, 1986, pp 30–42.
6. Kirklin JW, Barratt-Boyes BG. Clinical methodology of cardiopulmonary bypass. In: Cardiac Surgery. New York, John Wiley & Sons, 1986, pp 59–75.

Total Hemodilution in Children During Open Heart Surgery

J. M. Brito Perez, F. Villagra, J. P. Leon, R. Gomez, P. Diaz,
J. I. Diez, M. Salazar, S. L. Checa, P. A. Sanchez, A. Alonso,
and D. Vellibre

Introduction

Systematic total hemodilution is routinely employed during cardiac surgery in adults. It is seldom used in children, its use being usually reserved for some cases of Jehovah's witnesses.[1]

Material and Methods

From January 1986 to May 1988, 511 children have undergone operation with the aid of extracorporeal circulation. For the purposes of analysis of preoperative, intraoperative, and postoperative factors, these patients have been divided into four groups.

The first and second groups were made up of 316 patients weighing greater than 12 kg. Blood was added in the priming of the pump in 114 patients who served as a control group. The remaining 202 patients underwent bypass using total hemodilution. The third and fourth groups were composed of patients who all weighed less than 12 kg. A control group of 175 of these patients had unrestricted use of blood during the priming procedure. The remaining 20 patients underwent bypass by means of partial hemodilution, and the blood used in the priming was restricted to no more than 25% of its total volume.

The techniques used during extracorporeal circulation are shown in Tables 1 and 2. Priming of the extracorporeal circuit was reduced to the minimum deemed advisable, particularly in the group of patients undergoing priming by means of total hemodilution. In these patients, no blood was used in the priming, neither to refill nor during transfer of all the priming volume to the patient at the end of extracorporeal circulation. Once bypass was concluded, a normal circulating volume was maintained with the use of crystalloids or gelatin colloidal solutions, at a maximum dosage of 20 centiliters per kilogram of body weight. Mannitol (0.5–1 g/kg body weight) was routinely employed just prior to the conclusion of bypass in all the groups. We established certain minimal levels of the hematocrit as a safety measure. The values were 12% during bypass, 20% just after the end of the extracorporeal circulation, and 28% in the immediate postoperative period.

Table 1

Techniques of Extracorporeal Circulation

	With blood	With hemodilution
Reduced priming	yes	yes, extremely reduced
Priming	blood (1 unit) + Ringer	Ringer
Refilling	Ringer + ACD blood	Ringer
Priming transfer to the patients	no	yes
Plasma expanders post-ECC	ACD blood	none—gellatin colloids

ECC, extracorporeal circulation.

Table 2

Techniques of Extracorporeal Circulation: Children <12 kg Body Weight

	With blood	With partial hemodilution
Priming reduced	yes	yes, extremely reduced
Priming	blood (1 unit) (45%)	<25% blood
	Ringer	>75% Ringer
Refilling	50% blood	<25% blood
	50% Ringer	>75% Ringer
Plasma expanders post-ECC	blood	none or gellatin-colloids

ECC, extracorporeal circulation.

Table 3

Homogeneity of the Main Groups

Parameters	Priming with blood	With hemodilution	p
Age (years)	6.2 ± 3	4.7 ± 2	NS
Body weight (kg)	22.2 ± 10	15.9 ± 4	NS
Preop HCT (%)	41.5 ± 4	42.8 ± 6	NS
Preop creatinine (mg/dL)	0.54 ± 0.1	0.59 ± 0.1	NS
Preop proteins (g/dL)	6.8 ± 0.6	6.5 ± 1.2	NS
Prothrombin ACT (%)	87 ± 15	89 ± 18	NS
Cephaline	36 ± 3	35 ± 4	NS
Platelets ($\times 10^3$)	223 ± 81	245 ± 98	NS
Fibrinogen (mg/dL)	312 ± 40	322 ± 70	NS
Extracorporeal circulation (min)	50 ± 16	50 ± 26	NS
Aortic cross-clamping (min)	30 ± 16	32 ± 24	NS
Rectal temperature (° C)	31 ± 2	31 ± 2	NS
Perfusion pressure (mmHg)	43 ± 13	40 ± 11	NS
ECC flow (L/min/m²)	2 ± 0.3	2 ± 0.2	NS

NS, not significant (p > 0.05). HCT, hematocrit; ACT, activation; ECC, extracorporeal circulation.

The balance of fluids was calculated according to the initial volume needed for priming, the volume needed for refilling, the amount of absorbed cardioplegic solution, and the volumes of liquids and/or blood administered. On the output side, we noted any diuresis or hemorrhage, and calculated the amount of the priming volume which was not transferred to the patient. These volumes were all expressed in cc/kg body weight. Table 3 reflects the homogeneity of values for the children weighing more than 12 kg, showing the most relevant data together with their mean values and their standard deviations. There was no statistically significant difference ($p > 0.05$), whether these patients underwent bypass using a blood prime or hemodilution.

Results

Neither morbidity nor mortality were directly related to the use of hemodilution. Neurological problems were absent.

Sixty percent of the 202 patients undergoing total hemodilution received blood transfusions in the postoperative period, while the other 40% did not require any blood, always maintaining a hematocrit above 28%. The mean weight of those children requiring blood transfusion (14.2 ± 1.5 kg) was significantly lower ($p < 0.05$) than those in whom blood was unnecessary (19.7 ± 6.4 kg). The arterial pH, base excess, venous oxygen tension, and heart rates are shown in Table 4. Levels of creatinine in the blood and volumes of diuresis are represented in Figure 1. The fluid balance is represented in Figure 2, and the hematocrit values are shown in Table 5. The results of coagulation tests are represented in Figure 3.

The postoperative drainage was 9 ± 4 cc/kg body weight in the heavier patients having blood priming and 13 ± 9 cc/kg body weight in those in the heavier group undergoing total hemodilution ($p > 0.05$).

The mean cost per patient is detailed in Table 6. As may be seen, use of blood in our institution increases the cost more than sixfold.

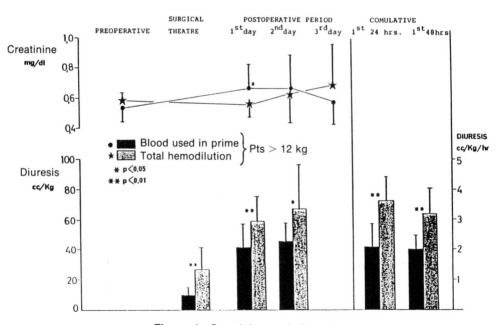

Figure 1. Creatinine and diuresis.

Table 4
Tissue Oxygenation

	Beginning ECC	End ECC	1st Postop day	2nd Postop day
Arterial pH (37° C)				
Blood	7.4 ± 0.08	7.4 ± 0.07	7.4 ± 0.08	7.4 ± 0.3
Hemodilution	7.4 ± 0.1	7.4 ± 0.09	7.4 ± 0.1	7.4 ± 0.3
Base excess				
Blood	1.7 ± 3	1.6 ± 4	−1.5 ± 3	1.5 ± 1
Hemodilution	0.8 ± 4	1.5 ± 3	0.37 ± 4	1.1 ± 2
Venous pO_2 (37) mmHg				
Blood		34.7 ± 8		
Hemodilution		42.7 ± 13		
Heart rate (beats/min)				
Blood			115 ± 15	119 ± 13
Hemodilution			131 ± 22	123 ± 17

ECC, extracorporeal circulation.

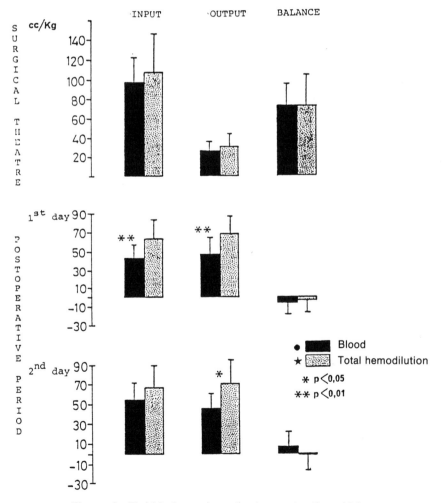

Figure 2. Fluid balance in patients greater than 12 kg.

Table 5

Hematocrit

	Blood	Hemodilution
Preoperative	41.5 ± 4	42.8 ± 6
Beginning of ECC	29 ± 5	22 ± 5
End of ECC	28 ± 4	21 ± 4
1st postop day	41 ± 3	32 ± 5
2nd postop day	39 ± 3	31 ± 5
3rd postop day	37 ± 3	31 ± 5
6th postop day	35 ± 3	33 ± 3
Blood transfused postoperatively (cc/kg)	25 ± 11	10 ± 7[a]

[a] Packed red cells.
ECC, extracorporeal circulation.

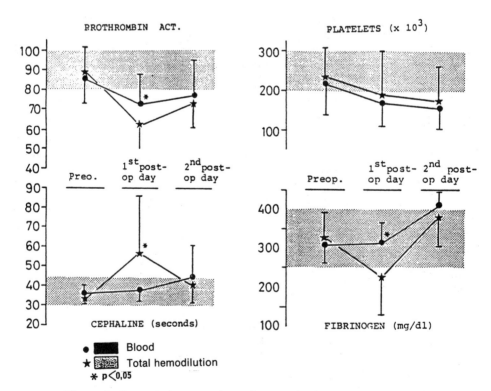

Figure 3. Coagulation tests in patients weighing more than 12 kg.

Table 6

Mean Cost per Patient

Concept	Blood	Hemodilut
Blood and/or hematic products	19.678 PTAS	3.714 PTAS
Prolonged hospitalization due to blood absence in blood bank	3.600	—
	23.278 PTAS	3.714 PTAS

PTAS, pesetas.

Discussion

The systematic practice of total hemodilution in children has not been recommended because of fears of inadequate tissue oxygenation,[2] excessive retention of fluid, and increases in postoperative hemorrhage.[3] Previous prospective studies of our group[4,5] show that systematic total hemodilution is feasible (and even advisable) in children weighing over 12 kg. Total hemodilution decreases the viscosity of the blood and increases the cardiac output, thus compensating for the diminished oxygen content per blood unit. Total hemodilution partially compensates for some of the theoretical disadvantages of hypothermia, such as the increase in blood viscosity and the decrease of regional flow.[1,6] Total hemodilution is also made possible by the use of oxygenators and appropriately tailored circuits which require low volumes of priming.

A hematocrit of 28% has usually been considered as the lowest safe limit during the postoperative period following cardiac surgery in children. Our own experience, and that of others, however, shows that a hematocrit of less than 23% may be equally safe in certain cases.[1,4,5–7]

Reduction in the cost of operation per patient and a decrease in the complications of transfusion, notably hepatitis,[8] represent further great advantages in the use of total hemodilution.

Our study shows, therefore, that total hemodilution is feasible and even advisable

in children weighing over 12 kg. In this group of patients, there was no hypoxemia, acidosis, or any other significant complications, and in addition, there was a lesser degree of hemolysis. Total hemodilution improved renal function and there was no greater retention of fluid than in the group of patients used as a control. Total hemodilution is also economically attractive and avoids complications of transfusion.

In children weighing under 12 kg, however, retention of fluid remains a significant problem.[7,9] Low weight, inadequate diuresis, longer times of extracorporeal circulation, and disproportion in the volume needed for priming compared with the body weight may explain this difference. Restriction in the use of blood, however, is associated with lesser hemolysis and, perhaps, fewer complications of transfusion.

Total hemodilution for children weighing more than 12 kg, therefore, is now employed routinely in our unit. Systematic total hemodilution in children under 12 kg deserves further investigation.

References

1. Henling CE, Carmichael MJ, Keats AS, Cooley DA. Cardiac operation for congenital heart disease in children of Jehovah's Witnesses. J Thorac Cardiovasc Surg 1985;89:914–20.
2. Kawamura M, Minamikawa O, Yokochi H, et al. Safe limit of hemodilution in cardiopulmonary bypass. Comparative analysis between cyanotic and acyanotic congenital heart disease. Jpn J Surg 1980;10:206–11.

3. Eernise JG, Brand A, van Driel OJR, Dirksen T. Prevention of bleeding tendency after open-heart surgery for tetralogy of Fallot. Scand J Thorac Cardiovasc Surg 1977;11:105–9.

4. Villagra F, de Leon JP, Vellibre D, et al. Hemodilucion total en ninos en la cirurgia correctora de las cardiopatias congenitas (I). Estudio prospectivo en ninos de peso superior a 12 kg. Rev Esp Cardiol 1987;40:28–34.

5. Villagra F, de Leon JP, Vellibre D, et al. Hemodilucion total en ninos en la cirugia correctora de las cardiopatias congenitas (II). Estudio prospectivo en ninos de peso superior a 12 kg. Rev Esp Cardiol 1987;40:35–40.

6. Utley JR, Wachtel C, Cain RB, et al. Effects of hypothermia, hemodilution and pump oxygenator on organ water content, blood flow and oxygen delivery and renal function. Ann Thorac Surg 1981;31:121–33.

7. Utley JR, Stephens DB. Fluid balance during cardiopulmonary bypass. In: Utley JR (ed), Pathophysiology and Techniques of Cardiopulmonary Bypass, vol. II. Baltimore, Williams & Wilkins, 1982, pp 23–35.

8. Barcena R, Suarez E, Gil Grande L, et al. Estudio propectivo de hepatitis postransfusionales no A no B: incidencias y factores de riesgo. Gastroenterol Hepatol 1982;6:571–5.

9. Aubert J, Pannetier A, Alfonsi R, Jarry JM. Safe bypass time in infants under three months of age. In: Parenzan L, Crupi G, Graham D (eds), Congenital Heart Disease in the First Three Months of Life. Medical and Surgical Aspects. Bologna, Patron Editore, 1981, pp 293–300.

Circulatory Arrest Versus Cardiopulmonary Bypass

J. L. Monro

Introduction

For more than 30 years, cardiopulmonary bypass has been the standard method of supplying the oxygen requirements of the body when open heart surgery is being performed. As cooling reduces oxygen consumption, it is usual to combine moderate hypothermia to about 28°C (Fig. 1a), which allows reduction in flow and short periods of arrest for up to 10 minutes.[1] It is an excellent technique and, with improvements, particularly in design of oxygenators, has become very safe. It is the technique of choice in older children. If the temperature is further reduced, intermittent circulatory arrest or low flow perfusion can be used to improve the operating conditions.

In infants, however, venous cannulas and blood in the heart can impair the operating conditions, and longer bypass times are less well tolerated. Twenty years ago, the results of open heart surgery in the first year of life were generally not good, and palliation rather than correction was often recommended. Reports from Kyoto University,[2] however, regarding the use of surface cooling and total circulatory arrest at 20°C and bypass rewarming achieved encouraging results. This technique was popularized by

Barratt-Boyes[3] whose results were better than those previously reported. Subsequently, many surgeons started to use this method.

The technique, nonetheless, is time-consuming (Fig. 1b). Surface cooling (which is usually achieved by placing ice bags on the patients) is quicker in small, lean babies. The cooling period can be lessened by the use of a water bath and vasodilator drugs. At about 28°C, the chest is opened and a single arterial and venous cannula inserted. The patient is rapidly cooled on bypass to a nasopharyngeal temperature of about 18°C. Bypass is stopped, the aorta is cross-clamped, and the heart allowed to drain. Cardioplegic fluid is infused through the ascending aorta and sucked from the right atrium.

During the period of arrest, with removal of the venous cannula, an excellent view is obtained of the inside of the heart which is still and free from blood. This allows ideal conditions for the repair, following which, with reinsertion of the venous cannula, the patient is rewarmed on bypass.

In order to shorten the rather time-consuming process of surface cooling, core cooling can be used (Fig. 1c).[4] The chest is opened at normal temperature and aortic and venous cannulas inserted with minimal

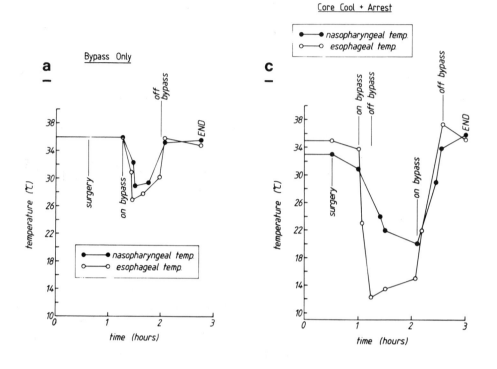

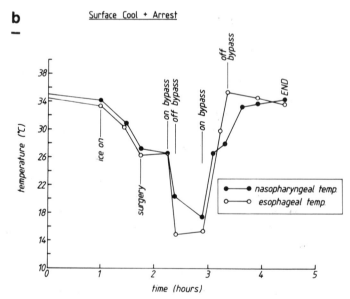

Figure 1. The temperature/time graphs of three infants undergoing correction of tetralogy of Fallot are shown, (a) in a 7-month-old infant simple cardiopulmonary bypass with moderate cooling is used; (b) surface cooling and total circulatory arrest with bypass rewarming is used in a 2-month-old infant; (c) core cooling, total circulatory arrest, and bypass rewarming was used in this 8-month-old infant. It can be seen that the technique of surface cooling is considerably more time-consuming, but total bypass times were 45, 33, and 52 minutes in patients a, b, and c, respectively.

disturbance. Cooling should probably take at least 20 minutes, as the nasopharyngeal temperature lags more behind the esophageal temperature than with surface cooling. Core cooling, therefore, is probably not so even or safe.[3] Once arrest is achieved, the process is the same as with surface cooling. It is clear when comparing these techniques that bypass alone is the most expedient. The introduction of the improved venous cannulas designed by Pacifico allows adequate exposure in most infants. In the smallest infants, however, the excellent operating conditions achieved with total circulatory arrest and removal of the venous cannula contribute greatly to the results achieved, particularly in those with complex conditions. Whether total circulatory arrest is achieved by core cooling or surface cooling is a matter of decision for the individual surgeon. Total bypass times, nonetheless, are considerably shorter with surface cooling, which, though more time-consuming, over all is probably safer.

The main concern about the use of total circulatory arrest is whether it causes brain damage. The evidence is confusing. It is known that oxygen consumption falls with temperature, but there is still considerable doubt as to what is a safe arrest period at a given temperature.[5] Certainly 30 minutes, and probably 40 minutes, are safe at 18°C. In practice, this has often been exceeded, particularly in the early years.[3] In studying 72 patients of the original group undergoing surgery by Barratt-Boyes, Clarkson[6] found a mean intelligence quotient of 92.9 at age 22 to 84 months, and concluded that the level of intelligence bore no relationship to the duration of circulatory arrest or other aspects of surgical technique.

Dickinson and Sambrooks[7] tested 38 patients 22–72 months following circulatory arrest after core cooling. They found a mean quotient of 99.2 but found no correlation between intelligence and age or weight at operation or the duration of circulatory arrest. They suggested a safe period of up to 60 minutes. Wells[8] and his colleagues tested 31 patients who survived operation at a mean age of 15 months using total circulatory arrest. Their mean quotient was 91 when tested between 3.5 and 5.5 years postoperatively at a mean age of 68 months. They compared this with a group of 19 patients having similar operations under cardiopulmonary bypass and with the siblings of each group, all of whom had somewhat higher levels of intelligence. Although the groups are small, and other factors could affect the differences, their work sounded a cautionary note. Many people have now stopped using circulatory arrest or else have reduced their time of arrest.

Clinical Experience

During the last 10 years, I have operated on 280 consecutive infants using surface cooling and total circulatory arrest, of whom 13.9% died within a month of operation. The mean period of arrest was 49 minutes, the mean weight 4.6 kg, and 34 patients weighed less than 3 kg. There were 55 neonates of whom 17 (32.3%) died within 1 month of operation. No death in this group was considered to be directly attributable to the technique. Rather, there would have been a higher mortality without it. Twelve patients had fits postoperatively, of whom three could be accounted for by postoperative hypoxic events. Three further patients who did not have fits have permanent cerebral damage attributable to postoperative hypoxic events. Four other patients are developmentally slow.

"Fitting" has been described as a complication occurring after total circulatory arrest in from 5 to 10% of patients.[5] As in our patients, there is usually no detectable long-term deficit. It is difficult to know how much preoperative neurological damage was present in these patients, many of whom were very acidotic or deeply cyanosed prior to surgery.

The risk of cerebral damage increases with the duration of arrest, and 54 of my

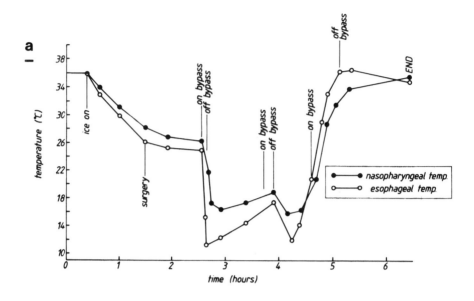

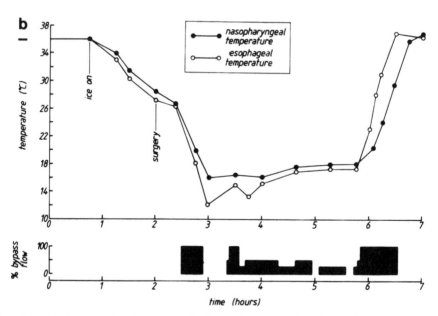

Figure 2. (a) This temperature/time graph shows two periods of circulatory arrest used for correction of a common arterial trunk with separate origins of the pulmonary arteries and interruption of the aortic arch between the left subclavian and common carotid arteries in a 2.3 kg neonate. The total bypass time was 54 minutes, with 16 minutes of recirculation between arrest periods of 54 and 40 minutes; (b) combination of circulatory arrest and low flow bypass have been used in this 3.3 kg infant undergoing anatomical correction of a double outlet right ventricle with subpulmonary ventricular septal defect (Taussig-Bing malformation).

patients (19.3%) had arrest periods of 60 minutes or more, of whom 45 (83.3%) survived. We have tested intelligence in 16 patients more than 5 years after surgery as infants with circulatory arrest for 60 minutes or more. The mean quotient was 98.1 and seemed to bear no relation to the duration of arrest. The mean age at operation of these 16 patients was 6.2 months. This is less than the 15 months of the group studied by Wells et al.[8] It may well be that these long periods of total circulatory arrest are tolerated better at a younger age. Since the report of Wells et al.,[8] however, we have tried to keep the arrest time nearer to 40 minutes.

Where a longer period is needed for the repair, two episodes of arrest can be used (Fig. 2a). This has been used in ten patients with two early deaths. At least 10 minutes of recirculation between periods of arrest is advisable but, if possible, we try not to use it at all.

For most of our 280 patients, fresh heparinized blood has been used in the bypass prime. More recently, however, we have used blood stored in saline, adenosine, glucose, and mannitol.[9] Short periods of bypass and avoidance of suckers in the open heart also contribute to the low hemolysis rate occurring with the use of circulatory arrest. We transfuse platelets routinely after rewarming, and only eight (2.9%) patients have been returned to the operating room because of problems due to bleeding.

Rather than arguments about circulatory arrest as opposed to bypass, it is likely that a combination of the techniques will provide the best operating conditions without risk of cerebral damage (Fig. 2b). It must be left to each individual surgeon to select which technique or combination is appropriate according to the complexity of the procedure to be performed.

References

1. Kirklin JW, Barratt-Boyes BG. Whole body perfusion during cardiopulmonary bypass. In: Cardiac Surgery. New York, John Wiley & Sons, 1986, pp 44–59.
2. Hikasa Y, Shirotani H, Satomura K, et al. Open heart surgery in infants with the aid of hypothermic anaesthesia. Arch Jpn Chir 1967; 36:495–508.
3. Barratt-Boyes BG, Neutze JM, Seelye ER, Simpson M. Complete correction of cardiovascular malformations in the first year of life. Prog Cardiovasc Dis 1972;15:229–53.
4. Hamilton D, Shackelton J, Rees GJ, Abbott T. Experience with deep hypothermia in infancy using core cooling. In: Barratt-Boyes BG, Neutze JM, Harris EA (eds), Heart Disease in Infancy. Baltimore, Williams and Wilkins, 1973, pp 52–64.
5. Kirklin JW, Barratt-Boyes BG. Hypothermia, circulatory arrest and cardiopulmonary bypass. In: Cardiac Surgery. New York, John Wiley & Sons, 1986, pp 30–43.
6. Clarkson PM, MacArthur BA, Barratt-Boyes BG, et al. Developmental progress following cardiac surgery in infancy using profound hypothermia and circulatory arrest. Circulation 1980;62:855–61.
7. Dickinson DF, Sambrooks JE. Intellectual performance in children after circulatory arrest with profound hypothermia in infancy. Arch Dis Child 1979;54:1–6.
8. Wells FC, Coghill S, Caplan HL, et al. Duration of circulatory arrest does influence the psychological development of children after cardiac operation early in life. J Thorac Cardiovasc Surg 1983;86:823–31.
9. Hogman CF, Akerblom O, Hedlund K, et al. Red cell suspension in SAG M Medium. Vox Sang 1983;45:217–23.

The Effects of Deep Hypothermic Cardiopulmonary Bypass and Total Circulatory Arrest on Cerebral Blood Flow in Infants and Children

W. J. Greeley, R. M. Ungerleider, L. R. Smith, and J. G. Reves

Introduction

Several studies have indicated that autoregulation of pressure and flow of cerebral blood and responses of the cerebral vasculature to arterial carbon dioxide tension are maintained in adults during cardiopulmonary bypass.[1,2] Techniques and management of cardiopulmonary bypass in infants and children, however, involve more extensive alterations in temperature, hemodilution, perfusion pressure, and rates of pump flow, together with periods of total circulatory arrest. In this article, we describe a study designed to examine the effect of deep hypothermic cardiopulmonary bypass with and without periods of total circulatory arrest on cerebral blood flow.

Materials and Methods

Patients

After approval of our institutional review board and informed parental consent, we studied 25 infants and children undergoing repair of congenital heart defects by means of deep hypothermic cardiopulmonary bypass. Their ages ranged from 2 days to 60 months. Fourteen patients underwent repair by means of deep hypothermic cardiopulmonary bypass combined with total circulatory arrest, while a further 11 patients underwent deep hypothermia alone.

Management of Cardiopulmonary Bypass

During cardiopulmonary bypass, nonpulsatile flow through a membrane oxygenator was maintained at the rate of 100 ml/kg/min. The pump oxygenator was primed with lactated Ringers, albumin, mannitol, and packed red blood cells in order to achieve a hematocrit of 20% $\pm$ 2% during the period of bypass. All patients were cooled with the perfusate to conditions of deep hypothermia (18–23°C). The pH was maintained between 7.35 and 7.40, and the tension of carbon dioxide between 35 and

40 mmHg, both uncorrected for temperature.

Cerebral Blood Flow

Cerebral blood flow was measured using clearance of xenon.[3,4] Five determinations were made in both groups at three predefined intervals during surgery: prior to bypass; during cardiopulmonary bypass at three stages (two cold and one rewarmed); and after cardiopulmonary bypass. The determinations of cardiopulmonary bypass for those having hypothermia and arrest were made at stable hypothermic conditions at 18°C before and after the period of circulatory arrest and again when the patients were rewarmed. Equivalent determinations were made at stable hypothermic conditions between 18 and 23°C at 5 and 25 minutes and when the patient was rewarmed in those not having an additional period of arrest. To examine the relationship of mean arterial pressure, tension of carbon dioxide, and hematocrit to cerebral blood flow during deep hypothermia (18–23°C), data from determinations made during bypass were pooled. The conditions were similar, and more observations could be examined. These same relationships were also examined at normothermic cardiopulmonary bypass during rewarming in those patients having hypothermia alone, providing a comparison of variables for deep hypothermic and normothermic bypass. To assess the effect of total circulatory arrest on cerebral blood flow, the group undergoing circulatory arrest was compared to the other patients treated under identical conditions excepting the use of total circulatory arrest.

Paired data for each group were compared for differences by two-tailed, paired t-tests, and variables were analyzed by stepwise linear regression.

Results

Figure 1 shows the parallel relationship of regional cerebral blood flow and nasopharyngeal temperature with time. There was also a highly significant correlation of the parameters during cardiopulmonary bypass ($p = 0.007$). There was a highly significant association between cerebral blood flow and mean arterial pressure during deep hypothermic cardiopulmonary bypass ($p = 0.027$) but not during normothermic bypass ($p = 0.57$). No significant association between regional cerebral blood flow and the level of carbon dioxide ($p = 0.16$) was found during deep hypothermic bypass. There was a significant association, however, of those parameters during normothermic bypass ($p = 0.02$).

Figure 2 demonstrates the relationship of regional cerebral blood flow with time for the two groups. As can be seen, all patients showed a significant decrease in cerebral blood flow at deep hypothermic conditions compared to baseline, prebypass levels. In those not undergoing a period of circulatory arrest, cerebral blood flow returned to baseline levels in the rewarming phase of bypass. Those patients, however, undergoing repair under deep hypothermia with total circulatory arrest had no significant increase in cerebral blood flow during rewarming either after the period of arrest or even after being weaned from cardiopulmonary bypass ($p = 0.013$). All patients survived their operations and were followed up for any evidence of short-term neurologic complications. No apparent neurologic sequels were seen in any patient, excepting one patient who developed choreoathetoid movements which resolved after 4 months.

Discussion

Several recent studies in adult patients[1,2,5,6] have demonstrated the preservation of autoregulation of pressure and flow and cerebrovascular response to carbon dioxide during moderate hypothermic (26–28°C) cardiopulmonary bypass. These studies demonstrate that flow of cerebral blood correlates well with nasopharyngeal

CEREBRAL BLOOD FLOW AND TEMPERATURE

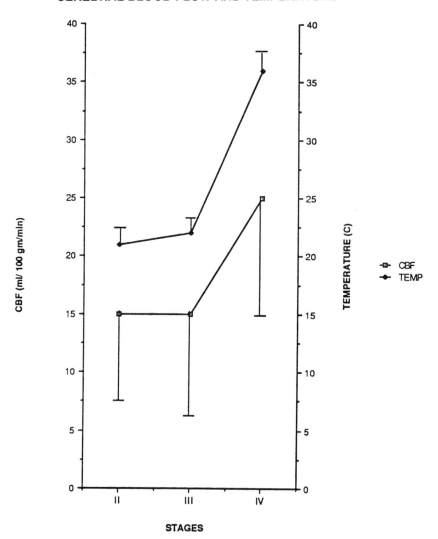

Figure 1. Cerebral blood flow (CBF) and nasopharyngeal temperature during various stages of bypass. Data are shown as mean ± standard deviation. Note the parallel relationship of flow and temperature with time.

temperature and is well maintained through a wide range of perfusion pressures. Infants and children undergoing repair of congenital heart defects are exposed to more extreme conditions of cardiopulmonary bypass. This study investigated the effects of deep hypothermic cardiopulmonary bypass and total circulatory arrest on cerebral blood flow with an attempt to account for the impact of variables such as temperature, perfusion pressure, and tension of carbon dioxide during deep hypothermia. Our study demonstrates that there is a significant decrease in regional cerebral blood flow during deep hypothermic cardiopulmonary bypass. The changes in regional flow during bypass are directly related to changes in temperature and, presumably, reflect reduced cerebral metabolism. This has certainly been shown to be the case in adults.[6]

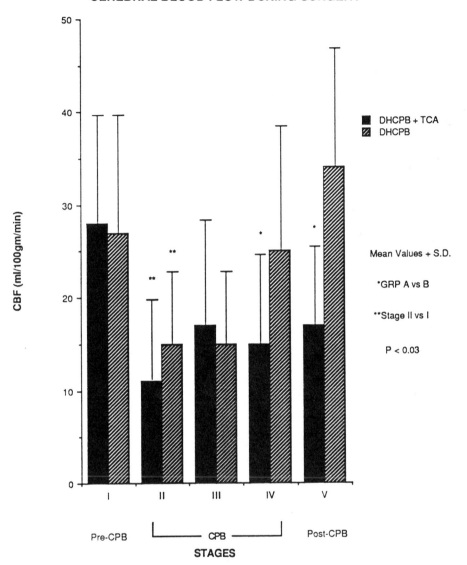

Figure 2. Cerebral blood flow measurements in the two groups of patients during all study intervals. There was a significant decrease in cerebral blood flow (CBF) in both groups during deep hypothermia (DH). There was a significant difference in flow between groups at the stages of rewarming and after completion of bypass. CPB, cardiopulmonary bypass.

Another major finding is that deep (unlike moderate) hypothermia abolishes autoregulation of pressure and flow. There is a significant association between regional flow and mean arterial pressure during deep hypothermic conditions (18–23°C), suggesting that blood flow is dependent on pressure at these low temperatures. During normothermic cardiopulmonary bypass, however, no correlation was found between cerebral blood flow and mean arterial pressure either in this study or in others.[1,2]

Previous studies in adult patients[1,6] have demonstrated the maintenance of the response of the cerebral circulation to changes in carbon dioxide tension during moderate hypothermic (26–28°C) cardiopulmonary bypass. Our data in infants and children during normothermic bypass similarly demonstrate this association. We observed no association, however, between cerebral blood flow and levels of carbon dioxide during deep hypothermic (18–23°C) cardiopulmonary bypass. The loss of cerebrovascular responses to changes in carbon dioxide under deep hypothermic conditions has never been demonstrated in humans. This, therefore, represents a new observation for which there is no apparent explanation.

Although current techniques of deep hypothermic cardiopulmonary bypass with total circulatory arrest have no apparent long-term neurologic or developmental sequels, little information is available with regard to the critical aspects of this technique. Several reports have documented the association of total circulatory arrest with transient dysfunction of the central nervous system.[7–9] The data from our study suggest that one possible mechanism causing such transient dysfunction is abnormal reperfusion following total circulatory arrest. In our study, cerebral reperfusion after deep hypothermia was significantly impaired if the patient was exposed to a period of total circulatory arrest. Whether such impaired cerebral reperfusion after deep hypothermic bypass with circulatory arrest can be altered by changing rates of flow or whether it is related in severity to the duration of the period of total circulatory arrest will be investigated by future studies. The clinical importance of these observations remains to be determined. Only one of our patients exhibited any signs of neurologic dysfunction in the postoperative period (transient choreoathetoid movements). The understanding of how cerebral reperfusion is affected by total circulatory arrest and how those changes can be best controlled, however, has far reaching implications.

In conclusion, changes in cerebral blood flow during cardiopulmonary bypass under deep hypothermia are primarily due to changes in temperature where reduced metabolic rate reduces cerebral blood flow. Autoregulation of pressure and flow is lost under these conditions. Furthermore, the association between arterial tension of carbon dioxide and cerebral blood flow seen during normothermia is lost with deep hypothermia. Finally, our study suggests that cerebral reperfusion is impaired after total circulatory arrest.

References

1. Govier AV, Reves JG, McKay RD, et al. Factors and their influence on regional cerebral blood flow during nonpulsatile cardiopulmonary bypass. Ann Thorac Surg 1984;38:592–600.
2. Brusino FG, Reves JG, Smith LR, et al. The effects of age on cerebral blood flow autoregulation during hypothermic cardiopulmonary bypass. J Thorac Cardiovasc Surg 1989;97:541–7.
3. Waltz AG, Wanek AR, Anderson RE. Comparison of analytic methods for calculation of cerebral blood flow after intracarotid injection of 133 Xe. J Nucl Med 1972;13:66–72.
4. Olesen J, Paulson OB, Lassen NA. Regional cerebral blood flow in man determined by the initial slope of the clearance of intraarterially injected 133 Xe. Stroke 1971;2:519–40.
5. Prough DS, Stump DA, Rou RC, et al. Response of cerebral blood flow to changes in carbon dioxide tension during hypothermic cardiopulmonary bypass. Anesthesiology 1986;64:576–81.
6. Murkin JM, Farrar JK, Tweed WA, et al. Cerebral autoregulation and flow/metabolism coupling during cardiopulmonary bypass: The influence of $PACO_2$. Anesth Analg 1987;66:825–32.
7. Messmer BJ, Schallberger U, Gattiker R, Senning A. Psychomotor and intellectual development after deep hypothermia and circulatory arrest in early infancy. J Thorac Cardiovasc Surg 1976;72:495–502.
8. Stevenson JG, Stone EF, Dillard DH, Morgan BC. Intellectual development of children subjected to prolonged circulatory arrest during hypothermic open heart surgery in infancy. Circulation 1974;50(suppl II):54–9.
9. Wells FC, Coghill S, Caplan HL, Lincoln C. Duration of circulatory arrest does influence the psychological development of children after cardiac operation in early life. J Thorac Cardiovasc Surg 1983;86:823–31.

Myocardial Protection in Immature Hearts

A. Corno

Introduction

Important differences have been demonstrated between neonatal and adult myocardium with regard to structure, metabolism, and function.[1] Because of these differences, the preservation of myocardial function in neonates during cardiac operations assumes even greater importance than in adults, since a perioperative insult is less tolerated and more difficult to treat.

Properties of the Neonatal Heart

In terms of structure, the neonatal heart has greater ratio of surface to wall thickness, smaller myocytes, a greater proportion of noncontractile mass (nuclei, mitochondria, surface membranes) to the number of myofibrils, underdevelopment of sarcoplasmic reticulum, and a decreased density of T-tubules and calcium pumps. The mitochondria have reduced number and mass, increased content of cytochrome, and increased aerobic capacity. The myocardium is also immature in terms of its autonomic innervation and reduced concentrations of epinephrine and norepinephrine.[1]

As far as metabolism is concerned, the mitochondria have increased activity of the cytochrome *c* oxidase and increased oxygen consumption per milligram of protein in presence of adenosine diphosphate. Further features of the myocardial metabolism are the facility for anaerobic rather than aerobic production of adenosine triphosphate, the dependence on carbohydrate rather than fatty acid as sources of energy, production of lactate, and abundant glycogen stores.[1] The neonatal heart is also different in terms of its calcium homeostasis. There is reduced myofibrillar calcium-activated adenosine triphosphate, a relatively slow rate of active transport of calcium in the vesicles of sarcoplasmic reticulum, increased dependency for calcium-induced release of calcium from sarcoplasmic reticulum in the vicinity of myofilaments, reduced intracellular concentrations of calcium, and increased dependency on extracellular calcium for excitation–contraction coupling.[2]

Functionally, there is reduced participation of the sarcoplasmic reticulum in myocardial activation and relaxation processes in the neonatal heart, a different length/tension relationship of the myofibrils, reduced maximal rate of development of tension as opposed to developed tension, and a reduced generation of contractile force at any given extracellular concentration of calcium.[1] The neonatal heart has reduced ventricular compliance (reduced influence of the filling volume on cardiac output) and increased influence of ventricular filling volume on the contralateral ventricular volume and pressure.[1] The consequence of these particular properties of the neonatal heart is a reduced functional reserve in both systole and diastole.[1]

The neonatal myocardium presents an increased inotropic response to exogenous calcium and a reduced response to inotropic agents.[3] In contrast, it a has greater tolerance to hypoxia, greater vulnerability to ischemia, and greater susceptivity to reoxygenation and injury produced by reperfusion.[4-6]

Experimental Studies

The methods of myocardial protection used in pediatric cardiac surgery include a single period or intermittent periods of ischemic arrest with topical cooling, hypothermic perfusion of the fibrillating heart, and/or use of crystalloid or blood cardioplegia.

Hypothermia, by reducing cardiac metabolism and by inhibiting glycolysis, is a protective factor during ischemia. In neonates, because of the greater ratio of surface to wall thickness, uniform cooling and adequate myocardial protection can be obtained very easily with isolated topical cooling.[7]

Continuous coronary perfusion is one of the methods of intraoperative myocardial protection, but hypothermia raises subendocardial coronary resistance, with the most disproportionate rise in resistance occurring in neonatal hearts.[8]

An experimental study[7] on the isolated neonatal piglet heart perfused with blood demonstrated the superiority of a cardioplegic solution consisting of cold blood supplemented with potassium (16 mmol/L). With this solution, given for 2 minutes at a pressure of 80 mmHg and repeated every 20 minutes for 2 hours, there was complete recovery of left ventricular performance.

The same study[7] confirmed the adequate myocardial protection provided in the neonatal heart by isolated topical cooling and the structural and functional damage due to the utilization of hyperosmolar solutions (450 mOsm/kg H_2O). The study further showed that either the crystalloid or the blood cardioplegic solutions provide a better myocardial protection with normal levels of calcium level (1.2 mmol/L) than with low levels (0.06 mmol/L). This fact, in contrast with both the experimental and clinical experience with adults, suggests that the increased sensitivity of the neonatal heart to the level of calcium in the cardioplegic solution may be due to the particular properties of calcium homeostasis in the neonate.[7]

Another experimental study[9] using the same isolated neonatal heart model perfused with blood demonstrated complete recovery of systolic function after long-term (12 hours) hypothermic storage by manipulating the storage solution and controlling the conditions of reperfusion.

The best functional recovery was obtained using a hyperosmolar, high glucose, intracellular solution for storage, followed by reperfusion with blood supplemented by glucose, aspartate and glutamate (28 mmol/L), superoxide dismutase and catalase (105,000 U/L). The last experimental study[10] demonstrated the recovery of 90% of the baseline stroke work index after 12 hours of hypothermic storage, by using reperfusion with leukocyte-depleted blood.

Conclusion

Because of the particular properties of the immature hearts, adequate myocardial protection in neonates may be obtained by using reduced periods of ischemia, topical cooling, blood cardioplegia with normal levels of calcium, or reperfusion with blood modified by various agents.

Acknowledgement: We thank Luana Castellacci for her help in preparing the manuscript.

References

1. Friedman WF. The intrinsic physiologic properties of the developing heart. Prog Cardiovasc Dis 1972;15:87–111.
2. Nishiota K, Nakanishi T, George BL, Jamarkani JM. The effect of calcium on the inotropy of catecholamine and paired electrical stimulation in the newborn and adult myocardium. J Moll Cell Cardiol 1981;13:511–20.
3. Parisi F, Corno A, La Vigna G, et al. Uso delle amine simpaticomimetiche nel neonato: Nostra esperienza. G Ital Cardiol 1984;14:586–8.
4. Chiu RCJ, Bindon W. Why are newborn hearts vulnerable to global ischemia? The lactate hypothesis. Circulation 1987;76:(suppl V):146–9.
5. Corno A, Laks H, Davtyan HG, et al. The effect of acute hypoxia and reoxygenation on function and metabolism of the isolated neonatal heart. J Am Coll Cardiol 1987;9:354–8.
6. Otani H, Engelman RM, Rousou JA, et al. The mechanism of myocardial reperfusion injury in neonates. Circulation 1987;76:(suppl V):161–7.
7. Corno A, Bethencourt DM, Laks H, et al. Myocardial protection in the neonatal heart. J Thorac Cardiovasc Surg 1987;93:163–72.
8. Buckberg GD. Heart function during and after extracorporeal circulation. In: Hagl S, Klovekorn WP, Mayr N, Sebening F (eds), Thirty Years of Extracorporeal Circulation. Munchen, Deutsches Herzzentrum, 1984, pp 157–77.
9. Davtyan HG, Corno A, Laks H, et al. Long-term neonatal heart preservation. J Thorac Cardiovasc Surg 1988;96:44–53.
10. Breda MA, Drinkwater DC, Laks H, et al. Prevention of reperfusion injury in the neonatal heart with leukocyte-depleted blood. J Thorac Cardiovasc Surg 1989;97:654–65.

Myocardial Protection in the Neonatal Rat Heart

M. V. Braimbridge, Y. Yano, F. Yamamoto, and E. Riva

Introduction

In 1975, we began to use what became known as the St. Thomas' Hospital cardioplegic solution clinically in the adult[1] and assumed, because in the smaller dog and rat heart it was also protective, that it would be equally effective in the infant. We were supported in this view by Kirklin et al.[2] They reviewed 335 cardiac operations in neonates and infants, comparing their series before 1977 using cold ischemic arrest with the later series in which cardioplegia was used. The probability of hospital death due to cardiac failure was directly related to the duration of ischemia when cold ischemic arrest was used, whereas with cardioplegia there was no correlation. Bull et al.,[3] however, reviewed 400 cardiac operations in neonates, infants, and children between 1974 and 1981, comparing cold ischemic arrest and cardioplegia, and showed no significant difference in mortality in neonates and infants.

Is myocardial protection during cardiac surgery, therefore, less successful in neonates and infants than in the adult? To answer this, it is important to define in experimental animals the same three age groups as in the human. We consider that the neonatal age for the rat is from birth to 1 week,

infancy is from 1 week to 1 month, and adulthood is over 1 month.

Vulnerability of Neonatal, Infant and Adult Rat Hearts to Ischemia

The vulnerability of the developing rat heart to ischemia was assessed by using isolated hearts from neonatal (3–6 days old), infant (20–25 days old), and adult (50–60 days old) Wistar rats. Retrograde aortic perfusion in the Langendorf mode with Krebs-Henseleit bicarbonate buffer was performed at 37°C with an isovolumic balloon in the left ventricle. Indices measured were left ventricular developed pressure, coronary flow, ventricular rate, and leakage of creatine phosphokinase during reperfusion. The effluent was collected throughout reperfusion and analyzed for creatine phosphokinase.

The experimental protocol provided 10 minutes for establishment of control conditions. Thereafter, St. Thomas' Hospital cardioplegic solution was infused for 2 minutes followed by between 0 and 100 minutes of global ischemia at 37°C. There followed 30 minutes of reperfusion, at the end of which time recovery was expressed as a percentage of control.

The St. Thomas' Hospital cardioplegic solution, which is now commercially available as Plegisol (Abbott Laboratories, Chicago), is (in mmol/L) sodium chloride 110.0, potassium chloride 16.0, magnesium chloride 16.0, calcium chloride 1.2, sodium bicarbonate 10.0; with pH adjusted to 7.8 and the osmolarity 324 mosm/L.

Results

There was no difference in recovery between the three groups with up to 40 minutes of ischemia (Fig. 1). After this time, the hearts from adults and infants continued to deteriorate until, at 80 and 100 minutes, there was no functional recovery. The neonatal hearts, however, still recovered to approximately 30% of control even after 100 minutes of normothermic ischemia. In assessment of leakage of creatine phosphokinase on reperfusion, there was increasing production during the recovery period for all hearts with increasing duration of ischemia but, after 40 minutes, the neonatal hearts separated out, so that at periods of 60 to 100 minutes there was a significant difference in leakage ($p < 0.05$ or less).

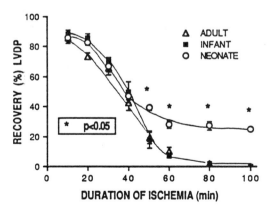

Figure 1. Percent recovery of left ventricular developed pressure (LVDP) in isolated adult (△), infant (■), and neonate (○) rat hearts perfused in the Langendorf mode after various durations of global ischemia at 37°C.

Susceptibility to Calcium-Mediated Injury

The aim of our second study was to investigate whether these differences in tolerance to ischemia reflected age-related susceptibility to injury mediated by calcium. Isolated hearts from neonatal rats (3–6 days old) were used with the same Langendorf preparation. The protocol was similar to that of the previous study, with 30 minutes of control perfusion, 2 minutes of infusion of St. Thomas' Hospital cardioplegic solution (in which the calcium concentration was varied from 0 to 2.4 mmol/L), 60 to 180 minutes of global ischemia at 37°C, and then 30 min of reperfusion, at the end of which recovery was expressed as a percentage of control.

Results

The effects of the different concentrations of calcium on postischemic recovery in these neonatal rat hearts were compared with a previous series performed with a preparation of the adult working heart after 35 minutes of normothermic ischemia.

In adults hearts, when there was no calcium in the solution, there was no recovery of function (Fig. 2a). With increasing concentrations of calcium, there was a bell-shaped curve with optimal recovery at 1.2 mmol/L. Leakage of creatine phosphokinase during reperfusion was massively increased to over 500 IU/15 min/g when there was no calcium in the solution followed by a tendency towards a bell-shaped curve with a minimum at 1.2 mmol/L.

In the neonatal hearts, the results were entirely different (Fig. 2b). Recovery of developed pressure within the left ventricle was 30% of control even when there was no calcium in the cardioplegic solution; in other words, there was no calcium paradox. There was also no suggestion of a bell-shaped curve of recovery at the different

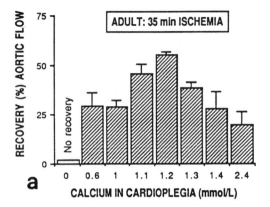

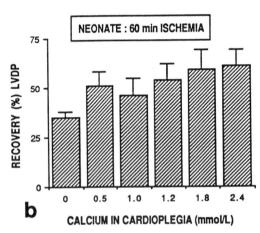

Figure 2. (a) Percent recovery of aortic flow in isolated rat hearts perfused in the working mode with St. Thomas' Hospital cardioplegic solution in which the calcium concentration was varied from 0 to 2.4 mmol/L, followed by 35 min of global ischemia at 37°C. (b) Percent recovery of left ventricular developed pressure (LVDP) in isolated neonatal rat hearts perfused in the Langendorf mode with St. Thomas' Hospital cardioplegic solution in which the calcium concentration was varied from 0 to 2.4 mmol/L, followed by 60 minutes of global ischemia at 37°C.

concentrations of calcium. Leakage of creatine phosphokinase with no calcium in the cardioplegic solution was only 100 IU/30 min/g and, again, there was no subsequent bell-shaped curve.

Discussion

These two studies show, firstly, that neonatal rat hearts are more tolerant than those of infants and adults to myocardial ischemia during normothermic cardioplegic arrest. Secondly, neonatal rat hearts are more tolerant than those of adults to calcium-mediated injury and, in particular, show no calcium paradox. We would make a plea for international agreement on the precise definition of "neonatal," "infant," and "adult" in the hearts of rats, pigs, and dogs and, in particular, that the terms "immature," "puppy," and "piglet" to cover both neonatal and infant periods should be abandoned.

References

1. Hearse DJ, Stewart DA, Braimbridge MV. Cellular protection during myocardial ischemia. The developement and characterization of a procedure for the induction of reversible ischemic arrest. Circulation 1976;54:193–202.
2. Kirklin JK, Blackstone EH, Kirklin JW, et al. Intracardiac surgery in infants under age of 3 months: Incremental risk factors for hospital mortality. Am J Cardiol 1981;48:500–6.
3. Bull C, Cooper J, Stark J. Cardioplegic protection of the child's heart. J Thorac Cardiovasc Surg 1984;88:287–93.

The Vulnerability of the Immature Myocardium to Ischemia and Its Responsiveness to Cardioplegic Protection

M. Avkiran and D. J. Hearse

Introduction

Despite the successful application of cold chemical cardioplegia cardiac surgery for adults,[1] current evidence suggests that myocardial protection provided by cardioplegia may be inadequate during the repair of congenital heart defects in children.[2,3] It is, therefore, necessary to determine whether the immature myocardium has a different susceptibility to ischemic damage than the adult, and to establish whether chemical cardioplegia can protect the immature myocardium from such damage. In this article, we describe investigations of the effects of the St. Thomas' Hospital cardioplegic solution on the functional recovery of isolated neonatal and adult rat hearts following normothermic global ischemia.

Methods

Neonatal (3–5 days old) and adult (84–112 days old) male Wistar rats were anes-

This work was supported in part by grants from the National Heart, Lung and Blood Institute (R01 HL 39457), the National Heart Research Fund and STRUTH.

thetized with diethyl ether. Following heparinization of the animal, the heart was removed and mounted on the perfusion apparatus via an aortic cannula. Perfusion of the coronary arteries was carried out according to the Langendorf technique, at a constant pressure of 40 mmHg for neonatal hearts and 75 mmHg for adult hearts. The perfusion medium was a modified Krebs-Henseleit bicarbonate buffer of the following composition (in mmol/L): sodium chloride 118.5, sodium bicarbonate 25.0, potassium chloride 4.8, magnesium sulfate 1.2, potassium biphosphate 1.2, calcium chloride 1.4, glucose 11.0. The buffer was continuously gassed with 95% oxygen + 5% carbon dioxide (pH 7.4 at 37°C). Each heart was housed in a thermostatically controlled heart chamber maintained at 37°C throughout the experiment.

Left ventricular pressure was recorded from an intraventricular balloon inflated to give an end-diastolic pressure of 2–8 mmHg. Left ventricular developed pressure, maximum rate of rise of left ventricular pressure (dP/dt), and ventricular rate were derived from the pressure signal. The rate of coronary flow was measured by timed collection of coronary effluent. The product of ventricular rate and developed pressure (rate-pressure product) was used as an index of cardiac work.

After control readings were taken, the aortic line was clamped and the heart infused for 2 minutes with either the St. Thomas' Hospital cardioplegic solution (composition in mmol/L: sodium chloride 110.0, potassium chloride 16.0, magnesium chloride 16.0, calcium chloride 1.2, sodium bicarbonate 10.0; pH adjusted to 7.8) or perfusion buffer. Normothermic global ischemia was then initiated and, following the ischemic period (30 minutes in the adult and 30, 60, 90, 120, or 150 minutes in the neonate), the heart was reperfused for 60 minutes with the perfusion buffer.

The recovery of function at the end of reperfusion was expressed as a percentage of preischemic control. Student's unpaired t-test was used for comparing recoveries in corresponding neonate and adult groups, and animals having cardioplegia or no cardioplegia at each duration of ischemia. Statistical significance was assumed at $p < 0.05$.

Results

The preischemic control values of left ventricular developed pressure, rate of rise of pressure, coronary flow, and ventricular rate were 121.0 ± 4.7 mmHg, 3,049 ± 187 mmHg/s, 10.9 ± 0.5 ml/min/g, and 288 ± 14 beats/min, respectively, in adult hearts (n = 10), and 50.9 ± 2.4 mmHg ($p < 0.05$), 1,388 ± 52 mmHg/s ($p < 0.05$), 18.6 ± 1.2 ml/min/g ($p < 0.05$), and 297 ± 7 beats/min, respectively, in neonatal hearts (n = 12). Consequently, the preischemic rate–pressure product was significantly lower in neonatal hearts (15.0 ± 0.5 × 10^3) than in adults (34.3 ± 1.2 × 10^3). Following 30 minutes of ischemia without cardioplegia, there was a significantly greater recovery of the rate–pressure product in neonatal hearts (78 ±

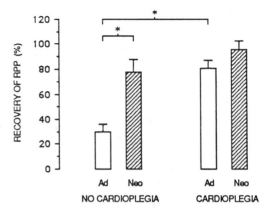

Figure 1. Recovery of the rate–pressure product (RPP) following 30 minutes of normothermic global ischemia and 60 minutes of reperfusion in adult (Ad, open columns, n = 5) and neonatal (Neo, hatched columns, n = 6) hearts, with or without a 2-minute preischemic infusion of the St. Thomas' Hospital cardioplegic solution. Vertical bars represent standard error of the mean; *$p < 0.05$.

10% vs. 30 ± 6% in adults), while infusion of cardioplegia improved recovery in both age groups (Fig. 1). As a result of the high recovery obtained in the absence of cardioplegia, however, the improvement in recovery to 96 ± 7% in neonatal hearts did not attain statistical significance. Left ventricular developed pressure and rate of rise also recovered to a significantly greater extent in neonates than in adults in the absence of cardioplegia (Table 1). Cardioplegia improved the recovery of left ventricular developed pressure and rate of rise in both age groups, the improvement again achieving statistical significance in adults but not in neonates. In the absence of cardioplegia, there was no difference in the recovery of coronary flow between the two age groups. The use of cardioplegia, however, resulted in an increased coronary flow during reperfusion in neonatal hearts. Ventricular rate returned to preischemic values in both age groups, and cardioplegia had no effect on its recovery.

In the absence of cardioplegia, 100% (5/5) of adult hearts and 67% (4/6) of neonatal hearts exhibited contracture during the is-

Table 1

Recovery of Functional Indices in Isolated Hearts from Adult and Neonatal Rats Following Various Durations of Normothermic Global Ischemia and 60 Minutes of Reperfusion

Ischemia (min)	Age	Recovery (%)									
		LVDP		dP/dt		Coronary flow		Heart rate		RPP	
		(−C)	(+C)	(−C)	(+C)	(−C)	(+C)	(−C)	(+C)	(−C)	(+C)
30	Ad	36 ± 7	86 ± 7	37 ± 9	94 ± 7	69 ± 5	77 ± 5	83 ± 7	94 ± 3	30 ± 6	81 ± 6
	Neo	80 ± 10[a]	89 ± 6	78 ± 9[a]	92 ± 7	85 ± 7	122 ± 14[a,b]	98 ± 3	107 ± 6	78 ± 10[a]	96 ± 7
60	Neo	66 ± 11	83 ± 8	67 ± 12	88 ± 8	97 ± 9	112 ± 19	94 ± 7	111 ± 4	64 ± 13	93 ± 9
90	Neo	53 ± 7	74 ± 6[b]	54 ± 7	75 ± 8	108 ± 17	144 ± 8	99 ± 6	93 ± 3	54 ± 8	71 ± 8
120	Neo	33 ± 6	58 ± 5[b]	30 ± 5	56 ± 5[b]	100 ± 4	148 ± 14[b]	75 ± 5	83 ± 8	24 ± 3	47 ± 5[b]
150	Neo	21 ± 4	41 ± 7[b]	19 ± 3	39 ± 6[b]	106 ± 9	132 ± 26	75 ± 3	79 ± 7	16 ± 3	33 ± 8[b]

(−C), no cardioplegia; (+C), cardioplegia; LVDP, left ventricular developed pressure; dP/dt, maximum rate of rise of pressure; RPP, rate—pressure product; Ad, adult (n = 5); Neo, neonate (n = 6).
[a] $p < 0.05$ compared to adult; [b] $p < 0.05$ compared to (−C).

chemic period of 30 minutes. The mean time to onset of ischemic contracture was significantly longer in neonatal hearts (23.8 ± 1.9 minutes) compared to adults (15.4 ± 1.1 minutes). None of the adult hearts and only one neonatal heart exhibited contracture during ischemia of 30 minutes in the presence of cardioplegia.

The effects of cardioplegia on the neonatal heart were also investigated with longer durations of normothermic ischemia (60, 90, 120, and 150 minutes). There was no significant difference in preischemic function between the groups of neonatal hearts (six in each group). Cardioplegia improved the recovery of contractile function and cardiac work with all durations of ischemia, the improved recovery becoming statistically significant with ischemic durations of 90 minutes or longer (Table 1). Thus, in the presence of cardioplegia, there was significantly greater recovery of left ventricular developed pressure after 90 minutes of ischemia and of left ventricular developed pressure, rate of rise of pressure, and the rate–pressure product after 120 and 150 minutes of ischemia. Cardioplegia tended to produce an increase in coronary flow during reperfusion after all durations of ischemia, the effect becoming significant after 120 minutes. The recovery of heart rate was not affected by cardioplegia.

In all 60 neonatal hearts studied, the incidence of ischemic contracture was 90% (27/30) without cardioplegia and 63% (19/30) with cardioplegia. Cardioplegia produced a significant delay in the onset of ischemic contracture from 24.7 ± 1.1 min to 37.0 ± 1.5 minutes, and a significant reduction in the magnitude of contracture from 14.9 ± 1.1 mmHg to 7.8 ± 0.9 mmHg.

Discussion

The results of this study are in agreement with increasing experimental evidence,[4–6] suggesting a greater resistance to ischemia in the neonatal heart. Thus, after 30 minutes of normothermic global ischemia in the absence of cardioplegia, contractile function recovered to more than 75% of preischemic control in the neonate, but to under 40% in the adult. The greater resistance of the neonatal heart was also confirmed by the longer time to onset of ischemic contracture at this age.

The well established protection by cardioplegia in the adult heart was again demonstrated in this study. Although cardioplegia appeared not to improve the recovery of contractile function to a significant extent in neonatal hearts after the shorter durations of ischemia, this was probably due to the excellent recoveries in the groups not receiving cardioplegia, leaving little scope for improved protection. Indeed the significant protective capability of cardioplegia in the neonatal heart was unmasked when hearts were subjected to prolonged durations of ischemia. Cardioplegia also delayed the onset and reduced the magnitude of ischemic contracture in neonatal hearts. Bove and colleagues,[7] using the rabbit, have also demonstrated recently significant protection with the St. Thomas' Hospital cardioplegic solution in the neonatal heart.

These findings contrast with the reported inadequacy of myocardial protection by cardioplegia during pediatric cardiac surgery.[2,3] Apart from possible species differences, one important distinction between most experimental studies and the clinical situation is the use of hearts from healthy animals in the former. Accelerated depletion of high-energy phosphates during ischemia and depressed recovery of cardiac function during reperfusion have been reported in surgically induced models of congenital heart disease.[8,9] It has also been suggested that chronically cyanotic patients may have an increased vulnerability to damage by free radicals.[10] It may not be age in itself, therefore, but other factors associated with the congenital defect that result in an increased susceptibility to damage induced by ischemia and reperfusion in children undergoing cardiac surgery.

Acknowledgments: We thank Dr. Emma Riva for helpful discussion and Mrs. Cathy Erlebach for secretarial assistance.

References

1. Hearse DJ, Braimbridge MV, Jynge P. Protection of the Ischemic Myocardium: Cardioplegia. New York, Raven Press, 1981.
2. Bull C, Cooper J, Stark J. Cardioplegic protection of the child's heart. J Thorac Cardiovasc Surg 1984;88:287–93.
3. Del Nido PJ, Mickle DAG, Wilson GJ, et al. Inadequate protection with cold cardioplegic arrest during repair of tetralogy of Fallot. J Thorac Cardiovasc Surg 1988;95:223–9.
4. Nishioka K, Jarmakani JM. Effect of ischemia on mechanical function and high-energy phosphates in rabbit myocardium. Am J Physiol 1982;242:1077–83.
5. Yano Y, Braimbridge MV, Hearse DJ. Protection of the pediatric myocardium: Differential susceptibility to ischemic injury of the neonatal rat heart. J Thorac Cardiovasc Surg 1987;94:887–96.
6. Bove EL, Stammers AH. Recovery of left ventricular function after hypothermic global ischemia: Age-related differences in the isolated working rabbit heart. J Thorac Cardiovasc Surg 1986;91:115–22.
7. Bove EL, Stammers AH, Gallagher KP. Protection of the neonatal myocardium during hypothermic ischemia: Effect of cardioplegia on left ventricular function in the rabbit. J Thorac Cardiovasc Surg 1987;94:115–23.
8. Silverman NA, Kohler J, Levitsky S, et al. Chronic hypoxemia depresses global ventricular function and predisposes to the depletion of high-energy phosphates during cardioplegic arrest: Implications for surgical repair of cyanotic congenital heart defects. Ann Thorac Surg 1984;37:304–8.
9. Del Nido PJ, Benson LN, Mickle DAG, et al. Impaired left ventricular post-ischemic function and metabolism in chronic right ventricular hypertrophy. Circulation 1987;76(suppl V):168–73.
10. Del Nido PJ, Mickle DAG, Wilson GJ et al. Evidence of myocardial free radical injury during elective repair of tetralogy of Fallot. Circulation 1987;76(suppl V):174–9.

Postischemic Metabolism of Infant Hearts Following Either Ischemic or Cardioplegic Arrest

C. J. Preusse, K. Kocherscheidt, A. Krian, J. Winter,
H. D. Schulte, and W. Bircks

Introduction

There is no longer any doubt that crystalloid cardioplegic solutions protect effectively adult hearts against intra- and postischemic damage. Different formulations of cardioplegic solutions are used routinely worldwide.[1] The protective properties of these various cardioplegic solutions in pediatric cardiac surgery, however, remain controversial.[2-5] Questions remain concerning the propriety of using the results of experimental investigations on immature animal hearts in direct relation to the heart of the child. We started, therefore, to investigate the metabolic and functional status of the hearts of infants during the early postischemic and postoperative period after different methods of myocardial protection. In addition to pure ischemic cardiac arrest, we have used the Bretschneider method for myocardial protection in our clinic for over a decade.[6-8]

Patients and Methods

The clinical data of the two groups undergoing investigation are summarized in Table 1. The period of ischemia was distinctly higher in the group receiving cardioplegia. After declamping of the aorta, it was necessary to defibrillate two of eight hearts (25%) of the group protected by ischemia, while the hearts of the patients in the other group returned to sinus rhythm spontaneously. On the other hand, two hearts protected by cardioplegia (8.3%) were treated with catecholamines after the period of ischemia.

We used the cold (5°–8°C) Bretschneider solution for cardioplegia.* Its composition (mmol/L) is as follows: sodium (15), potassium (10), magnesium (4), histidine (180), histidine-HCL (18), tryptophan (2), ketoglutarate (1), and mannitol (30). Further details of its clinical application have been given elsewhere.[6,7] In contrast to other methods for myocardial protection, we perfuse the infant hearts only once with a volume of about 300 ml at a perfusion pressure of 30–40 mmHg. Pure ischemic cardiac arrest was performed by cross-clamping the aorta at a blood temperature of 18° to 20°C.

---

* Manufactured by Dr. F. Kohler, D-6146 Alsbach.

Table 1

Clinical Data of Patients Undergoing Cardiac Surgery Treated with Different
Methods of Myocardial Protection

	Cardioplegia		Ischemia	
Number of patients	24		8	
Diagnoses	VSD	7	ASD	4
	Fallot's tetralogy	7	VSD	2
	ASD	4	aortic valve stenosis	1
	complete transposition	3	pulmonary valve stenosis	1
	mitral valve stenosis	1		
	pulmonary valve stenosis	1		
	Bland-White-Garland	1		
Sex	13 m		5 m	
	11 f		3 f	
Age	× 20.8 months		× 36.6 months	
Weight	× 9.2 kg		× 12.4 kg	
Time of ischemia	× 77.5 min		× 15.0 min	
Intraoperative defibrillations	0		2	
Intraoperative catecholamine support	2		0	

VSD, ventricular peptal defect; ASD, atrioventricular septal defect.

For evaluation of metabolic recovery, we measured the arterial and coronary venous concentrations of the activity of potassium, lactate, and creatine kinase at intervals up to 20 minutes during the early postischemic phase of total bypass.

Results

All hearts were revived in both groups and no low cardiac output syndrome occurred postoperatively. The analysis of the postischemic washout of potassium in respect to its re-uptake showed that, within 5 minutes of unclamping the aorta, re-uptake of potassium was discovered in both groups. In the group undergoing pure ischemic arrest, it could be found within 2 minutes, while the re-uptake in the group receiving cardioplegia started after 4 minutes. In the latter group, a continuous uptake of potassium was detected during the total period of measurement indicating a resynthesis of glycogen.

Independent from the mode of protection, all hearts showed loss of creatine kin-ase after the period of ischemia. The average loss of creatine kinase was 42 U/L/min in the group undergoing pulse ischemia, while it was 84 U/L/min in the other group.

It must be remembered, nonetheless, that the period of ischemia was five times longer in the group having cardioplegia. The loss of creatine kinase, therefore, was relatively higher in the group protected purely by cold ischemia, although, in absolute terms, it was only half of that seen in those having cardioplegia. The most surprising results were detected when analyzing the postischemic washout and uptake of lactate (Fig. 1). Lactate was taken up after about 15 minutes of reperfusion in the hearts arrested by cardioplegia while, in the other group, a permanent washout of lactate could be measured even after 20 minutes of reperfusion with blood.

Discussion

In contrast to other methods of myocardial protection, it is our policy to perfuse the infant hearts only once, except when electrical and mechanical evidence of ven-

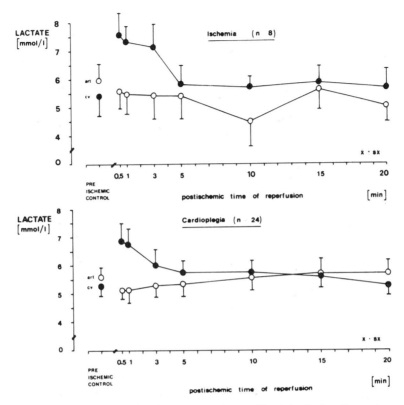

Figure 1. Arterial and coronary venous concentrations of lactate during the early postischemic period after different methods of myocardial protection (upper curves: pure ischemia; lower curves: myocardial protection with the Bretschneider solution).

tricular activity can be recognized.[6] In this fashion, we have been able to protect infant hearts for more than 2½ hours. Among the patients receiving cardioplegia, there were three cases with complete transposition that had been arrested for 167 ± 9 minutes ($\bar{x}$ ± SEM). These patients were weaned from bypass without problems.

The lack of effectiveness of myocardial protection reported in infant hearts[2,3] may depend on the formulation of the solution being used. Most of the investigators have used the St. Thomas' solution in their clinical and experimental studies. This solution contains procaine and magnesium at a high concentration. This can be harmful for infant and neonatal hearts because the diameter of their muscle fibers is only about half that of adult hearts. This causes an increased diffusion and uptake per unit weight together with an added risk of toxicity.

The metabolic recovery of the hearts treated with cardioplegia was excellent, even after long periods of cardiac arrest. Within 20 minutes of unclamping the aorta, the washout of potassium and lactate changed into uptake. So, with the solution of Bretschneider, there is no critical limit after 80 minutes of ischemia, as opposed to Bull et al.[3] having found such a limit with another cardioplegic solution.

The postischemic loss of myocardial enzyme is dependent on the time of ischemia and on the method of myocardial protection in both groups. The loss of creatine kinase in the group protected only by cold ischemia, however, was relatively higher in relation to the time of ischemia. Bull et al.[3] found that the release of creatine kinase remained unchanged from control values even after 120 minutes of ischemia, while Bjork and Bomfim[9] found an increasing leakage of creatine kinase-MB up to 120 minutes after unclamping the aorta. The metabolic recovery related to the postischemic uptake of lactate was excellent in those protected by cardioplegia. In the other group, in contrast, a continuing washout was recognized. Such a permanent washout of lactate may be caused by reduced permeation from the intra- to the extracellular space and/or by lasting anaerobic glycolysis.

In conclusion, we have the impression that arrest by cardioplegia is superior to that produced by pure ischemia on the basis of analysis of our metabolic and functional investigations. The Bretschneider method used is as effective in infant hearts as in adult ones. The need postoperatively for catecholamines in this group depends mostly on the myocardial disease. The incidence of catecholamine support, nonetheless, was distinctly lower than that reported by others.[4]

References

1. Buckberg GD. A proposed "solution" to the cardioplegic controversy. J Thorac Cardiovasc Surg 1979;77:803–13.

2. Magovern JA, Walter EP, Miller CA, et al. The immature and the mature myocardium: responses to multidose crystalloid cardioplegia. J Thorac Cardiovasc Surg 1988;95:618–24.

3. Bull C, Cooper J, Stark J. Cardioplegic protection of child's heart. J Thorac Cardiovasc Surg 1984;88:287–93.

4. Schachner A, Vladutin A, Montes M, et al. Myocardial protection in infant open heart surgery. Scand J Thorac Cardiovasc Surg 1983; 17:101–7.

5. Bove EL, Stammers AH, Gallagher KP. Protection of the neonatal myocardium during hypothermic ischemia. J Thorac Cardiovasc Surg 1987;94:115–23.

6. Preusse CJ, Schulte HD, Bircks W. High volume cardioplegia. Ann Chir Gynaecol 1987;76:39–45.

7. Schulte HD, Preusse CJ, Groschopp C, et al. Crystalloid cardioplegia—Experience with the Bretschneider solution. In: Engelman RM, Levitsky S (eds), A Textbook of Clinical Cardioplegia. Mt. Kisco, New York, Futura Publishing Co., 1982, pp 199–210.

8. Bretschneider HJ, Gebhard MM, Preusse CJ. Cardioplegia: Principles and problems. In: Sperelakis N (ed), Physiology and Pathophysiology of the Heart. Boston, The Hague, Martinus Nijhoff, 1984, pp 605–16.

9. Bjork VO, Bomfim V. Cardioplegia in pediatric cardiac surgery—Repair after infancy. In: Engelman RM, Levitsky S (eds), A Textbook of Clinical Cardioplegia. Mt. Kisco, New York, Futura Publishing Co., 1982, pp 365–71.

Clinical Experience with Blood Cardioplegia in Infants and Children
Perioperative Risk Factors for Mortality

H. Laks, A. Billingsley, D. Drinkwater, B. George, J. Pearl, and A. Wu

Introduction

Several studies[1-6] have examined the effectiveness of cold crystalloid cardioplegia in pediatric patients. To date, however, there has not been a large clinical review examining the use of cold blood cardioplegia. In this article, we describe our experience with the use of cold blood cardioplegia in pediatric cardiac surgery, and identify perioperative variables which contribute to the increased risk of mortality.

Methods

From 1982 to 1987, myocardial protection by means of cold blood cardioplegia was evaluated in 280 children undergoing selected cardiac procedures with relatively long ischemic times. These included 92 Fontan procedures, 92 repairs of tetralogy of Fallot, 76 Senning operations, and 20 arterial switch procedures. Ages ranged from 1 day to 16 years, with a mean of 38 months. Fifty-seven percent (159) of the patients were less than 24 months of age. Preoperative, intraoperative, and postoperative variables were identified by univariate analysis to select those factors significantly associated with mortality. Further evaluation by multivariate analyses was then used to determine independent risk factors for mortality.

Preoperative variables evaluated for increased risk included age at operation, weight, primary diagnosis, preoperative medications (digoxin, Lasix, Inderal, prostaglandin E_1, and inotropes), and preoperative condition defined as stable or unstable. Those patients who were considered stable were in good medical condition and underwent elective operation, while those who were unstable required inotropes and/or mechanical ventilation and underwent emergency operation. Intraoperative variables included ischemic cross-clamp time, difficulty in weaning from cardiopulmonary bypass, hypotension (a systolic blood pressure of less than 80 or a diastolic pressure of less than 50), rhythm off bypass, a single period of circulatory arrest, use of a warm blood cardioplegic reperfusate, and use of inotropes (low dose: 0–5 μg/min; medium dose: 5–10 μg/min; or high dose: greater than 10 μg/min). Postoperative variables included the use of inotropes, postoperative rhythm, left and right atrial pressures, hypotension, low cardiac output, low urine output, congestive heart failure, bleeding, pleural effusion, and time required for the toe temperature to approach within 5° C of the rectal temperature.

Statistical Analysis

A univariate analysis was initially used to select those variables associated with increased mortality (chi-square or t-test p value of < 0.10). A multivariate, simultaneous analysis utilizing logistic regression and linear discriminant analysis was then used to identify a subset of variables which were independently associated with increased mortality.

Technique of Cardioplegic Administration

A cardioplegic solution with a high or low concentration of potassium containing tromethamine buffer, citrate-phosphate-dextrose, and nitroglycerin, was mixed with blood in a 1:4 ratio, producing a solution with a pH of 7.6–7.7, calcium of 0.5–0.8 mEq/L, potassium of 10–20 mEq/L, and nitroglycerin of 15–25 μg/L (Table 1). In neonates undergoing circulatory arrest, the citrate-phosphate-dextrose dose was either reduced or eliminated. A high potassium solution, 30 cc/kg, at 4°C and 120 mmHg mean pressure was initially administered, followed by subsequent doses of low potassium cold blood cardioplegia every 20 minutes at 15 cc/kg and 80 mmHg mean pressure. A final dose of warm blood cardioplegia at 37°C and 50 mmHg mean pressure was given. If the heart was felt to have sustained significant ischemic injury, a warm last dose of cardioplegia enriched with

glutamate and aspartate was given. Ventricular distension was carefully avoided, as we have found that pressures of 120 torr resulted in significant injury to the neonatal ventricle.

Results

The overall early (<30 days) operative mortality in this series was 7.1% (20/280) with 60% (12/20) of deaths due to cardiac failure. Of the 12 deaths, two were due to coronary arterial problems, including injury to the right coronary artery in a reoperation for the Fontan procedure and difficulties with an anomalous left anterior descending artery in repair of tetralogy of Fallot. Three of the deaths were in patients undergoing the arterial switch procedure in whom problems with the coronary arteries may have played a role. This gave seven patients (35%) in whom isolated myocardial dysfunction was the cause of death. The operative mortality of the different operations was 10.9% (10/92) for the Fontan procedure, 3.9% (3/76) for Senning's operation, 15% (3/20) for arterial switch procedures, and 4.3% (4/92) for repair of tetralogy of Fallot. Of the patients, 82.1% had excellent postoperative hemodynamic function as determined by measurements of cardiac function and peripheral perfusion.

Variables Not Associated with Increased Mortality by Univariate Analysis

Variables not associated with increased mortality (p > 0.10) by univariate analysis included the age of the patient and preoperative use of digoxin, intraoperative or postoperative rhythm, the length of the period of circulatory arrest, use of intraoperative or postoperative low dose inotropes, or the use of warm blood cardioplegic reperfusate.

Table 1

UCLA Blood Cardioplegia

Pediatric-unmodified	Final solution
500 ml D5.25 NS	$K = 10$–20 mEq/L
50 cc CPD	$Na = 115$ mEq/L
200 cc THAM	$Cl = 100$–105 mEq/L
30–60 mEq KCl	$Ca^{++} = 0.5$–0.8 mM/L
45–100 µg/L NTG	$Osm = 305$–315 mOsm/kg
	$pH = 7.6$–7.7
	$NTG = 15$–25 µg/L

Mixed with blood in 1:4
  ratio

Pediatric modified
Addition of 250 cc .23 molar glutamate
                          .23 molar aspartate

Circulatory arrest
500 cc NS
45 mEq KCl
200 cc THAM
No CPD

NS, normal saline; CPD, citrate-phosphate-dextrose; THAM, tromethamine buffer; NTG, nitroglycerin.

Table 2

Independent Risk Factors by Multivariate Analysis[a]

Risk factor	Logistic coefficient (± SD)	% Mortality
Preop		
Diagnosis of PAIVS	5.1 ± 1.8	28.6%
Inotropes	3.7 ± 1.8	42.9% (6.2%)[b]
Intraop		
Hypotension	3.0 ± 1.0	38.9% (5.0%)
Postop		
Hypotension	5.0 ± 1.5	36.0% (0.9%)
CHF	3.0 ± 1.1	40.0% (4.6%)
Low cardiac output	0.3 ± 1.0	42.5% (1.2%)
High RAP	0.8 ± 0.04	

[a] $p < 0.01$.
[b] Percent mortality in patients without variable.
PAIVS, pulmonary atresia with intact ventricular septum; CHF, congestive heart failure; RAP, right atrial pressure.

Variables Associated with Increased Mortality Using Multivariate Analysis (Table 2)

Those risk factors identified by multivariate analysis to be independently associated with mortality (and their relative scores where 0 is no risk) were the diagnosis of pulmonary atresia (5.1 ± 1.8); the use of inotropes (3.7 ± 1.8); intraoperative hypotension (3.0 ± 1.0); postoperative hypotension (5.0 ± 1.5); congestive heart failure (3.0 ± 1.0); low cardiac output (3.0 ± 1.0); and high right atrial pressures (0.08 ± 0.04). Using these nine variables, 80% (16/20) deaths and 96.9% (251/259) of survivals were correctly predicted.

Discussion

In contrast to previous studies,[1,7] the age of our patients was not associated with increased risk, perhaps due to recent advances in pre- and postoperative intensive care, improved understanding and treatment of specific congenital anomalies, and improved techniques for myocardial protection. Although an unstable preoperative condition was associated with increased risk on univariate analysis, it was not found to be an independent risk factor when evaluated by multivariate analysis. Prolonged periods of cross-clamping, initially identified as a risk factor for mortality by univariate analysis, also failed to emerge as an independent risk factor on subsequent multivariate analysis. Low dosages of inotropes, given both intraoperatively and in the immediate postoperative period, were also not associated with increased risk. Postoperative hypotension, congestive heart failure, low cardiac output, and high right atrial pressures were all independently associated with increased mortality. Low output of urine, bleeding, pleural effusion, and prolonged toe temperature time, which were initially identified as

univariate risk factors, were not found to be independent risk factors after multivariate analysis. Finally, the use of inotropes in medium to high doses also did not emerge as an independent risk factor.

The overall mortality in our study was 7.1% (20/280). Of the deaths, 35% (7/20) were due to isolated myocardial dysfunction. The identification of the use of inotropes preoperatively as a significant risk factor for mortality indicates the importance of the preoperative status of the patient. Of these patients, 16.1% and 7.1% required inotropes given in medium and high doses postoperatively. These results, and the fact that the period of cross-clamping was not a predictor for increased mortality, suggest that, although cold blood cardioplegia provides excellent myocardial protection in the majority of patients, it has not eliminated myocardial dysfunction as a cause of postoperative mortality.

References

1. Kirklin JD, Blackstone EH, Kirklin JW, et al. Intracardiac surgery in infants under age 3 months: Incremental risk factors for hospital mortality. Am J Cardiol 1981;48:500–6.
2. Bull C, Cooper J, Stark J. Cardioplegic protection of the child's heart. J Thorac Cardiovasc Surg 1984;88:287–93
3. Roe BR, Hutchinson JC, Fishman NH, et al. Limits of myocardial protection with potassium cardioplegia. Ann Thorac Surg 1978; 26:507–14.
4. Katz NM, Kirklin JW, Pacifico AD. Concepts and practices in surgery for total anomalous pulmonary venous connection. Ann Thorac Surg 1978;25:479–87.
5. Alfieri O, Blackstone E, Kirklin J, et al. Surgical treatment of tetralogy of Fallot with pulmonary atresia. J Thorac Cardiovasc Surg 1978; 76:321–34.
6. Crawford FA, Barnes TY, Heath BJ. Potassium-induced cardioplegia in patients undergoing correction of congenital heart defects. Chest 1980;72:316–20.
7. Castaneda AR, Lamberti J, Sade RM, et al. Open-heart surgery during the first three months of life. J Thorac Cardiovasc Surg 1974;68:719–31.

Clinical Experience with the HTK Cardioplegic Solution for the Correction of Congenital Heart Defects

H. Korb, A. Borowski, M. M. Gebhard, A. Hoeft, and E. R. de Vivie

Introduction

It is now generally accepted that myocardial protection by cardioplegia is an inevitable prerequisite for any complex and long-lasting cardiac surgical intervention. Compared to adult hearts, however, a differential susceptibility to ischemic injury has been suggested for the infant hearts.[1] It has even been suggested, recently, that about half the hospital deaths in children after pediatric cardiac surgery can be attributed to inadequate myocardial protection.[2] The cardioplegic solutions currently in widespread clinical use are based essentially on three ionic principles. The first is to increase the concentration of extracellular myocardial potassium as, for example, in the cardioplegic solution promoted by Kirklin. The second is to increase the extracellular myocardial concentration of ionized magnesium, as in the St. Thomas' cardioplegic solution in which it is supplemented by the local anesthetic drug procaine. The third principle is simultaneously to reduce the extracellular myocardial concentration of sodium and ionized calcium to values corresponding to those found in the cytoplasm, as in the Bretschneider HTK cardioplegic solutions.

Experimental comparison of these three principles has demonstrated that the reduction of extracellular sodium and ionized calcium is the superior method for myocardial protection when it is combined with the highest possible artificial buffering of the myocardial extracellular compartment by supplementing the osmotic margin of the solution with the buffer system histidine/histidine-HCl. This is realized in the Bretschneider HTK solution which has the following formula (mmol/L): 15 sodium chloride, 4 magnesium chloride, 180 histidine, 18 histidine-HCl, 2 tryptophan, 1 K-ketoglutarate, 30 mannitol. The pH is 7.1 at 25°C; osmolality is 314 mosmol/kg. The solution is prepared by Dr. F. Kohler Chemie, Alsbach/Bergstrasse, West Germany.[3]

When given in the dog heart, in single as well as multiple doses and at identical

231

Table 1

Duration of Reperfusion Times Necessary for Postoperative
Functional Stability

Groups (n = 361)	Ischemic time $\bar{x}$	Reperfusion time $\bar{x}$ (range)	Relation rep/isch time
Up to 60 min (n = 155; 43%)	42 min	23 min (5–68)	1:0.54
60–90 min (n = 114; 31%)	78 min	37 min (5–79)	1:0.47
90–120 min (n = 55; 15%)	101 min	38 min (10–85)	1:0.37
120–150 min (n = 26; 7%)	132 min	40 min (10–78)	1:0.30
150–220 min (n = 11; 3%)	173 min	51 min (19–89)	1:0.29

rep, reperfusion; isch, ischemic.

temperatures, the HTK solution prolongs the ischemia tolerance by a factor of 5 or 6 in comparison to aortic cross-clamping provided by the low-buffered solutions of Kirklin or St Thomas'. In comparison to a histidine-free, low sodium and low calcium solution, tolerance is increased by a factor of 2.[4–6]

Based on these convincing experimental results, we started to use the HTK cardioplegic solution for myocardial protection in pediatric cardiac surgery. In this article, we describe our clinical experience in terms of the duration of time of reperfusion and the number of defibrillations required to achieve stable postoperative function and electrical activity.

Patients Studied

From January 1985 to January 1988, a total of 361 patients (222 males and 139 females) underwent correction of congenital heart defects on cardiopulmonary bypass. The spectrum covered practically the whole range of congenital malformations, ranging from simple closure of an atrial septal defect to the switch procedure for complete transposition. Of the patients, 102 were aged less than 1 year, 75 between 1 and 3 years, 57 between 3 and 5 years, and 127 were older than 5. The mean age at operation was 5.4 years.

Operative Procedures

After lowering the body temperature to between 20 to 25°C and applying topical cooling to the heart, 30 ml/kg body weight of the 4°C cold cardioplegic solution was infused (by gravity in 83% of the cases and in 17% by means of a pressure and volume controlled roller-pump). Care was taken that perfusion was maintained for at least 5 minutes for optimal equilibration of the histidine buffer in the extracellular space. The maximal initial perfusion pressure was 60 mmHg. Diastolic arrest of the heart occurred after about 21 seconds without prior ventricular fibrillation.

Results

We selected five groups on the basis of the period of ischemia. One hundred fifty-

Table 2

Number of Defibrillations Necessary for Postoperative Electrical Stability

Group (n = 361)	Defibrillation (12.5/25 Watts)				
	1	2	3	4	Total
Up to 60 min (n = 155; 43%)	34 (21.9%)	9 (5.8%)	7 (4.%)	6 (3.8%)	56 (36.1%)
60–90 min (n = 114; 31%)	20 (17.5%)	8 (7.0%)	4 (3.5%)	6 (5.2%)	38 (33.3%)
90–120 min (n = 55; 15%)	10 (18.1%)	2 (3.6%)	1 (1.8%)	5 (9.0%)	19 (34.5%)
120–150 min (n = 26; 7%)	3 (11.5%)	2 (7.6%)	—	—	5 (19.2%)
150–220 min (n = 11; 3%)	4 (36.3%)	—	1 (9.0%)	—	5 (45.4%)
Total					123 (33.7%)

five patients (43%) had less than 60 minutes of ischemia. In 114 patients (31%), ischemia lasted between 60 and 90 minutes, and in 55 patients the ischemia time was from 90 to 120 minutes (15%). In 26 patients, ischemia continued for between 120 and 150 minutes (7%), while in the remaining 11 patients ischemia lasted for between 150 and 220 minutes (3%) (Table 1). All hearts recovered, with proportionally increasing periods of reperfusion of 23, 37, 38, 40, and 51 minutes for the corresponding periods of ischemic arrest. No intraoperative cardiac pump failure occurred, and all children could be weaned from cardiopulmonary bypass.

The data demonstrate that the surgical procedure could be performed in the majority of cases within a period of ischemia lasting up to 120 minutes. In at least 10% of the children, however, the period of ischemia lasted longer than 2 hours with, in 11 children, an ischemic time of more than 150 minutes being required. This is far beyond the resuscitation time which can theoretically be achieved with either the solutions advocated by Kirklin or the St. Thomas' group. Even in patients with prolonged periods of ischemia, the hearts recovered functionally with average periods of reperfusion

of 40 and 51 minutes, respectively. It is remarkable that there is no close correlation between the periods of ischemia and reperfusion. Indeed, in the patients undergoing ischemia for times between 60 and 150 minutes, the periods of reperfusion were nearly identical.

The number of defibrillations necessary postoperatively to achieve electrical stability is shown in Table 2. The onset of rhythmic myocardial activity occurred spontaneously in 70% of all the children. Electrical stability was reached with only one defibrillation in 21% of those undergoing ischemia for less than 1 hour, in 17% of those with from 60 to 90 minutes of ischemia, in 19% of those with 90 to 120 minutes ischemia, in 12% of those with ischemia lasting between 120 and 150 minutes, and in 35% of those with ischemia of more than 150 minutes. Only 1 of 10 patients needed more than one electrical shock. Considering that, in the latter cases, the average core temperature was about 30°C while rewarming was still in progress, the data give strong evidence for an excellent electrophysiological outcome even after long-lasting periods of ischemia.

Discussion

Our clinical results demonstrate conclusively that the use of the Bretschneider HTK cardioplegic solution provides adequate myocardial protection in pediatric cardiac surgery. It guarantees a short postischemic recovery period for functional and electrical stability even when correcting complex malformations requiring long periods in the operating room.

References

1. Yano Y, Braimbridge MV, Hearse DJ. Protection of the pediatric myocardium. Differential susceptibility to ischemic injury of the neonatal rat heart. J Thorac Cardiovasc Surg 1987;94:887–96.

2. Bull C, Cooper J, Stark J. Cardioplegic protection of the child's heart. J Thorac Cardiovasc Surg 1984;88:287–93.

3. Gebhard MM, Bretschneider HJ, Gersing E, Schnabel P. Bretschneider's histidine-buffered cardioplegic solution: Concept, application and efficiency. In: Roberts A (ed), Myocardial Protection in Cardiac Surgery. New York, Marcel Dekker, 1987, pp 95–107.

4. Schnabel P, Gebhard MM, Pomykaj T, et al. Myocardial protection: Left ventricular ultrastructure after different forms of cardiac arrest. Thorac Cardiovasc Surg 1987;35:148–56.

5. Gebhard MM, Preusse CJ, Schnabel P, Bretschneider HJ. Different effects of cardioplegic solution HTK during single or intermittent administration. Thorac Cardiovasc Surg 1984;32:271–6.

6. Gebhard MM, Gersing E, Brockhoff CJ, et al. Impedance spectroscopy: A method for surveillance of ischemia tolerance to the heart. Thorac Cardiovasc Surg 1987;35:26–32.

VII

Miscellaneous

7.1

Introduction

G. Crupi and R. H. Anderson

This, the final section of our volume, is made up of those articles which did not conveniently fit into any of our other sections. Its title of "miscellaneous" should not detract from the important contents of the various sections. Some have been grouped together with a theme, that of obstruction of the aortic outflow tract at either valvar, subvalvar, or supravalvar level. Thereafter, the conditions discussed range from His bundle tachycardia occurring in the postoperative period to the morphological features of hearts with isomerism of their atrial appendages and visceral heterotaxy.

The Surgical Treatment of Critical Congenital Valvar Aortic Stenosis
Results Up to Twenty-Five Years After Surgery

J. Ostermeyer, D. Horstkotte, W. Bircks, and F. Loogen

Introduction

Aortic valvar stenosis is one of the most frequent congenital cardiovascular malformations. The natural history of these patients is influenced by the site of stenosis, its severity at birth, the degree of left ventricular dysfunction, the presence of associated cardiovascular lesions, and a variety of other parameters and variables.[1-4] In patients with significant (or even critical) obstruction and severe clinical symptoms, a surgical intervention has to be performed for prognostic reasons.

Material and Methods

Between 1960 and 1983, 133 patients underwent surgery for relief of critical congenital valvar stenoses. Primary valvar replacement was performed in 8 of these (6%) in whom repair was considered not feasible. Of the remaining 125 patients who had aortic valve commissurotomy, 3 (2.4%) were lost for follow-up. A total of 122 patients, 71 male and 51 female, were available for long-term follow-up which totalled more than 19,500 months.

The mean age at the initial operation was 12.7 ± 2 years. Fourteen patients (11.5%) underwent surgery within the first year of life, and a total of 56 patients (45.9%) required operation within their first decade.

The mean systolic transvalvar pressure gradient was 92 ± 43 mmHg. The most frequent preoperative symptoms were dyspnea, syncope or fatigue, signs of congestive heart failure, failure to grow, and chest pain. At least one of these symptoms was present in more than 50% of the patients.

Hospital mortality was higher than 22% in those patients operated before 1965. Between 1965 and 1969, the operative mortality decreased to 14%, and in the early 1970s it fell to approximately 11%. Between 1975 and 1980, mortality was 4.4%. Among those patients operated upon after 1980 there was no perioperative death. There were 15 early postoperative deaths (12.3%). Eight of these patients underwent surgery during the first 3 months of life, and their lesion was associated with other cardiac defects such as endocardial fibroelastosis, coarctation, aortic atresia, sub- or supravalvar aortic stenosis, or persistent patency of the arterial duct.

Other modes of early postoperative death were severe aortic incompetence after valvotomy, sepsis, endocarditis, and respiratory failure.

There were 10 late deaths, 2 occurring at reoperation. The cumulative survival at 25 years after surgery (hospital mortality included) was 76.2%. The mortality was predominantly related to the early postoperative period. Late survival was similar to that of the general population matched for age, sex, and race.

The most frequent complications after the initial operation were bacterial endocarditis and malignant ventricular tachyarrhythmias (including ventricular fibrillation and sudden cardiac death). Pacemaker implantation was performed in three patients with complete postoperative atrioventricular block. Reoperation was required in two patients because of residual mitral lesions.

The cumulative rates of aortic reoperation were 9% at 10 years, 24% at 20 years, and 32% at 25 years after the initial operation. Therefore, more than two-thirds of all patients were free of reoperation after 25 years of follow-up. Complications after reoperation for valve replacement (n = 22) were death (n = 2), severe hemorrhage due to anticoagulation (n = 1), chronic intravascular hemolysis (n = 1), and thromboembolism (n = 1).

Cumulative event-free rates (including deaths, reoperations, endocarditis, thromboembolism, hemorrhage, malignant ventricular tachyarrhythmias, and left heart failure) revealed event-free rates of 72% at 10 years, 47% at 20 years, and 44% at 25 years postoperatively.

Following the initial operation, 60% of the survivors were symptom-free, 34% were symptomatic but not limited in their day-to-day activities, and 6% were symptomatically limited. At the end of 25 years of follow-up, 46% of the survivors were still asymptomatic, 23% were symptomatic but not significantly limited, and 31% had had a reoperation or reported symptoms with limitations in their activities.

Therapeutic Implications

The long-term follow-up herein reported of a substantial number of patients with congenital valvar aortic stenosis shows that aortic valve commissurotomy can be initially performed with a low risk, satisfactory clinical results, and acceptable long-term mortality and morbidity. The long-term prognosis was influenced more significantly by complications such as infective endocarditis and ventricular tachyarrhythmias than by mortality and morbidity related to reoperation or a progression of the valvar stenosis. Further follow-up will show if patients treated with balloon valvoplasty will have comparable long-term results as those undergoing aortic commissurotomy.

References

1. Hossack KF, Neutze JM, Lowe JB, Barratt-Boyes BG. Congenital valvular aortic stenosis. Natural history and assessment for operation. Br Heart J 1980;43:561–7.
2. Braverman IB, Gibson S. The outlook for children with congenital aortic stenosis. Am Heart J 1957;53:452–87.
3. Cohen LS, Friedman WF, Braunwald E. Natural history of mild congenital aortic stenosis. Am J Cardiol 1972;30:1–7.
4. Lambert EC, Wagner HR, and the Natural History of Congenital Heart Disease Study Group. The collaborative study of the natural history of some congenital cardiac defects. Birth Defects 1972;8:57–62.

Open Repair of the Stenotic Aortic Valve in Newborns and Early Infancy

P. Bardos and B. J. Messmer

Introduction

Aortic valve stenosis occurs with an incidence of 3–5.5% in children with congenital heart disease.[1] About 10% of this group develop intractable congestive heart failure soon after birth and need urgent surgical intervention.[2,3]

Two types of basic interventions are used; closed transventricular commissurotomy[4] or open commissurotomy of the stenotic valves either using normothermia or inflow occlusion with moderate hypothermia.[5] Extracorporeal circulation with deep hypothermia and circulatory arrest is a further option.[6] The surgical procedure generally involves splitting of the fused commissures without opening a rudimentary commissure (if present). Morphologically, the subcommissural tissue represents a part of the stenosis and should also be removed, as should any myxoid deformation or thickened fibrous tissue attached to the leaflets of the valve. We believe that excision should be as complete as possible. To be efficient, this technique needs a bloodless operating field. In an 8-year period, 24 consecutive newborns (20 boys and 4 girls) with an age of 1.0 ± 1.0 months (ranging 2 days to 3.4 months) and weights of 3,730 ± 760 g under-

went open repair of critical aortic stenosis. They form the basis of this report.

Case Material

Isolated valvar stenosis was present in 13 cases (54%), while 11 patients (46%) had associated lesions (Table 1). Five children (20%) had severe deformations of the mitral valve. Two of these patients needed replacement of the valve because of persistent mitral insufficiency 6 and 10 weeks, respectively, after the first operation. In three cases, reconstruction of the mitral valve was carried out. Five children died in hospital (20%). Two of them died because of persistent left ventricular failure. Another one with hypoplastic left ventricle, a severe parachute deformity of the mitral valve, and endocardial fibroelastosis died 20 days after the operation. A further patient died because of persistent mitral insufficiency. The fifth child underwent successful replacement of the mitral valve but died 2 months later because of thrombosis of the prosthesis. For the whole group, the period of aortic cross-clamping was 36 ± 12 minutes.

Emergency operations were necessary in nine infants. Early mortality was not sig-

Table 1

Associated Defects

	Patients	%
Patency of the arterial duct	9	37
Mitral valve disease	5	20
Subaortic stenosis	3	12
Atrial septal defect	3	12
Coarctation	1	4

nificantly affected by the period of aortic cross-clamping, urgency of surgery, or age. Associated disease of the mitral valve was the only risk factor for mortality.

Seven patients underwent reoperation (Table 2). Two of these had replacement of their mitral valves early after initial operation because of persistent mitral insufficiency. Two infants needed a second commissurotomy of the stenotic aortic valve after 1 and 3 years, respectively. One child required replacement of a failed bioprosthesis in mitral position. Subaortic stenosis associated with mitral insufficiency and coarctation were also indications for reo-

Table 2

Reoperations

	No.
Mitral insufficiency	2
Aortic restenosis	2
Subaortic stenosis and mitral insufficiency	1
Mitral prosthetic dysfunction	1
Coarctation	1

peration in one case each. The actuarial survival after 5 years is 67%.

One child died 5 months after initial surgery, and he also had severe valvar and subvalvar stenosis. The left ventricular shortening fraction which was estimated by echocardiography in 14 patients always showed normal contractility after the operation.

Discussion

Open repair of the stenotic aortic valve in neonates and infants is a lifesaving operation with both immediate and long-term benefits. Associated disease of the mitral valve remains the most important risk factor for increased early and late mortality and morbidity.

References

1. Nadas AS, Fyler DC. Aortic stenosis. Pediatric Cardiology, 3d ed. Philadelphia, W. B. Saunders, 1972, pp 474–94.
2. Campbell M, Kauntze R. Congenital aortic valvular stenosis. Br Heart J 1953;15:179–94.
3. Rowe RD, Freedom RM, Mehrizi G, Bloom A. The Neonate with Congenital Heart Disease, 2nd ed. Philadelphia, W. B. Saunders, 1981, pp 562–71.
4. Trinkle JK, Norton JB, Richardson JD, et al. Closed aortic valvulotomy and simultaneous correction of associated anomalies in infants. J Thorac Cardiovasc Surg 1975;69:758–62.
5. Keane JF, Bernhard WF, Nadas AS. Aortic stenosis surgery in infancy. Circulation 1975; 52:1138–43.
6. Breckenridge IM, Oehlert H, Graham GR, et al. Open heart surgery in the first year of life. J Thorac Cardiovasc Surg 1973;65:58–64.

Discrete Subvalvar Aortic Stenosis
Surgical Approach, Associated Findings, and Late Results

J. Anderson

Introduction

Discrete subvalvar aortic stenosis is often the cause of severe left ventricular outflow tract obstruction. The distinctive feature of this entity is the focal presence of a fibromuscular shelf immediately beneath the uninvolved ventriculo-aortic junction. Diffuse muscular hypertrophy is not present in this entity. Treatment has typically been that of direct excision of the fibromuscular shelf through the aortic root with the addition of a ventricular myotomy or myectomy at the time of the procedure. The risk of morbidity and mortality for this operation is usually low.[1] The reoperation rate, however, has been variable depending on the length of late follow-up. Delayed appearance of discrete subvalvar aortic stenosis following the repair of a separate cardiovascular defect has also been described.[2,3] Discovery of other separate obstructive lesions of the left ventricular outflow tract at the time of resection of the discrete subvalvar stenotic lesion has also contributed to recurrence of obstruction necessitating reoperation.

Description

From 1974 through 1988, 31 patients were diagnosed as having severe left ventricular outflow tract obstruction due to discrete subvalvar aortic stenosis. Of the 31 patients, 12 (39%) had no other cardiac defects. Nineteen patients (61%) presented with previously repaired or concomitant associated cardiovascular abnormalities. Within those with isolated stenosis, 9 patients had undergone previous repair of aortic coarctation (3 had also spontaneous closure of a ventricular septal defect). Four patients required open valvotomy, and one patient, closed transventricular valvotomy for aortic valvar stenosis. Two patients had previously undergone repair of complete atrioventricular septal defect and one patient had undergone repair of an ostium primum atrial septal defect with closure of the "cleft" in the left atrioventricular valve. Ligation of a patent arterial duct had been performed in two patients. A total of six patients had spontaneous closure of a ventricular septal defect. Several patients in this series had multiple congenital anomalies. Shone's

242

syndrome and congenital rubella syndrome was present in two patients each. Noonan's syndrome, Vater's syndrome, and Trisomy 18 were each present in a single patient. Three patients had Trisomy 21.

The mean age of surgery was 8 years for the entire group (range 6 months to 22 years). For those with isolated stenosis, the mean age was 11.4 years. The mean age was 4.7 years for those with associated lesions. Mean weight for the total group was 24.7 kg (range 4.5 kg to 84 kg), 43.3 kg for those with isolated stenosis, and 13.7 kg for those with associated lesions.

Methods

Surgical repair with excision of the fibromuscular shelf was electively performed in all patients. When the obstructive lesion extended on to the anterior (aortic) leaflet of the mitral valve, it was carefully shaved so as to avoid injury to the leaflet. A myotomy was placed in the ventricular septum immediately beneath the commissural junction of the left and right coronary leaflets (Fig. 1). Repair of a malformed aortic valve was required in 8 patients. Valvotomy was performed in 3 patients with a three-leaflet valve and in 1 with a four-leaflet valve. A valvoplasty for a prolapsing leaflet was required in the remaining 4 patients, 2 of these having a bicuspid valve. A three-leaflet aortic valve was present in 23 patients (74%), and a bicuspid aortic valve in 5 (16%). The remaining 3 patients had either a four-leaflet or a dysplastic/unclassified valve.

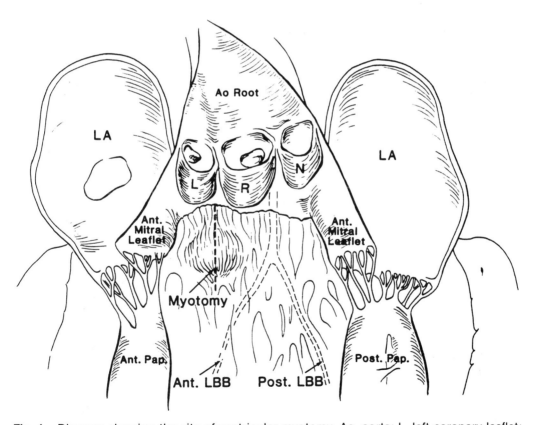

Fig. 1. Diagram showing the site of ventricular myotomy. Ao, aorta; L, left coronary leaflet; R, right coronary leaflet; N, noncoronary leaflet; LA, left atrium; Ant. Pap., anterior papillary muscle; Post. Pap., posterior papillary muscle; Ant. LBB, anterior left bundle branch; Post. LBB, posterior left bundle branch.

Table 1

Discrete Subvalvar Aortic Stenosis: Reoperation for Late Left Ventricular Outflow Tract Obstruction

Diagnosis	Initial procedure	Aortic valve architecture	Reop. interval (months)	Recurrent gradient (mmHg)	Reop. procedure
1. DSS, SC VSD	MR & My	3 leaflet	35	68	MR & My
2. DSS, SC VSD, COA repair	MR & My	3 leaflet	81	54	MR & My
3. DSS	MR & My	3 leaflet	60	80	MR & My
4. DSS, AVS, PDA Lig., SC VSD	MR & My Aortic valvotomy	Bicuspid	50	75	MR & My
5. DSS, AVS	MR & My Aortic valvotomy	3 leaflet	72	128	MR & My
6. DSS, COA repair	MR & My	Bicuspid	14	80	LV-AO valved conduit
7. DSS, AVS, transv.	MR & My Aortic valvoplasty	Bicuspid	69	100	LV-AO valved conduit
8. DSS, COA repair, SC VSD	MR & My	3 leaflet	73	98	MVR for endocarditis

DSS, discrete subaortic stenosis; SC VSD, spontaneous closure VSD; COA, coarctation; AVS, aortic valve stenosis; MR & My, membrane resection & myotomy; PDA Lig., ligation of patent arterial duct; LV-AO, left ventricle to aorta.

Results

Two patients with associated cardiac lesions died postoperatively. Age at surgery was 6 months and 10 months, respectively. Both patients had undergone ligation of a patent arterial duct and repair of aortic coarctation earlier in life. Both also had important deformities of their mitral valve, and died early postoperatively of low cardiac output state and pulmonary venous hypertension.

One patient developed complete heart block following resection of the subaortic shelf at reoperation and required insertion of a permanent pacemaker. Other postoperative complications included reexploration for bleeding (one case), pneumothorax requiring chest tube drainage in one patient, superficial wound infection (one case), and postpericardiotomy syndrome requiring aspirin therapy in two cases and steroid therapy in one.

Complete follow-up is available in all patients for a mean of 62 months, ranging from 4 months to 136 months. Echo-Doppler evaluation of the outflow tract was performed in 22 of the 29 patients (76%), late postoperatively, at a mean of 48.3 months. This showed a mean peak systolic gradient of 23.4 mmHg, ranging from 0 to 70 mmHg.

Doppler evaluation of the function of the aortic valve revealed most patients to have either trivial or mild aortic valvar regurgitation. A moderate regurgitation was present in only three patients. Eighty-six percent of the patients were free of reoperation at 60 months of follow-up. Late reoperation for recurrent left ventricular outflow tract obstruction (Table 1) was required in seven (24%) patients. Three of them had initially had isolated stenosis (25%), while an associated cardiac lesion (23.5%) was present in the remaining four. In two of the latter patients the reoperation required insertion of an apical conduit between the left ventricle and the aorta. Both of these patients have a bicuspid aortic valve and a small ventriculo-aortic junction. A separate patient with associated lesions required reoperation at 73 months for replacement of the mitral valve due to endocarditis. This patient also had recurrent left ventricular outflow tract obstruction at the time of surgery, which was relieved by replacement of the valve. The mean interval from the initial operation was 57 months, ranging from 14 to 81 months. There was only one late death which occurred (3.4%) 90 months postoperatively due to end-stage left ventricular failure following a late episode of viral myocarditis.

Discussion

Although the surgical treatment for discrete subvalvar aortic stenosis has been well described and is quite standardized, recurrence remains a serious problem.[4,5] Two-thirds of our patients had other associated cardiac anomalies which had either been previously repaired elsewhere or were present at the time of resection of the subvalvar stenotic lesion. All our patients with a previous history of ventricular septal defect presented at the time of surgery with spontaneous closure of that defect.[6-8] These patients (4 of 6) were at a high risk for the development of recurrent discrete subvalvar aortic stenosis. The reoperation rate was also high in the presence of a bicuspid aortic valve (3 of 5) or of a previous repair of aortic coarctation (3 of 7).

The subvalvar obstructive shelf may be less localized on rare occasions, while the stenotic area can also extend for a various length in the subaortic region (tunnel subaortic stenosis). Two of our patients with this type of obstruction required reopera-

tion following initial resection of the subaortic shelf and ventricular myotomy. Relief of the obstruction to the left ventricular outflow tract in those patients who also had a bicuspid aortic valve and a small ventriculo-aortic junction was achieved by placement of a conduit from the left ventricular apex to the aorta.

Five of the 31 patients in this series had aortic valvar stenosis. One patient had previously undergone closed transventricular aortic valvotomy, while the remaining four patients required valvotomy at the time of surgery. The development of discrete subaortic stenosis following repair of complete atrioventricular septal defect or closure of the "cleft" in the left atrioventricular valve had been previously described[2,3] and occurred in three patients in our series. Mitral valvar stenosis in two patients and a parachute mitral valve in one patient were perhaps the most severe associated anomalies observed. The two patients with mitral valvar stenosis, the youngest in our series, were also those who died early postoperatively. Aortic incompetence is also frequently associated with discrete subvalvar aortic stenosis.[9,10] Four patients in this series required aortic valvoplasty for repair of severe prolapse of the leaflets of the aortic valve at the time of subaortic membrane resection. These were the only instances of severe aortic valvar regurgitation observed in our series. Additional late follow-up with echo-Doppler evaluation of the left ventricular outflow tract showed that the majority of our patients have only a trivial regurgitation across the aortic valve.

In summary, satisfactory early and late relief of left ventricular outflow tract obstruction due to discrete subvalvar obstruction can be obtained by resection of the obstructive shelf combined with ventricular myotomy. Operative mortality is low and is related to severe associated cardiovascular defects and younger age at initial surgery. There is a greater incidence of recurrent left ventricular outflow tract obstruction in patients with a history of spontaneous closure of ventricular septal defect, presence of a bicuspid aortic valve, or previous repair of aortic coarctation. Late follow-up reveals the majority of patients to have good aortic valvar function.

References

1. Champsaur G, Trusler GA, Mustard WT. Congenital discrete subvalvar aortic stenosis. Surgical experience and long-term follow-up in 20 pediatric patients. Br Heart J 1973;35:443–6.
2. Ben-Shachar G, Moller JH, Castaneda-Zuniga W, Edwards JE. Signs of membranous subaortic stenosis appearing after correction of persistent common atrioventricular canal. Am J Cardiol 1981;48:340–4.
3. Gow RM, Freedom RM, Williams WG, et al. Coarctation of the aorta or subaortic stenosis with atrioventricular septal defect. Am J Cardiol 1984;53:1421–8.
4. Katz NM, Buckley MJ, Liberthson RR. Discrete membranous subaortic stenosis. Report of 31 patients, review of the literature, and delineation of management. Circulation 1977; 56:1034–8.
5. Newfeld EA, Muster AJ, Paul MH, et al. Discrete subvalvular aortic stenosis in childhood. Study of 51 patients. Am J Cardiol 1976;38:53–61.
6. Chung KJ, Fulton DR, Kriedberg MB, et al. Combined discrete subaortic stenosis and ventricular septal defect in infants and children. Am J Cardiol 1984;53:1429–32.
7. Lauer RM, Du Shane JW, Edwards JE. Obstruction of left ventricular outlet in association with ventricular septal defect. Circulation 1960;22:110–25.
8. Manouguian S, Kirckhoff PG, Koncz J, et al. Ventricular septal defect associated with fibrous subvalvar aortic stenosis: Diagnostic problems and surgical management. Thoraxchirurgie 1975;23:444–7.
9. Kelly DT, Wulfsberg BA, Rowe RD. Discrete subaortic stenosis. Circulation 1972;46:309–22.
10. Feigl A, Feigl D, Lucas RV Jr, Edwards JE. Involvement of the aortic valve cusps in discrete subaortic stenosis. Pediatr Cardiol 1984;5:185–9.

Late Results After Resection of Discrete and Tunnel Subaortic Stenosis

A. Mazzucco, G. Stellin, U. Bortolotti, E. Tiso, M. Rubino, G. Faggian, A. Milano, and V. Gallucci

Introduction

Satisfactory relief of fixed subaortic stenosis can be accomplished with a very low surgical risk.[1-3] The effect of a simultaneous myotomy in association with the excision of the obstructing fibrous tissue remains uncertain. Furthermore, very little is known about the long-term fate of the incompetent aortic valve which may progressively worsen if the stenosis is not resected.

In order to provide further data on these issues, and to assess the long-term surgical results, we have reviewed our experience with resection of subaortic stenosis.

Material and Methods

From May 1969 through December 1987, 84 consecutive patients (51 male and 33 female) underwent surgical resection of subaortic stenosis. Sixty-six of them were under the age of 18 years (range 6 months to 18 years) with a mean age of 12 years. This subgroup forms the basis of the present study (Fig. 1). Excluded were children with hypertrophic cardiomyopathy and complex congenital malformations presenting with a pure muscular subaortic obstruction.

Preoperative Data

Exertional dyspnea was reported preoperatively in 17 children, with palpitation in 8 and fatigue in 5. Eight children complained of syncopal episodes, while three have had chest pain. Aortic valve endocarditis had been reported in 1 patient. The remaining 39 children were asymptomatic.

All the patients underwent a complete cardiac catheterization prior to surgery. This disclosed a peak transaortic pressure gradient of 85 ± 43 mmHg (range 20–205 mmHg). Aortograms showed incompetence of the aortic valve in 45 cases (68%). This was secondary to healed endocarditis in one. In the remainder, it was most likely the result of leaflet injury caused by the turbulence of the bloodstream, due to the subvalvar narrowing. Associated cardiovascular lesions were present in 37 children (56%).

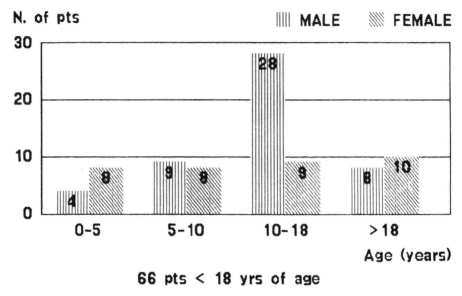

Figure 1. Graphic representation of patient population according to age and sex.

These consisted mostly of obstructive lesions in the left heart, such as aortic valvar stenosis, mitral valvar stenosis, aortic isthmic coarctation, or septal defects.

At surgery, a discrete obstruction of varying thickness was present in 63 cases, while in 3 it was more diffuse, constituting a fibromuscular tunnel. Early in our experience, the subaortic stenosis was excised by sharp resection, and a myotomy with or without myectomy was routinely performed. More recently, since September 1983, the obstruction was removed by blunt resection after finding a plane of cleavage between the fibromuscular ring and the muscular tissue of the left ventricle, much as described by McKay and Ross.[4] Small tendinous cords, usually connecting the obstructive shelf to the aortic and/or mitral valve, were carefully peeled off the endocardium to obtain a complete excision of the entire anomalous tissue.

Results

There were two hospital deaths (3%). These occurred early in our experience, one from intractable ventricular fibrillation in a patient with marked ventricular hypertrophy and preoperative heart failure and the other from low output syndrome in a 3-year-old boy. The latter patient died because of massive mitral regurgitation following a commissurotomy aimed to correct severe stenosis of a dysplastic mitral valve.

Atrioventricular conduction disturbances requiring insertion of a permanent pacemaker occurred perioperatively in two children. Replacement of the aortic valve because of intraoperative injury was needed in one. Low output syndrome occurred in another, successfully treated by prolonged inotropic support. Seven patients underwent concomitant replacement of the aortic valve because it was deformed by associated lesions.

There were two late deaths. One of these occurred suddenly at home after initial resection of a discrete stenosis together with replacement of the mitral valve because of congenital dysplasia. The other died of low output syndrome at reoperation performed 12 years later because of recurrent tunnel subaortic stenosis.

Seven patients required late reopera-

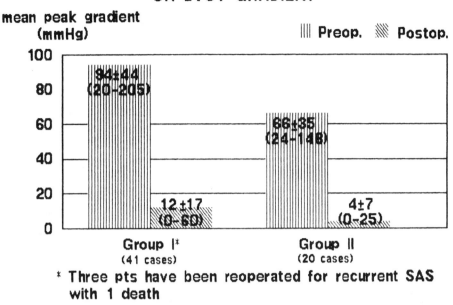

Figure 2. Long-term effect of surgery on the gradient across the left ventricular outflow tract. Graphic representation of the pre- and postoperative gradient of patients treated with two different techniques. Group 1: those undergoing sharp dissection with or without myotomy; Group 2: those undergoing blunt enucleation of the obstructive shelf; LVOT, left ventricular outflow tract; SAS, subaortic stenosis.

tion. This was for recurrent subaortic stenosis in three, recurrent valvar stenosis or regurgitation in three, and mitral regurgitation in one.

Out of sixty-two survivors, 60 children are asymptomatic 3 months to 19 years after surgery (mean 154 months). One patient complains of exertional dyspnea because of recurrent aortic and mitral valve stenosis. The other has signs of moderate to severe valve incompetence, having undergone a valvoplasty of a prolapsing aortic valve leaflet and closure of a subpulmonary ventricular septal defect. He is now scheduled for reoperation.

In order to assess function of the aortic valve late postoperatively and to determine whether resection of the subaortic stenosis had any influence in the progression of the preoperative regurgitation, we have re-evaluated 61 patients, during the follow-up, by means of a cardiac catheterization and/or cross-sectional and Doppler echocardiography. Among 44 children who have not undergone surgical maneuvers on the aortic valve, incompetence remained unchanged in 25, while it decreased from mild to nil in 17 and from moderate to mild in 2.

The subaortic residual gradient was also re-evaluated, showing a similar stepdown in the groups treated with different surgical techniques (Fig. 2).

Discussion

Surgical resection of subaortic stenosis has been generally reported as an effective and safe procedure in relieving obstruction of the left ventricular outflow tract.[1-6] Controversy remains, nonetheless, on which type of surgical technique should be employed to avoid the long-term recurrence of obstruction.[1,5,7] Our data provide the opportunity to compare, in the long range, the results obtained with two different surgical techniques: sharp excision of the obstruction associated with myotomy and/or myectomy versus simple but complete blunt enucleation. From our experience, comparing patients who showed similar preoperative gradients (Fig. 2), it appears that the surgical technique does not influence the reduction of the transaortic pressure gradient. Therefore, we currently favor the enucleation technique which, besides providing satisfactory relief of the obstruction by removing the entirety of the fibrous tissue, most likely eliminates also the potential for recurrence. Furthermore, we believe that routine resection of the underlying hypertrophied left ventricular muscle is unnecessary unless obvious localized septal hypertrophy is identified in the relaxed heart. Indeed, this procedure exposes the patient to an undue risk of injury to the left bundle branch, damage to the leaflets of the aortic and mitral valves, and induces the potential for postoperative left ventricular arrhythmias.

Varying degrees of aortic valvar incompetence are frequently associated with subaortic stenosis.[1-3,5,6] Wright et al.,[2] reporting their results with surgical treatment of subaortic stenosis, observed that valvar incompetence was present in 47% of their patients. According to Kirklin and Barratt-Boyes,[3] trivial or mild valve incompetence is present in almost two-thirds of the patients having subaortic stenosis. In our experience, excluding those patients with associated congenital malformations of the aortic valve, incompetence was observed in 68%. Most probably it results from the jet effect created by the increased velocity of the blood passing through the subvalvar area.[8] In agreement with previous observations,[2,3] the present study indicates that valvar incompetence occurs most likely as a

consequence of an unresected subaortic stenosis and it stops (or disappears) once the obstructing tissue is removed (Fig. 2). Therefore, in accordance with others,[2] we believe that, in order to prevent the onset or the progression of valvar incompetence, early treatment of the lesion is justified, regardless of the magnitude of the pressure gradient across the outflow tract.

Three patients undergoing sharp dissection and none of those having blunt enucleation underwent reoperation because of recurrent subaortic stenosis. Furthermore, 35% of the patients treated by dissection versus 50% of those undergoing blunt enucleation were free from aortic regurgitation at long-term follow-up. Even though the data are too small to reach a statistically significant difference, it is our impression that simple but complete enucleation of the obstructing fibrous shelf produces better long-term results since recurrence is prevented and the integrity of the aortic valve is preserved.

References

1. Cain T, Campbell D, Paton B, Clarke D. Operation for discrete subvalvular aortic stenosis. J Thorac Cardiovasc Surg 1984;87:366–70.
2. Wright GB, Keane JF Nadas AS, et al. Fixed subaortic stenosis in the young: Medical and surgical course in 83 patients. Am J Cardiol 1983;52:830–5.
3. Kirklin JW, Barratt-Boyes BG. Congenital discrete subvalvular aortic stenosis. Cardiac Surgery, New York, John Wiley & Sons, 1986, pp 988–1001.
4. McKay R, Ross DN. Technique for the relief of discrete subaortic stenosis. J Thorac Cardiovasc Surg 1982;84:917–20.
5. Ashraf H, Cotroneo J, Dhar N, et al. Long term results after excision of fixed subaortic stenosis. J Thorac Cardiovasc Surg 1985;90:864–71.
6. Moses RD, Barnhart GR, Jones M. The late prognosis after localized resection for fixed

(discrete and tunnel) left ventricular outflow tract obstruction. J Thorac Cardiovasc Surg 1984;87:410–20.

7. Lavee J, Porat L, Smolinsky A, et al. Myectomy versus myotomy as an adjunct to membranectomy in the surgical repair of discrete and tunnel subaortic stenosis. J Thorac Cardiovasc Surg 1986;92:944–9.

8. Newfeld EA, Muster AJ, Paul MH, et al. Discrete subvalvular aortic stenosis in childhood. Study of 15 patients. Am J Cardiol 1976;38:53–61.

Obstruction of Coronary Flow Due to Hypoplasia of the Left Sinus of Valsalva Subsequent to Repair of Fixed Subaortic Stenosis

J. Mulet, C. Barriuso, C. Mortera, G. Fita, and C. Gomar

Coronary arterial obstruction is well recognized to be associated with supravalvar aortic stenosis[1] and congenital aortic regurgitation.[2] This seems to be caused by hypoplasia of the sinus of Valsalva[3] with adherence of the leaflet to the aortic wall. An abnormal aortic valve is present in 20–25% of patients with fixed subaortic stenosis, but obstruction to coronary arterial flow is rare.[3]

We report here two patients who, after repair of fixed subaortic stenosis, showed signs of left coronary arterial hypoperfusion on discontinuation of cardiopulmonary bypass. The left sinus of Valsalva was hypoplastic in both cases, with only a slitlike opening between an adherent small leaflet and the aortic wall. Adequate left ventricular function was obtained after widening the opening of the aortic sinus.

Case 1

An 8-year-old girl was admitted after two episodes of syncope. She had a powerful left ventricular apex, and a loud ejection murmur was heard at the left sternal edge. Electrocardiography showed left ventricular hypertrophy, and the chest roentgenogram was unremarkable. Echocardiography revealed a typical subaortic shelf, and the gradient measured by Doppler across the obstruction was estimated to be 60 mmHg. No other anomalies were seen. Surgical correction was achieved through a median sternotomy with the aid of cardiopulmonary bypass. Crystalloid cardioplegia and topical cooling were used for myocardial protection. The ascending aorta was opened through a hockey-stick incision, revealing a three-leaflet aortic valve with a hypoplastic left sinus which was only 3 mm long, leaving a very small passage to the orifice of the left coronary artery which was placed far down the wall of the sinus (Fig. 1). Resection of the fibrous tissue under the aortic leaflets was done in the usual fashion. Following routine closure of the aortotomy, the patient could not be weaned off bypass, and repeated attempts with pharmacological support were unsuccessful. The aorta was

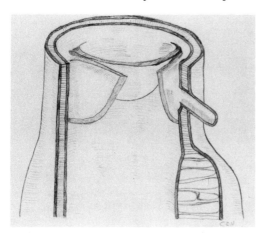

Figure 1. Artist's reconstruction of the surgical findings, emphasizing the short distance between the aortic wall and the free edge of the leaflets.

therefore reopened, the left leaflet was partially detached, and the central portion of its free edge was resected. This maneuver increased the aperture of the sinus, allowing eventually a clear visualization of the left coronary ostium. Cardiopulmonary bypass was then successfully discontinued with the aid of an epinephrine infusion, but the sternal incision could not be closed. Delayed closure was performed on the third postoperative day. Recovery was slow and complicated by a peripheral neuropathy which impaired her gait. Late postoperative echocardiography showed adequate left ventricular function. A subaortic gradient of 30 mmHg was measured by Doppler without signs of aortic regurgitation.

Case 2

A 6-year-old girl was found to have a systolic murmur during a routine physical examination. Chest roentgenogram was normal and electrocardiography showed left ventricular hypertrophy. Cross-sectional echocardiography showed a typical subaortic fibrous shelf with a gradient measured by

Doppler of 70 mmHg which was confirmed by cardiac catheterization. An ascending aortogram demonstrated trivial aortic insufficiency and thickening of the leaflets but no valvar stenosis. A left superior caval vein was also present. Cardiopulmonary bypass and myocardial protection were utilized as described earlier. At surgery, the aortic valve and subvalvar region were exposed: the morphology of the left sinus was similar to case 1 (Fig. 1), but the aortic leaflets were thicker and less pliable. After closure of the aortotomy, the heart was defibrillated, but again bypass could not be discontinued. It was clearly apparent that the left ventricular myocardium was underperfused. The aorta was again cross-clamped and cardioplegia reinfused, complemented with topical cooling. The left leaflet of the aortic valve was treated in the same way as in the first case. Its commissures were partially detached from the aortic wall and the nodule of Arantius was resected. Cardiopulmonary bypass could then be easily disconnected. Recovery was uneventful and, at follow-up after 2 years, the echocardiogram showed a normal left ventricle and a subaortic gradient of 25 mmHg as measured by Doppler.

Comment

Congenital obstruction of the left ventricular outflow tract is a complex anomaly. All its components can participate in the production of the stenosis. Frequently, more than one element causes the obstruction and dynamic obstruction is well recognized, thus explaining why the surgical results are not uniformly good. Coronary arterial ostial obstruction has been found in association with supravalvar stenosis[1] and in a rare case of congenital aortic regurgitation.[2] Harlan and colleagues[3] have stressed the importance of using an extended aortoplasty repair to improve late results when aortic stenosis is complicated by hypoplasia of the left sinus of Valsalva. The configuration they de-

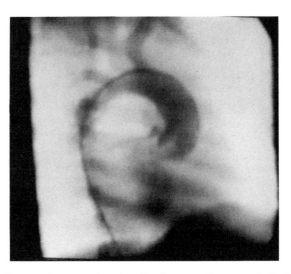

Figure 2. Ascending aortogram showing the long and narrow left sinus of Valsalva.

scribed is similar to one of our two cases, but the stenosis in their cases was located at the level of the aortic leaflets, and all of their 13 patients had bicuspid valves. One of their patients had the "extended aorto-plasty" performed some time after a repair of subaortic stenosis, supposedly without in-traoperative coronary flow obstruction.

It is difficult to explain why the obstruc-tion occurred on cardiopulmonary bypass and did not manifest itself prior to surgery. Closure of the aortic valve, and clearing of the coronary ostia, is facilitated by vortex formation in the aortic sinus. The shape of the sinuses is also important for the mech-anism of valvar closure. During bypass, with arterial return through the ascending aorta, the flow dynamics and the formation of vor-tices are distorted. These changes, in the presence of a slitlike opening of the left sinus, could prevent the blood from reach-ing the coronary arterial orifice.

Thubrikar and colleagues[4] have made studies using fluoroscopy of the aortic root and noted that it increased 15.7% ± 4% in diameter during systole. The tension gen-erated by this increase in diameter could well function like the closing mechanism of a coin-purse. The taut and unelastic free edge of the leaflet would close against the aortic wall under the distention created by the continuous flow from the pump.

The solution proposed for this problem is simple and has proved effective. Extended aortoplasty seemed to us to be too laborious and would prolong dangerously the time of aortic cross-clamping. It is possible that our patients will need replacement of their aor-tic valve in the future but, as stated by Har-lan and colleagues,[3] patients treated by ex-tended aortoplasty may also have to undergo surgery of the aortic valve.

Preoperative identification of this anomaly is essential to assure a successful repair for these patients. Ascending aortog-raphy (Fig. 2) and high resolution cross-sec-tional echocardiography should be planned accordingly.

References

1. Martin MM, Lemer JH, Shafer E, et al. Obstruc-tion to left coronary artery blood flow sec-ondary to obliteration of the coronary ostium in supravalvular aortic stenosis. Ann Thorac Surg 1988;45:16–20.
2. Line DE, Babb JD, Pierce WS. Congenital aortic

valve anomaly. Aortic regurgitation with left coronary artery isolation. J Thorac Cardiovasc Surg 1979;77:533–5.

3. Harlan JL, Clark EB, Doty DB. Congenital aortic stenosis with hypoplasia of the left sinus of Valsalva. Anatomic reconstruction of the aortic root. J Thorac Cardiovasc Surg 1985; 89:288–94.

4. Thubrikar MJ, Nolan SP, Aouad J, Deck JD. Stress sharing between the sinus and leaflets of canine aortic valve. Ann Thorac Surg 1986;42:434–40.

Anastomosis of the Right Internal Mammary Artery with the Right Coronary Artery in an Eight-Year-Old Girl After Correction of a Severe Supravalvar Stenosis of the Ascending Aorta

P. Schupbach, P. Gersbach, I. W. Weber, F. Stoker, and
U. Althaus

Case Report

An 8-year-old Libyan girl was admitted to our center on an emergency basis with dyspnea due to severe heart failure. She was known to have severe supravalvar aortic stenosis with cardiomegaly and was able to walk only 20 meters before the onset of dyspnea.

Echocardiography and cardiac catheterization confirmed cardiomegaly and revealed a very low ejection fraction, left ventricular end-diastolic pressure of 30 mmHg, and a gradient of 80 mmHg between left ventricle and ascending aorta. The angiogram (Fig. 1) showed severe supravalvar aortic stenosis immediately above the origin of the coronary arteries which extended to the level of the brachiocephalic artery. With the exception of anemia, routine preoperative laboratory investigations showed no abnormalities.

With the aid of extracorporeal circulation and temporary circulatory arrest, the ascending aorta was enlarged using a tear-drop shaped Dacron patch. Special attention was directed to the right coronary artery, which arose immediately proximal to the narrowest part at the beginning of the stenotic aortic segment. Patch enlargement was extended into the aortic arch between the brachiocephalic trunk and the left carotid artery. Recovery of the heart after bypass was satisfactory with the need for small doses of dopamine. Severe heart failure with ventricular fibrillation occurred suddenly 1 hour after weaning from the bypass during closure of the chest. The heart was easily resuscitated by direct massage and reestab-

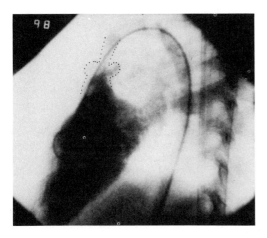

Figure 1. Cineangiogram in the ascending aorta showing severe supravalvar stenosis with an intact right coronary artery.

lishment of bypass. The deterioration was presumed to be due to traction or kinking of the initial segment of the right coronary artery close to its origin from the aortic sinus, following the enlargement of the ascending aorta with concomitant ischemia of its myocardial territory. The right internal mammary artery was, therefore, detached from the chest wall and anastomosed with the right coronary artery. A considerable disproportion was noted between the limited length of the thorax (and internal mammary artery) and the size of the heart as compared to adults. Recovery was more satisfactory after the additional procedure, and digital aortography 14 days following the operation revealed patency of the internal mammary and right coronary arteries with good flow (Fig. 2). The girl was able to run and to climb stairs prior to leaving our hospital.

Comment

Surgical correction of severe supravalvar stenosis of the ascending aorta produced a severe complication, probably due to stretching or kinking of the initial part of the right coronary artery. This resulted in critical ischemia of the myocardium supplied by the right coronary artery which was treated by direct revascularization using a graft of the right internal mammary artery. Similar successful revascularizations of injured or malformed coronary arteries have been described previously in children.[1-4] We noted a proportional shortness of the pedicle of the internal mammary artery due to the shape of the chest and the size and the position of the heart in children.

Kirklin and Barratt-Boyes[5] describe two different incisions for opening the ascending aorta for patch enlargement in patients with supravalvar aortic stenosis. The first is carried down into the noncoronary sinus and the other runs into the right coronary sinus. Both incisions are extended to the right of the orifice of the coronary artery. If the narrowest part of the stenosis is close to the arterial origin, considerable risk exists for injury of the initial segment of the right coronary artery subsequent to enlargement of the stenosis with a patch. The risk of stretching the initial segment of the right coronary artery can be diminished if an incision is se-

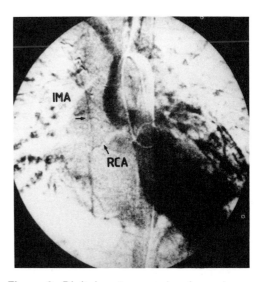

Figure 2. Digital aortogram showing enlargement of the ascending aorta by a patch graft and anastomosis of the internal mammary (IMA) and right coronary (RCA) arteries.

lected which extends into the right coronary sinus on the left of the right coronary artery[6] or, alternatively, if the right coronary artery is carefully dissected. This maneuver, however, may present a greater risk of direct injury to the orifice of the right coronary artery. In our own case, it was not possible to inspect directly the right coronary artery and the aortic valve. Thus, we preferred to open the aorta by cutting into the noncoronary sinus.

References

1. Allen HD, Moller JH, Formanek A, Nicoloff D. Atresia of the proximal left coronary artery associated with supravalvular aortic stenosis. J Thorac Cardiovasc Surg 1974;67:266–71.

2. Fortune RL, Baron PJ, Fitzgerald JW. Atresia of the left main coronary artery: Repair with left internal mammary artery bypass. J Thorac Cardiovasc Surg 1987;94:150–1.

3. Hirose H, Kawashima Y, Nakano S, et al. Long-term results in surgical treatment of children 4 years old or younger with coronary involvement due to Kawasaki disease. Circulation 1986;73(suppl I):77–88.

4. Cooley DA, Duncan JM, Gillette PC, McNamara DG. Reconstruction of coronary artery anomaly in an infant using the internal mammary artery: 10-year follow-up. Pediatr Cardiol 1987;8:257–9.

5. Kirklin JW, Barratt-Boyes BG. Congenital aortic stenosis. In: Kirklin JW, Barratt-Boyes BG (eds), Cardiac Surgery. New York John Wiley & Sons, 1986, pp 1001–7.

6. Stark J, de Leval M. Left ventricular outflow tract obstruction. In: Stark J, de Leval M (eds) Surgery for Congenital Heart Defects. London, New York, Grune & Stratton, 1983, pp 447–9.

Reconstruction of the Right Ventricular Outflow Tract Using Autologous Pericardial Trifoliate Valve Incorporating Construction of Sinuses of Valsalva

I. Chiu, S. Chao, M. Wu, J. Wang, C. Hung, and H. Lue

Introduction

Whether to use a conduit or an artificial valve in the reconstruction of the right ventricular outflow tract remains a problem. Xenograft valves are known to degenerate and inevitably calcify when implanted in children. The homograft also has the problem of calcification, albeit mainly in the aortic wall,[1] but supply of such valves is difficult and inconsistent outside the Western countries. As an alternative, therefore, we have attempted to reconstruct the pulmonary valve inside either the patient's own pulmonary trunk or a pericardial conduit by using autologous pericardium in trifoliate fashion with concomitant formation of the commissures and sinuses of Valsalva. We have now used this approach in our first patient with a good short-term result.

Case Report

A 7-year-old girl weighing 20 kg was admitted for repair of Fallot's tetralogy complicated by so-called absence of the leaflets of the pulmonary valve. Correction was performed using cardiopulmonary bypass with moderate hypothermia. A rectangular shape of pericardium was cleaned as far as possible from fatty tissue and then immersed in 0.6% glutaraldehyde for 5 minutes. This was followed by washing the strip in 5% magnesium chloride dissolved in normal saline. Afterwards, the pericardium was sandwiched in a precut number 20 plastic patchholder and tailored into a trifoliate semilunar pattern (Fig. 1A). The sites of the planned commissures were marked by six separate sutures. The pulmonary trunk was huge, distal to the ventriculo-arterial junction, and was aneurysmally dilated. The

259

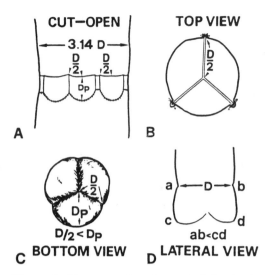

Figure 1. The geometry of an arterial valve is shown in various projections. The diameter is 3.14 times the length (D) of each leaflet. The depth of each leaflet (Dp) is greater than half the circumferential attachment of the leaflet (D/2). The diameter at the level of the commissures (ab) is less than the diameter of the ventriculo-arterial junction (cd).

ventricular septal defect, which was perimembranous and excavating the apical trabecular septum, was repaired using a Teflon patch inserted through the right atrium using a continuous suture. The pulmonary trunk and ventriculo-arterial junction were transected. Neither leaflets of the pulmonary valve nor sinuses of Valsalva were seen. The autologous pericardial patch was sutured onto the ventriculo-arterial junction using a running 5–0 Prolene suture. The stenotic junction was augmented by a transjunctional patch tailored from a Gore-Tex vascular graft, combining the pericardial patch within the suture line. Two commissures were reconstructed initially by burying the rectangular part between the leaflets into the wall of the pulmonary trunk (Fig. 1B). There the edges of the pulmonary trunk and the Gore-Tex patch (Fig. 2) were combined to augment the bulging contour of the anterior sinus of Valsalva. The remainder of the tear-drop shaped transjunctional patch was sutured as usual. The aorta was cross-clamped for 95 minutes during the procedure, after which the heart beat resumed spontaneously. Bypass was discontinued and the pressure within the pulmonary trunk was measured at 35/23 mmHg, and the $P_{RV/LV}$ ratio was 0.6. This was considered as a satisfactory result. The child was extubated the following morning and the postoperative recovery was uneventful. At follow-up, echocardiography and cardiac catheterization revealed a mild residual gradient of 14 mmHg across the new ventriculo-arterial junction. The newly constructed pulmonary valve was pliable without evidence of either regurgitation or stenosis. The child was discharged on a dosage of 200 mg aspirin daily. Subsequent follow-up using color Doppler revealed a competent pulmonary valve 7.5 months after operation, and the patient continued to be well at 11 months' follow-up.

Discussion

Usually, when the semilunar arterial valves are depicted in textbooks,[2] the depth of each leaflet appears to be shorter than or equal to half the length of the coapting part of each leaflet. In contrast, if one reconstructs the opened great vessel and inspects the bulging portion of the sinus of Valsalva from below (Fig. 1), it makes sense that nature creates the valve and sinus of Valsalva such that the depth is not shorter than half the length of each leaflet. In other words, the suspended part at the commissure is narrower than the bulging bottom portion (Fig. 1D). In this way, the ventriculo-arterial valve can be competent without having tendinous cords. Based on these observations, we found that anchoring the commissure as described, along with reconstruction of the sinus of Valsalva, makes the arterial valve consistently competent.

The essential role of the sinus of Valsalva in the normal mechanism of closure of the aortic valve has been shown by Bellhouse and Bellhouse[3] and has been applied

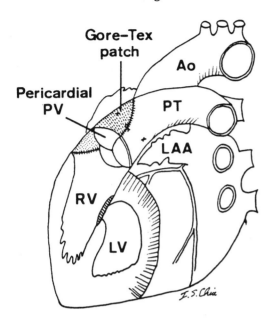

Figure 2. A diagrammatic representation of the completed procedures. Ao, aorta; PT, pulmonary trunk; LAA, left atrial appendage; PV, pulmonary valve; RV, right ventricle; LV, left ventricle.

to monocusp reconstruction of the right ventricular outflow tract in seven patients.[4] Our method of reconstruction is similar to that of Batista et al.,[5] described in their clinical experience using a stentless pericardial aortic monopatch for replacement of the aortic valve. They, nonetheless, sutured the patch into the ventriculo-arterial junction without appreciating the role played by the sinuses of Valsalva.

To date, the reconstruction of the diseased aortic valve has been less satisfactory than that for the mitral valve. Better understanding of the mechanism of closure of the semilunar valve and the role of the sinuses of Valsalva might improve the surgical results for repair of the aortic valve in the future. The use of an autologous pericardial conduit incorporating a bileaflet valve[6,7] has been reported with good long-term follow-up. The trifoliate valve should be more physiological and natural than a bicuspid valve. Technical problems in dividing the pericardium into three portions can be solved by

using a precut plastic patch-holder of different sizes. The significance and long-term effect of glutaraldehyde immersion followed by chemical treatment with magnesium chloride to prevent calcification of pericardial valve remains to be clarified.[8] Be that as it may, the bulging contour of the sinus of Valsalva might prevent the direct contact and adhesion of pericardium with the vessel wall, while the continuous washout by the vortices within the sinus should prevent the deposition of fibrin and later fibrosis and retraction.[4]

In conclusion, reconstruction of a trifoliate arterial valve together with its sinuses of Valsalva has been used in a single patient with tetralogy of Fallot and absence of the leaflets of the pulmonary valve. Its long-term fate awaits further evaluation.

References

1. Saravalli OA, Somerville J, Jefferson KE. Calcification of aortic homografts used for reconstruction of the right ventricular outflow tract. J Thorac Cardiovasc Surg 1980;80:909–20.
2. Wilcox BR, Anderson RH. Surgical Anatomy of the Heart. Edinburgh, Churchill-Livingstone, 1985, p 3.2
3. Bellhouse B, Bellhouse F. Fluid mechanics of model of a normal and stenosed aortic valves. Circ Res 1969;25:693–704.
4. Revuelta JM, Ubago JL, Duran CMG. Composite pericardial monocusp patch for the reconstruction of right ventricular outflow tract. Clinical application in 7 patients. Thorac Cardiovasc Surg 1983;31:156–9.
5. Vilela Batista RJ, Dobrianskij A, Comazzi M Jr, et al. Clinical experience with stentless pericardial aortic monopatch for aortic valve replacement. J Thorac Cardiovasc Surg 1987; 93:19–26.
6. Ishizawa E, Horiuchi T, Okada Y, et al. Late results of reconstruction of the right ventricular outflow tract using a valve-bearing tube graft made of autologous pericardium. J Jpn Assoc Thorac Surg 1978;26:385–7.
7. Schlichter AJ, Kreutzer GO. Autologous pericardial valved conduit (APVC). Rev Latina Cardiol Cir Cardiovasc Infantil 1985;1:43–8.
8. Carpentier A, Nashref A, Carpentier S, et al. Prevention of tissue valve calcification by chemical technique. In: Cohn LH, Gallucci V (eds), Cardiac Bioprostheses. New York, Yorke Medical Books, 1982, pp 320–7.

Successful Repair of a Congenital Diverticulum of the Right Ventricle in a Three-Month-Old Baby

I. L. Hartyanszky, T. Verebely, K. Kadar, V. Oprea, and I. Palik

Introduction

Congenital diverticulums of the left or right ventricle are very rare cardiac anomalies.[1,2] According to Arnold, the first case was described by O'Bryan in 1837.[3] During the last 150 years, fewer than 20 cases were reported involving the right ventricle.[3-8] Most early cases involved autopsy studies but, from 1944, when the first successful resection of a left ventricular diverticulum was carried out by Roessler,[9] correct diagnosis facilitated by cardiac catheterization and echocardiography has been reported in an increasing number of cases, and some patients underwent successful surgical correction.[1,7]

The diverticulum is a localized protrusion from the free wall of a ventricle and generally has a narrow connection with the ventricular cavity. The lesion is often associated with other congenital intracardiac diseases, and the left ventricular apical type in particular occurs as part of a syndrome of midline thoracoabdominal defects.[10] When seen in the right ventricle, the diverticulum can involve the outflow tract, the anterior wall, or the apical region.

Although the natural history of ventricular diverticulums has yet to be clarified, some reports have suggested that the lesion can be progressive and have a poor prognosis. Heart failure, thrombosis, coronary insufficiency, cardiac rupture, arrhythmias, and infective endocarditis have all been mentioned as causes of death.[1,4]

We present here a 3-month-old baby with midline thoracoabdominal defects, a congenital apical diverticulum of the right ventricle, and tetralogy of Fallot, in whom the reconstruction of the midline defects and removal of diverticulum were performed at the same operation.

Case Report

In June 1986, a 1-month-old baby with multiple congenital malformations was seen at the Hungarian Institute of Cardiology. He was the product of a normal full-term pregnancy and delivery. On admission there was mild cyanosis, and a systolic ejection heart murmur was heard. An umbilical hernia of about 6 cm in length was present in which

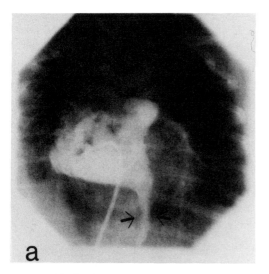

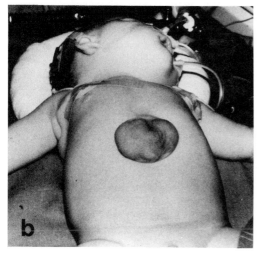

Figure 1. These pictures taken prior to operation show (a) an angiocardiogram revealing the right ventricular apical diverticulum (arrows) and (b) the baby with the intact omphalocele.

a pulsating mass was palpable extending from the xiphoid area to the umbilicus. The linea alba was also found to be deficient. Cross-sectional and Doppler echocardiography revealed the presence of tetralogy of Fallot complicated by a congenital diverticulum of the right ventricular apex. The diagnosis was confirmed at cardiac catheterization. Angiocardiography revealed a long, cone-shaped, pulsating diverticulum which

extended from the apex of the right ventricle towards the umbilicus (Fig. 1). The wall of the diverticulum contracted synchronously with the ventricular myocardium.

Although the clinical symptoms of tetralogy of Fallot were not severe, there was a possibility of infection of the omphalocele. Furthermore, operation was indicated since thrombosis or rupture of the diverticulum through the omphalocele could have produced ventricular fibrillation. The boy was now 3 months old and weighed 5,100 g. He was operated on without extracorporeal circulation. There was a huge intact omphalocele 6 cm in diameter (Fig. 1), and prominent cardiac pulsations were palpable and visible in the midepigastrium along its superior border. The omphalocele was excised, revealing a 6-cm long finger-like, actively contracting diverticulum, which extended through the diaphragmatic defect of the pericardial cavity and had a narrow connection to the right ventricular apex. A partial occluding clamp was applied to the right ventricular apex, the diverticulum was then excised, and the area was closed with mattress sutures. The defects of the diaphragm and the abdominal wall were both closed with a number of sutures. The diverticulum had a narrow cavity without obvious clots (Fig. 2) and a well-developed muscular

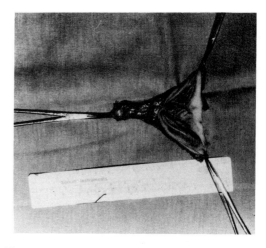

Figure 2. The right ventricular diverticulum after its removal at surgery.

wall. The postoperative period was uneventful, and the patient continues to do well 18 months after his operation. He is now scheduled for repair of the tetralogy of Fallot. Cross-sectional echocardiography and angiography reveals no residual diverticular extension of the right ventricle.

Comment

Surgery is indicated for right ventricular diverticulums because of their poor prognosis and known risk factors for complications.

If the diverticulum is part of the recognized syndrome of midline thoracoabdominal defects, it should be resected at the same procedure used for correction of the diaphragmatic and abdominal defects. This can safely be done in infancy.

To the best of our knowledge, this is the first report of a right ventricular diverticulum as part of Cantrell's syndrome. Our patient is also the youngest baby with such a lesion to undergo successful surgery.

References

1. Okereke OUJ, Cooley DA, Frazier OH. Congenital diverticulum of the ventricle. J Thorac Cardiovasc Surg 1986;91:208–14.
2. Hamaoka K, Onaka M, Tanaka T, Onouchi Z. Congenital ventricular aneurysm and diverticulum in children. Pediatr Cardiol 1987; 8:169–75.
3. Arnold J. Ueber angeborene Divertikel des Herzens. Wirchows Arch Pathol Anat 1984;137:318–29.
4. Cumming GR. Congenital diverticulum of the right ventricle. Am J Cardiol 1969;23:294–7.
5. Carter JB, Van Tassel RA, Moller JH, et al. Congenital diverticulum of the right ventricle. Association with pulmonary stenosis and ventricular septal defect. Am J Cardiol 1971;28:478–82.
6. Bharati S, Rowen M, Camarata SJ, et al. Diverticulum of the right ventricle. Arch Pathol 1975;99:383.
7. Magrassi P, Chartrand C, Guerin R, et al. True diverticulum of the right ventricle: Two cases associated with tetralogy of Fallot. Ann Thorac Surg 1980;29:357–63.
8. Freedom RM, Culham JAG, Moss CAF. Diverticulum of the right ventricle. In: Freedom RM, Culham JAG, Moss CAF (eds), Angiocardiography of Congenital Heart Disease. New York, Macmillan, 1984, pp 126–7.
9. Roessler W. Erfolgreiche operative Entfernung eines ektopischen. Herzdivertikels an einem Neugeborenen. Dtsch Z Chir 1944;258:561.
10. Cantrell JR, Haller JA, Ravitch MM. A syndrome of congenital defects involving the andominal wall, sternum, diaphragm, pericardium and heart. Surg Gynecol Obstet 1958; 107:602–14.

Severe Major Airway Compression Due to Absent Leaflets of the Pulmonary Valve with an Intact Ventricular Septum and Patency of the Arterial Duct

L. Levinsky, A. Schachner, T. Schonfeld, J. Ben-Ari,
M. Berant, and M. J. Levy

Severe major airway obstruction due to absence of the leaflets of the pulmonary valve and concomitant dilatation of the pulmonary arteries is a well-recognized entity. Most previously described cases involved the presence of a ventricular septal defect and the absence of an arterial duct. In this article, we describe a case with severe obstruction of the major airway in which the ventricular septum was intact and the arterial duct present and patent.

Case Report

A male infant was referred to our hospital at the age of 4 days. He was the product of a normal full-term pregnancy and delivery, being the son of healthy parents of Bedouin origin. Immediately after delivery he was noted to be in respiratory distress and required intubation and ventilation.

On examination, he was not cyanosed, but the upper part of body and face were edematous. The blood pressure was 70/40 mmHg. There was a systolic and diastolic murmur over his precordium, heard maximally at the upper left sternal border. Air entry was markedly diminished over the right lung, and there were crepitations over both lung fields. The liver was enlarged 4 cm below the right costal margin. Chest roentgenogram (Fig. 1A) showed that the lung fields were largely obscured by marked enlargement of the heart and pulmonary arteries. Bronchoscopy revealed extreme anterior narrowing of the trachea. Echocardiography showed a large right ventricle, which appeared to be shifted towards the right, a relatively small ventriculo-pulmonary junction with remnants of valve tissue, and gross dilatation of the pulmonary trunk and its two branches. There was also a moderate-sized patent arterial duct.

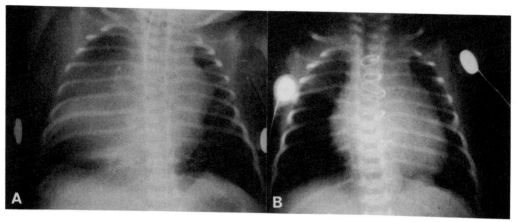

Figure 1. The frontal chest radiograph soon after birth (A) showed a markedly enlarged heart and obscuration of the right lung field. Eight days after surgery (B), the cardiac silhouette was much smaller and both lung fields are now seen.

The electrocardiogram showed right axis deviation and right ventricular hypertrophy. Cardiac catheterization confirmed the absence of the leaflets of the pulmonary valve and aneurysmatic dilatation of the pulmonary trunk and right pulmonary artery.

The left pulmonary artery was not seen but was later proved to be present by means of a lung scan. Simultaneous right heart angiography and bronchography (Fig. 2A) showed a horizontal right ventricle whose outflow tract appeared to be compressing

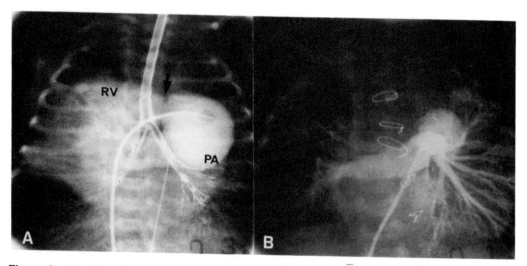

Figure 2. Injection of contrast medium in pulmonary trunk preoperatively (A) shows filling of the right ventricle which lies in a horizontal position. The outflow tract of the right ventricle is situated anterior to the trachea and carina. The arrow points to the relatively narrow ventriculo-pulmonary junction. The aneurysmatic pulmonary trunk compresses and distorts the left bronchus. The right bronchus is compressed by the enlarged right pulmonary artery. The left pulmonary artery is not shown. Two months after surgery (B), injection of contrast medium in the pulmonary trunk reveals a significant reduction in its size although there is marked narrowing of peripheral pulmonary arteries. RV, right ventricle; PA, pulmonary trunk.

the lower trachea and carina. The aneurysmatically dilated pulmonary trunk compressed and distorted the left bronchus, while the right bronchus was compressed by the enlarged right pulmonary artery. There was a gradient of 40 mmHg between the right ventricle and the pulmonary trunk.

An attempt to wean the baby from the respirator failed, and higher inspiratory pressures were needed to ventilate the baby, who showed a tendency to retain carbon dioxide. At 7 days of age the baby underwent surgical correction. The operative approach was through a median sternotomy. The pulmonary trunk was 4 cm in diameter, and the right ventricle lay horizontally and completely hid the right atrium. With the aid of cardiopulmonary bypass and deep hypothermia, the pulmonary trunk was reconstructed by excising a segment of its anterior wall. The aneurysmectomy was not continued into the pulmonary arteries. Residual dysplastic valve tissue was excised from the posterior aspect of the ventriculo-arterial junction. The incision in the pulmonary trunk was then extended down across the junction into the infundibulum which was widened with tissue excised previously from the pulmonary trunk. The ventriculo-arterial junction then accepted a dilator of 12 mm diameter. The patient was weaned from bypass with the aid of dopamine. He was initially cyanotic with a PO_2 of 50 mmHg, presumably due to right-to-left shunting through a patent oval foramen. Postoperatively, the infant could be ventilated with lower inspiratory pressures and the cyanosis gradually lessened. He was extubated 1 week after surgery when the chest x-ray (Fig. 1B) showed a much smaller cardiac silhouette with both lung fields visible.

Repeat bronchoscopy revealed marked reduction in the tracheal compression. The baby was discharged home 2 weeks after surgery. At follow-up 6 months after surgery, he is well and thriving. Cardiac catheterization performed 2 months after surgery (Fig. 2B) showed a normal position of the heart. The right outflow tract was wide. The pulmonary arteries had been significantly reduced in size, although there was a mild narrowing just proximal to the bifurcation. There was marked narrowing of the peripheral pulmonary arteries, a common finding in this lesion.

Discussion

Severe obstruction of the upper airway in the newborn is not a common finding.[1] Most cases of tracheal compression in infants are caused by either a vascular ring or a pulmonary sling. Tracheobronchial compression caused by aneurysmatic pulmonary arteries in association with so-called absent pulmonary valve is a rare entity. There have been nearly 170 cases reported in the literature,[2] most of which were associated with a ventricular septal defect and stenosis either at the level of the ventriculo-arterial junction or, less commonly, at the infundibulum.[3] Congenital absence of the leaflets of the pulmonary valve with an intact ventricular septum is particularly rare. It has been found as an isolated anomaly, in association with atrial septal defect or associated with Marfan's syndrome.[2]

There are several theories concerning the etiology of the aneurysmal dilatation of the pulmonary trunk and arteries. One theory suggests that heart failure and pulmonary arterial dilatation may result from increased right ventricular stroke volume due to pulmonary regurgitation and left-to-right shunt through the ventricular septal defect.[4-6] Emmanouilides et al.[3] observed, however, that the massive dilatation of the pulmonary trunk and its branches is primarily a prenatal phenomenon and, thus, should be attributed to stenosis at the pulmonary ventriculo-arterial junction associated with regurgitation. The arterial duct was absent in all four cases reported by Emmanouilides et al.[3] They, therefore, suggested that there may be a pathogenetic relation between the agenesis or hypoplasia of the duct and the aneurysmatic dilatation of the pulmonary arteries. This was because, in fetal life, absence of the duct would prevent run-off of the increased right ventricular stroke volume into the systemic circuit and, in the presence of the high resistance of the fetal lung, would result in dilatation of the pulmonary arteries. The findings in our case, and in the case described by Thanopoulos et al.[2] demonstrate unequivocally that agenesis of the duct is not essential in the etiology of dilatation of the pulmonary arteries. Thanopoulos and his colleagues[2] opined that stenosis at the level of the pulmonary ventriculo-arterial junction in association with increased right ventricular stroke volume was the essential feature for the genesis of the aneurysmal dilatation of the pulmonary arteries.

Infants with absence of the leaflets of the pulmonary valve with bronchial obstruction are known to have a poor prognosis. Results of surgery have been poor until recently, with a reported mortality rate of up to 60%.[7]

Palliative surgery has been performed in infants, consisting either of ligation or banding of the pulmonary trunk and insertion of a shunt. Ilbawi et al.[8] have reported a successful outcome in two infants operated at 2 and 3 days of age. Two other infants, however, operated on after several weeks of unsuccessful prolonged medical treatment and positive pressure ventilation, died. Dunnigan et al.[7] and Stellin et al.[9] have recommended definitive surgery to relieve the tracheobronchial obstruction by means of plication of the pulmonary arteries under deep hypothermia and circulatory arrest with patch closure of the ventricular septal defect. The latter authors operated on 6 infants, 2 of whom died. Karl et al.[10] used a similar technique for reducing the size of the pulmonary arteries, but they interposed an aortic homograft between the right ventricle and the pulmonary arteries. Only 4 of 9 infants below 1 year of age survived surgery, while there was no mortality in a group of 10 older children.

Our case is one of the youngest survivors of definitive surgical repair. In fact, it is quite impossible to take into consideration any type of palliative procedure when the ventricular septum is intact. This finding is undoubtedly very rare with absence of the leaflets of the pulmonary valve, as with patency of the arterial duct.

References

1. Kilham H, Gillis J, Benjamin B. Severe upper airway obstruction. Pediatr Clin North Am 1987;34:1–14.
2. Thanopoulos BD, Fisher EA, Hastreiter AR. Large ductus arteriosus and intact ventricular septum associated with congenital absence of the pulmonary valve. Br Heart J 1986;55:602–4.
3. Emmanouilides GC, Thanopoulos B, Siassi B, Fishbein M. "Agenesis" of ductus arteriosus associated with the syndrome of tetralogy of Fallot and absent pulmonary valve. Am J Cardiol 1976;37:403–9.
4. Stafford EG, Mair DD, McGoon DC, et al. Tetralogy of Fallot with absent pulmonary valve. Surgical considerations and results. Circulation 1973;47(suppl III):24–30.
5. Onesti SJ, Hamed HS. Absence of the pulmonary valve associated with ventricular septal defect. Am J Cardiol 1958;2:496–501.
6. D'Cruz IA, Arcilla RA, Agusstsson MH. Dilatation of the pulmonary trunk in stenosis of the pulmonary valve and of the pulmonary arteries in children. Am Heart J 1964;68:612–6.
7. Dunnigan A, Oldham HN, Benson DW. Absent pulmonic valve syndrome in infancy. Surgery recommended. Am J Cardiol 1981;48:117–22.
8. Ilbawi MN, Fedorchik J, Muster AJ, et al. Surgical approach to severely symptomatic newborn infants with tetralogy of Fallot and absent pulmonary valve. J Thorac Cardiovasc Surg 1986;91:584–9.
9. Stellin G, Jonas RA, Goh TH, et al. Surgical treatment of absent pulmonary valve syndrome in infants. Relief of bronchial obstruction. Ann Thorac Surg 1983;46:468–75.
10. Karl TR, Musumeci F, de Leval M, et al. Surgical treatment of absent pulmonary valve syndrome. J Thorac Cardiovasc Surg 1986;91:590–7.

His Bundle Tachycardia
An Important Cause of Postoperative Mortality and Morbidity

J. A. Till, E. Rowland, and M. L. Rigby

Introduction

His bundle tachycardia is an unusual but important cause of early postoperative mortality and morbidity.[1] The diagnosis can usually be made from the surface electrocardiogram, and the arrhythmia is classically characterized by atrioventricular dissociation with a rapid narrow QRS complex. The QRS rate is greater than the sinus rhythm. Thus, a high rate is combined with loss of atrioventricular synchrony and, as a consequence, cardiac output may be severely compromised. The proposed mechanism of the tachycardia is an ectopic focus in the His bundle, giving rise to a QRS complex which is similar to that seen during sinus rhythm.[2,3] The underlying cellular events involved are not known, but delayed afterdepolarizations have been implicated.[4] In the postoperative setting, a wide QRS complex is not unusual as a consequence of ventriculotomy or rate-related bundle branch block. Occasionally, retrograde ventriculoatrial conduction occurs, giving rise to atrioventricular dissociation and thus complicating the diagnosis. The etiology of the tachycardia remains unexplained, but trauma to the His bundle during surgery is suspected. Most cases have occurred subsequent to closure of a ventricular septal defect[5] High doses of catecholamines used to support ventricular function have also been implicated in the pathogenesis.[6]

Case Material

We have reviewed the last 14 cases of His bundle tachycardia seen at our institution in an attempt to identify etiological factors and examine management. The children were aged between 6 months and 21 years (median 2.25 years). They had a wide range of anatomical defects, and a range of surgical procedures were performed. Three had undergone a Fontan procedure (one for tricuspid atresia and two for double inlet left ventricle). Three had undergone correction of tetralogy of Fallot, two for double outlet right ventricle and one for common arterial trunk. Two children had had a Mustard procedure for correction of complete transposition with ventricular septal defect; one had closure of ventricular septal defect with straddling atrioventricular valve; one had placement of a conduit from the right ventricle to the pulmonary trunk in treatment of pulmonary atresia with intact septum and one a conduit from the left ventricle to the pulmonary trunk for congenitally corrected transposition with pulmonary stenosis. Only one child did not have a ventricular septal defect.

The tachycardia was recognized in the majority of children within 3 hours of surgery, the rate characteristically increasing as the child warmed. In 5 of 14 cases, however, the tachycardia was not present until later in the postoperative course, developing between 6 and 30 hours following surgery. In all of these cases, high doses of catecholamines (usually adrenaline) were being given and may have played a role in the development of the arrhythmia. In 10 cases, the diagnosis was made from the surface electrocardiogram. In the other 4, an atrial electrogram recorded from an epicardial electrode proved useful in confirming the relationship between atrial and ventricular excitation. The maximum rate of tachycardia varied between 160 to 380 beats per minute. In all cases, the tachycardia caused a fall in blood pressure associated with an increased requirement for inotropic support.

There was no set protocol for treatment, and a wide range of drugs were used. Digoxin was given to six children but failed to affect the arrhythmia. Amiodarone was used in seven and resulted in a significant slowing of the tachycardia rate in four (Fig. 1). Adenosine was given as a rapid intravenous bolus to three. In two, it failed to affect the arrhythmia but appeared transiently to terminate the tachycardia in one child. Encouraged by this unexpected finding, an infusion of adenosine was tried, but this resulted in only a small reduction in tachycardia rate and a significant fall in both systolic and diastolic blood pressure. We believed this to be a result of the vasodilator properties of adenosine unmasked from automatic regulation in the unconscious patient.[7] Flecainide used in two children resulted in slowing of rate in one but not the other. Ajmaline briefly terminated the His bundle tachycardia in one child, but ventricular flutter ensued. Verapamil was unsuccessful in one as was disopyramide in one.

His bundle tachycardia is to be an "automatic" tachycardia and, as such, would be expected to be unresponsive to overdrive pacing. This proved to be the case in three of our patients. Recently, induced hypothermia has been described as a successful technique to reduce the tachycardia rate in three children.[8] Cooling to 32°C was at-

Intravenous amiodarone 5 mg/kg

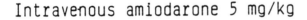

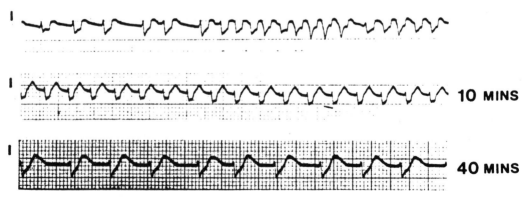

Figure 1. Successive electrocardiograms in an 8-month-old child with His bundle tachycardia following total correction of tetralogy of Fallot. The tracings show the fall in the rate of tachycardia following administration of intravenous amiodarone over 30 minutes.

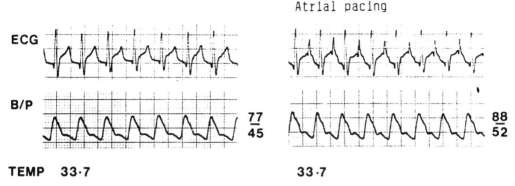

Figure 2. Electrocardiogram and blood pressure tracings before and after institution of atrial pacing at a rate coincident with that of the His bundle in a 9-month-old child following total correction of tetralogy of Fallot. Systolic blood pressure increases immediately from 77 to 88 mmHg and diastolic pressure from 45 to 52 mmHg. The temperature was 33.7°C.

tempted in three of our cases and successfully decreased the rate of tachycardia in two. Atrial pacing at a rate coincident with that of the His bundle was utilized in six children (Fig. 2). This restored atrioventricular synchrony and was associated with an immediate increase in blood pressure in all six. This, in turn, was associated with a decrease in the requirement for catecholamines.

Three children died. One died when an episode of ventricular tachycardia degenerated to ventricular fibrillation from which he could not be resuscitated. Two died in low cardiac output. Eleven children survived and the His bundle tachycardia resolved spontaneously between 1 and 8 days.

Nine of the 11 resumed sinus rhythm, while 2 continued in a slower junctional rhythm. Of the 11 survivors, 3 developed renal failure requiring dialysis or hemofiltration, 2 suffered neurological damage, and 1 underwent an episode of severe limb ischemia which later necessitated amputation. Hospital stay was prolonged. Time on intensive care ranged from 6 to 29 days (median 12), and total hospital stay ranged between 12 to 66 days (medium 25).

Discussion

Our results are similar to those of others, although Grant et al.[9] in their recent review reported digoxin as their single most effective agent. Six of eight of their group responded with a reduction in rate with the new class 1c agent, propafenone. We have not used propafenone but have used a similar agent, flecainide, in two cases. This reduced the rate in one but, as described by the previous authors,[10] great care in administering the drug is required because of its negative inotropic properties.

The results in our group mirror those in other reported series and remain poor. Ours was a retrospective review, but our experience indicates that early recognition and treatment of the arrhythmia is important. We would recommend atrial pacing at a rate coincident with that of the His bundle to restore atrioventricular synchrony, combined, in those children with a very high rate, with either cooling or amiodarone.

References

1. Krongrad E. Postoperative arrhythmias in patients with congenital heart disease. Chest 1984;85:107–13.
2. Coumel P, Fidelle JE, Attwel P, et al. Tachycardias focales Hissienes congenitales. Arch Mal Coeur 1985;69:899–909.
3. Waldo AL, Krongrad E, Kupermith J, et al. Ventricular pared pacing to control rapid ventricular heart rate following open heart surgery. Circulation 1976;53:176–181.

4. Rosen MR, Fisch C, Hoffman BF, et al. Can accelerated atrioventricular junctional escape rhythm be explained by delayed alterdepolarisations. Am J Cardiol 1980;45:1272–84.

5. Garson A, Gillette PC. Junctional ectopic tachycardia in children: Electrocardiography, electrophysiology and pharmacologic response. Am J Cardiol 1979;44:298–302.

6. Garson A. Arrhythmias. In: The electrocardiogram in infants and children: A systematic approach. Philadelphia, Lea & Febiger, 1983, pp 195–375.

7. Biaggioni I, Olafsson B, Robertson RM, et al. Cardiovascular and respiratory effects of adenosine in conscious man. Evidence for chemoreceptor activation. Circ Res 1987; 61:779–86.

8. Bash SE, Shah JJ, Albers WH, Geiss DM. Hypothermia for the treatment of postsurgical greatly accelerated junctional ectopic tachycardia. J Am Coll Cardiol 1987;10:1095–9.

9. Grant JW, Serwer GA, Armstrong BE, et al. Junctional tachycardia in infants and children after open heart surgery for congenital heart disease. Am J Cardiol 1987;59:1216–18.

10. Garson A, Moak JP, Smith RT, Norton JB. Usefulness of intravenous propafenone for control of postoperative junctional ectopic tachycardia. Am J Cardiol 1987;59:1422–4.

7.12

Morphological Features in Situs Ambiguus (Atrial Isomerism)

A. L. Calder

Complex congenital cardiac defects are frequent in patients with so-called situs ambiguus, the categorization which includes the asplenia (right atrial isomerism) and polysplenia syndromes (left atrial isomerism). The complex combinations of malformations, in particular anomalies of the systemic and pulmonary venous connections, may preclude surgical correction. To ascertain which features would be helpful in diagnosis, the morphology of 43 necropsied cases with situs ambiguus was analyzed (Tables 1–4, Figs. 1 and 2). Not all features could be evaluated in each patient.

Asplenia Syndrome

Twenty-six patients with congenital absence of the spleen (plus four patients with right isomerism of the atrial appendages and of the bronchi) are included in this group. Their ages ranged from stillborn to 4 years (median 6 weeks). The sex ratio was 15 male and 13 female, while 2 were of unknown sex.

The lung lobation was variable (Table 1). The bronchial lengths were in the range for right bronchi[1] in 88% and the relationship to the pulmonary arteries was of the bilateral right-sided type in 90% (Table 1).

The ratio of left-to-right bronchial lengths was asymmetrical in 28%. The shape of the atrial appendage was symmetrical in 97%, but the morphology of the atrial septum could not be used to determine atrial arrangement (Table 2). The systemic and pulmonary venous connections were variable (Table 3, Fig. 1). The coronary sinus was absent in 25 patients (89%).

Polysplenia Syndrome

Twelve patients with multiple spleens plus one patient with left isomerism of both the atrial appendages and of the bronchi are included. Their ages ranged from stillborn to 47 years (median 6 weeks). The sex was male in six and female in seven. The lungs were bilaterally bilobed in 92% (Table 1). The lengths of the bronchi were too variable to be useful, but the ratio of their lengths and their relationship to the pulmonary arteries could be used to identify the bronchial arrangement (Table 1). The morphology of the atrial appendages and the atrial septal structures were not diagnostic of the atrial arrangement in polysplenia (Table 2). The systemic and pulmonary venous connections are listed in Table 4 (Fig. 2). The cor-

Table 1
Thoracic Situs

	Asplenia	No.	%	Polysplenia	No.	%
Lung lobation:	Bilat. trilobed	20	78	Bilat. bilobed	11	92
	Normal	3	11	Bilat. trilobed	1	8
	Bilat. bilobed	2	7			
	R. tri., L. quad.	1	4			
Bronchial lengths:	Bilat. right	21	88	Bilat. left	6	50
	Indeterminate	3	12	Bilat. right	3	25
				Normal	1	8
				Mirror-image	1	8
				Indeterminate	1	8
Ratio L/R bronchi:	<1.8	17	72	<1.5	12	100
	>1.8	7	28			
Relationship of	Eparterial	18	90	Hyparterial	10	84
bronchi to PA:	Normal	1	10	Normal	1	8
				Mirro-image	1	8

Table 2
Atrial Situs

Asplenia	No.	%	Polysplenia	No.	%
Appendages					
Bilateral RAA	29	97	Bilateral LAA	6	46
Normal	1	3	Normal	5	39
			Mirror-image	2	15
Septum					
Absent	14	47	Indeterminate	6	55
Indeterminate	9	30	Absent	3	27
Lateralized	7	23	Lateralized	2	18

Table 3
Asplenia Syndrome

Systemic veins	No.	%
Bilateral SCV*	6	20
Symmetrical	6	20
Asymmetrical	4	13
Normal	4	13

Pulmonary veins	No.	%
TAPVC	25	89
Normal	2	7
To ipsilat. atria	1	4

* SCV, superior caval vein.

Table 4
Polysplenia Syndrome

Systemic veins	No.	%
Absent ICV	7	54
Normal	5	38
Bilat. ICV	1	8

Pulmonary veins	No.	%
To ipsilateral atria	7	54
Normal	4	31
TAPVC	2	15

ASPLENIA

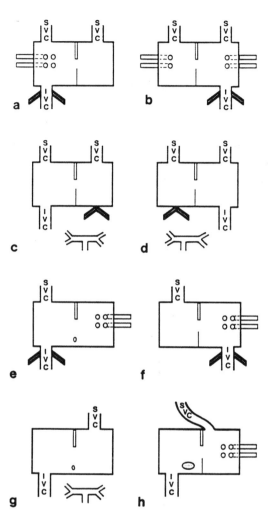

Figure 1. Illustrations of the anomalies of systemic and pulmonary venous drainage in cases with the congenital asplenia syndrome (right isomerism of the atrial appendages). In (a) to (d) the superior caval venous drainage is symmetrical; in (e) to (h) the superior and inferior caval venous connections are asymmetrical. The hepatic veins are represented by hatched areas, pulmonary veins by gray or dashed areas, coronary sinus by a gray oval, septum secundum by a narrow bar, septum primum by a straight line, and fibrous strand or remnant of atrial septum by a clear small oval. In (a), bilateral superior caval, inferior caval and hepatic veins drain to ipsilateral atria. In (c), bilateral superior caval and inferior caval veins are connected to right-sided atrium with totally anomalous pulmonary venous connection. In (d), the connections are similar to (c), with the inferior caval and hepatic venous connections inverted. In (e), the venous connections appear normal but the coronary sinus is absent. In (f), the superior and inferior caval and the hepatic veins connect to contralateral atria; the pulmonary veins connect to the left-sided atrium. In (g), the left-sided superior caval vein connects to the left-sided atrium, the right-sided inferior caval vein to the right-sided atrium with totally anomalous pulmonary venous connection. In (h), a right-sided superior caval vein and the pulmonary veins connect to the left-sided atrium while the inferior caval vein and the coronary sinus drain to the right-sided atrium.

POLYSPLENIA

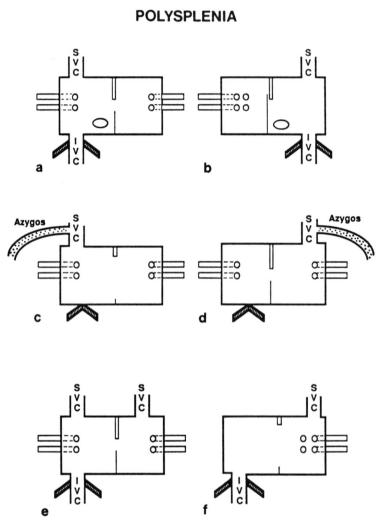

Figure 2. Anomalies of the systemic and pulmonary venous connection in cases with the polysplenia syndrome (left isomerism of the atrial appendages). Abbreviations as in Fig. 1. In (a), the superior caval, inferior caval, hepatic veins and coronary sinus drain to the right-sided atrium; the pulmonary veins connect to ipsilateral atria. In (b), pulmonary and systemic venous connections are as in situs inversus (mirror image atrial arrangement). In (c) and (d), the suprarenal to hepatic portion of the inferior caval vein is absent; the azygos or hemiazygos continuation of the vein drains to the right-sided superior caval vein, the hepatic veins connect to the right- or left-sided atrium, and the pulmonary veins drain to ipsilateral atria. In (e), bilateral superior caval and pulmonary veins connect to ipsilateral atria, the inferior caval with hepatic veins to the right-sided atrium. In (f), superior caval and pulmonary veins connect to the left-sided atrium; the inferior caval with hepatic veins to the right-sided atrium.

onary sinus was absent in five patients (38%).

Comment

The diagnosis of situs ambiguus may be suspected when bronchial isomerism is identified on chest-roengtenogram.[1-3] The types of systemic venous drainage, which may provide a clue to differentiate between the asplenia and polysplenia syndromes,[4] can be assessed with angiocardiograms[5] or echocardiography.[6] Because no single feature is completely reliable (Tables 1–4), all the data available are used to establish the diagnosis.[7] Surgical treatment using a total cavopulmonary shunt operation[9] may be precluded in patients with symmetrical connections of the superior caval and pulmonary veins (Figs. 1b, 2a, 2e).

References

1. Partridge JB, Scott O, Deverall PB, Macartney FJ. Visualization and measurement of the main bronchi by tomography as an objective indicator of thoracic situs in congenital heart disease. Circulation 1975;51:188–196.

2. Deanfield JE, Leanage R, Stroobant J, et al. Use of high kilovoltage filtered beam radiographs for detection of bronchial situs in infants and young children. Br Heart J 1980;44:577–583.

3. Soto B, Pacifico AD, Souza AS, et al. Identification of thoracic isomerism from plain chest radiograph. Am J Roentgenol 1978;131:995–1002.

4. Stanger P, Rudolph AM, Edwards JE. Cardiac malpositions. An overview based on study of sixty-five necropsy specimens. Circulation 1977;56:159–172.

5. Elliott LP, Cramer GG, Amplatz K. The anomalous relationship of the inferior vena cava and abdominal aorta as a specific angiocardiographic sign in asplenia. Radiology 1966; 87:859–863.

6. Huhta JC, Smallhorn JF, Macartney FJ, et al. Cross-sectional echocardiographic diagnosis of systemic venous return. Br Heart J 1982; 48:388–403.

7. Brandt PWT, Calder AL. Cardiac connections: the segmental approach to radiologic diagnosis in congenital heart disease. Current Problems in Diagnostic Radiology 1977;7:1–35.

8. Kawashima Y, Kitamura S, Matsuda H, et al. Total cavopulmonary shunt operation in complex cardiac anomalies. A new operation. J Thorac Cardiovasc Surg 1984;87:74–81.

9. Fontan F, Baudet E. Surgical repair of tricuspid atresia. Thorax 1971;26:240–248.

Coronary Arterial Bypass Grafting Using an Internal Mammary Artery as a More Effective Procedure for Treatment of the Coronary Arterial Lesions after Kawasaki Disease

F. Yamamoto, T. Yagihara, K. Ohara, H. Kishimoto, F. Isobe,
K. Nishigaki, T. Fujita, A. Suzuki, Y. Ono, M. Okuno,
and T. Kamiya

Introduction

Bypass grafting for coronary arterial lesions secondary to Kawasaki disease was first applied by Kitamura and his associates with autologous saphenous vein grafts. The patency rate was reported to be poor, and the first successful case of grafting with the internal mammary artery was reported by the same group to be advantageous compared to saphenous vein grafts. This clinical study describes several problems of bypass grafting for coronary arterial lesions secondary to Kawasaki disease.

Materials and Methods

Two patients who underwent coronary arterial bypass grafting for coronary arterial lesions secondary to Kawasaki disease were electively re-evaluated. The efficacy of grafting was analyzed by coronary angiography and exercise or dipyridamole load myocardial imaging by thallium cardiac scintigraphy at periods of 1 month and 1 year after the operations. The results of these investigations were compared with preoperative findings. The patency rate of internal mammary arterial and saphenous venous grafts was also investigated at 1 month and at 1 year after operation. Four hearts from cases (3 cases who had not received and 1 case who had received coronary arterial bypass grafts) who died of cardiac complications secondary to Kawasaki disease were examined by postmortem angiography and histological evaluation.

Results

There were no deaths in the 22 patients, but a 1-year-old boy who had an emergency

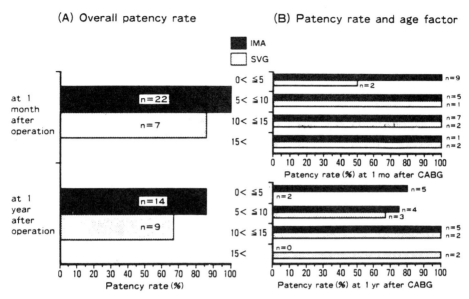

Figure 1. Graft materials and patency rate. (A) Difference of overall patency rate in internal mammary artery (IMA) and saphenous vein grafts (SVG). (B) Patency rate in internal mammary artery and saphenous vein grafts, according to age at operation. Patency rate was compared at 5-year intervals. CABG = coronary artery bypass grafting.

operation, due to acute narrowing of a stenotic lesion complicated by percutaneous angioplasty, died of occlusion of an aneurysm at the anastomotic site in the left anterior descending artery 3 months after the emergency operation. Thirty-two grafts (23 of internal mammary artery and 9 of saphenous vein) were implanted in the 22 patients. Overall patency rates of these grafts at 1 month and at 1 year after surgery are shown in panel A of Fig. 1, while the difference in patency rate with age at 5-year intervals is shown in panel B. Patients below the age of 10 years showed obstruction in 2 internal mammary and 4 saphenous vein grafts. Because of this age factor, the size of the internal mammary and the coronary arteries, which were measured during operation, was compared in patients below and over 10 years of age. Patients below the age of 10 years had significantly smaller diameters, expressed as a mean ± SD of their internal mammary and coronary arteries, than patients more than 10 years old [diameter below age 10 years: internal mammary artery = 1.38 mm ± 0.26 (n = 13), cor-

onary arteries = 1.57 ± 0.31 (n = 18); diameter over age 10 years: internal mammary artery = 1.96 mm ± 0.09 (n = 7), coronary arteries = 1.93 mm ± 0.28 (n = 11)]. The same analysis was performed by comparing the diameters of the internal mammary and coronary arteries between patients below and over 5 years of age. Significant differences were found. Figure 2 shows the change with exercise myocardial imaging at 1 month and at 1 year after operation compared with preoperative evaluation. Improvement occurred in 64% at one month and 67% at one year as compared with preoperative findings. Among 10 patients who had improved at 1 year, two showed marked deterioration as compared to findings at 1 month, due to closure of saphenous vein grafts. Most patients, however, showed significant improvement when compared with preoperative findings. Four patients showed improved findings at 1 month and, in these, the beneficial effect of coronary arterial bypass grafting was maintained for at least 1 year after operation. In 4 cases with unchanged findings, an inappropriate

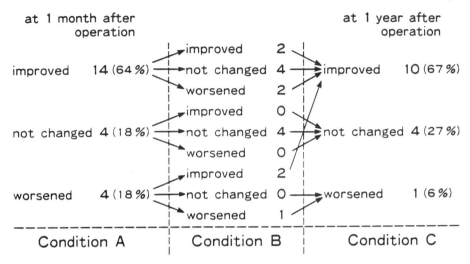

Figure 2. Evaluation with exercise or dipyridamole load myocardial imaging of Thallium scintigraphy. The results of condition A and C was obtained to compare the preoperative findings with the condition of myocardial imaging at one month or at one year after coronary artery bypass grafting. The results of condition B was obtained by comparing the results at one month with that at one year after coronary arytery bypass grafting. Myocardial imaging was performed in 22 patients before and at one month after grafting. In 15 out of 22 patients, this examination was performed one year after grafting, as well as at one month after grafting.

anastomotic site was found in 2 cases, technical error had occurred in 1 case, while the reason for the lack of improvement was unknown in the fourth case (the internal mammary artery in this case was aneurysmal but not stenotic). One case with deterioration, demonstrated by scintigraphy at 1 month and further worsening at one year, had stenosis at the anastomotic site. To evaluate lesions with increasing stenosis, we studied the 4 cases who died of cardiac complication secondary to Kawasaki disease (1 case died three months after coronary artery bypass grafting with a patent internal mammary artery) by using microscopy and postmortem angiography. Pathological changes (such as endothelial hypertrophy, increase of collagen fiber in media, and duplication of internal elastic lamina) without any angiographic change were recognized at several locations within the coronary arterial tree, in all cases. The case treated with bypass grafting revealed patency of the internal mammary arterial graft, but showed further narrowing of the stenotic lesion distal to the site of an-

astomosis with deposition of fresh thrombus.

Discussion

Many problems remain unsolved in the surgical treatment of coronary arterial lesions due to Kawasaki disease, despite improvements in surgical technique. Most patients who need bypass grafting are young, and it is difficult to best treat them on subjective symptoms, such as chest pain or other symptoms typically seen in adults. Differences also exist in the extent of involvement of the right and left coronary arteries in the disease process. Furthermore, some of the patients undergoing bypass grafting still, occasionally suffer sudden cardiac death. Several points, therefore, require special attention. The first is the material used for grafting. Indeed, this study demonstrated poorer patency rates following use of the saphenous vein as compared with the internal mammary artery in patients below 10 years of age. Furthermore, flow increased with time in internal mammary arterial grafts, as shown in 11 out of 14 internal mammary arterial grafts studied by angiography 1 year after operation. It is unclear, nonetheless, whether this increase in flow guarantees prevention of myocardial ischemia in all conditions. Also, the structural changes caused in the internal mammary artery by Kawasaki disease are not completely known. Other arteries, such as the common iliac artery, occasionally exhibit dilated or stenotic lesions. We found at least one instance of aneurysmal change in an internal mammary artery that resulted in its closure. This may discourage the use of the internal mammary artery since, unlike the saphenous vein, it is susceptible to the degenerations produced by Kawasaki disease after its use as a bypass graft. The second problem is the size of the internal mammary artery relative to the coronary arteries when bypass grafting is performed in young patients. Our data showed a significant difference in the size of these arteries in patients below and over 10 years of age, as well as in patients below and over 5 years of age. These discrepancies may cause difficulties for the surgeon in performing the arterial anastomosis. However, the use of absorbable and interrupted sutures may, at least partly, reduce the size of the problem. The third point is the indication for bypass grafting, especially in young patients. Clear-cut indications have yet to be established, and the criteria used for adults with atherosclerotic lesions are not always applicable. Currently, coronary artery grafting is used to bypass specific lesions, due to Kawasaki disease, in the presence of ischemic findings demonstrable by exercise or dipyridamole loading myocardial imaging. Stenoses detected by angiography in the absence of ischemia do not constitute absolute indication to perform elective bypass grafting, particularly if the characteristic clinical course of Kawasaki disease is carefully considered. This is characterized by recanalization of occlusive lesions, especially those found in right coronary arteries. Eventually, coronary artery bypass grafting, even with patent grafts, does not always give excellent clinical results, despite improvements in myocardial imaging. Most of our cases showed considerable improvement following grafting at 1 year after operation, but some of them had deteriorated. One of the reasons underscoring such deterioration is the progression of stenotic lesions distal to the anastomotic site. This feature was obvious in our autopsied cases, which indicated the silent worsening of stenotic lesions over long periods after bypass grafting. These findings, which can be lethal, should always be born in mind by the surgeon who is forced to perform bypass grafting by the progression of Kawasaki's disease.

References

1. Kitamura S, Kawashima Y, Fujita T, et al. Aortocoronary bypass grafting in a child with coronary artery obstruction due to mucocutaneous lymph node syndrome. Report of a case. Circulation 1976;53:1035–40
2. Kitamura S, Kawachi K, Oyama C, et al. Severe Kawasaki heart disease treated with an internal mammary artery graft in pediatric patients. A first successful report. J Thorac Cardiovasc Surg 1985;89:860–6
3. Kamiya T, Suzuki A. Ischemic disease in Kawasaki disease. In: Shulman T (ed), Kawasaki Disease. New York, Alan R. Liss, Inc.; 1987,pp 347–55.

Tissue Regeneration after Reconstruction of the Pericardium with Synthetic Absorbable Patches

T. Malm, S. Bowald, and A. Bylock

Introduction

Resternotomy is an operative procedure that carries an increased morbidity and mortality due to pericardial adhesions. There is evidence of an increasing number of reoperations in cardiac surgery over the last decade. In order to facilitate reoperation, we decided to study the effect of absorbable pericardial patches in an animal model in terms of adhesions, tissue regeneration, and frequency of infections. We employed two different versions of the synthetic absorbable patch.

Material and Methods

Twenty-five young sheep, age 6 weeks to 6 months, were used. They were anesthetized using intravenous thiopentalsodium for induction, intubated, and ventilated with 50% oxygen and 50% nitrous oxide together with 0.5–2% Halothane. A left-sided thoracotomy was performed, and a piece of pericardium excised over a part of the left and the right ventricles and the pulmonary trunk. A 5 × 3 cm patch was cut into an ellipse-shaped configuration and sutured with absorbable suture using a running technique. All animals received 0.2 ml/kg Penovet (Penicilline) im. prior to surgery. Postoperatively, the animals were provided a standard diet and routine care. They were sacrificed at varying intervals ranging from 2 months to 12 months. The patches were resected immediately after death, photographed and grossly examined. Specimens were fixed in glutaraldehyde and sectioned for light and scanning electron microscopy. For light microscopy, the specimens were sectioned longitudinally to include both the suture line and the central parts of the patch, as well as a part of the native pericardium. The blocks were embedded in paraffin, and sections of 5 μm in thickness were stained with hematoxyline, eosin, and Elastic van-Gieson stains. Sections were also taken for scanning electron microscopy.

Results

There was no perioperative mortality, but one animal died a week after the thoracotomy. The cause was cardiac herniation due to rupture of the suture line. No infections or postoperative hemorrhage were noted. At two months, the patches exhibited smooth surfaces on both their pleural and epicardial surfaces, but loose strings were seen extending between the patches and the epicardium. After four and five months, no such adhesions were seen. After two months, the patch was three to four times thicker than native pericardium due to hydrolysis of cellular compounds. The synthetic bases of the patch were insulated and surrounded by giant cells, macrophages, and fibroblasts, as well as fibrocytes. The thickened tissue lost water in time, and became thinner. Even after 6 months, however, it was possible to recognize the synthetic material as small islands surrounded by giant cells. The epicardial surface of the patch was completely smooth and covered by epithelial cells on fibrous laminas, showing close similarity to the surface of native pericardium. The smoothest part was found toward the epicardium.

At four to five months, there was ingrowth of small vessels over the surface and into and through the patch. No difference was noted histologically when the two different types of absorbable patches were compared. Scanning electron microscopy showed mesothelial cells in one specimen after five months.

Discussion

These preliminary results demonstrate that, absorbable patches made from synthetic material and used in this animal model to partially replace the pericardium did not produce any problems either postoperatively or in the intermediate follow-up. The regenerated tissue showed microscopic similarities with native pericardium. Further studies are needed to characterize the biochemical quality of the regenerated tissue, and to further investigate the resemblance between the regenerated tissue and native pericardium.

Double-Chambered Right Ventricle

C. A. Dietl, A. R. Torres, M. E. Cazzaniga, and R. G. Favaloro.

Introduction

The right ventricle may be divided into two discrete components by anomalous muscle bundles[1] or by a muscular shelf, secondary to hypertrophy of the septomarginal trabeculation.[2] Either of these eventualities create a two-chambered right ventricle in which the proximal portion (or inflow) is at high pressure, while the distal portion (or outflow) is at low pressure chamber.[3] The obstruction is proximal to the infundibulum and is anatomically distinct from tetralogy of Fallot,[3] although a two-chambered arrangement can coexist with tetralogy. The anomalous muscle bundles originate at the supraventricular crest or the subjacent ventricular septum, and insert into the free wall near the apex of the right ventricle.[2,4] In some instances, a muscular shelf with a discrete ostium separates the proximal and distal ventricular chambers.[5] A ventricular septal defect is present in most cases and usually communicates with the high-pressure inflow portion of the right ventricle.[1,3,6,7] A double-chambered right ventricle can be associated with various other intracardiac defects, including double-outlet right ventricle,[5,7] subaortic stenosis,[6,7,8] prolapse of the aortic valve,[6,9] atrial septal defect,[6] and pulmonary atresia and Ebstein's malformation.[6] Clinically, some patients may present with exercise intolerance and, if the shunt is large, there is growth failure with frequent respiratory infections during infancy.[3,10] Other may be asymptomatic[6] or simulate acyanotic tetralogy of Fallot.[1] In some cases, progressive right ventricular obstruction has been demonstrated by serial cardiac catheterizations.[7,10] The anomalous bands may be detected by cross-sectional echocardiography.[7] Angiocardiography, nonetheless, is the ideal diagnostic technique, with the contrast medium being injected in the inflow portion of the right ventricle in order to visualize the obstruction proximal to the infundibulum.[3] Double-chambered right ventricle is amenable to surgical correction either by using a "classical" transventricular approach [1,5,7,10] or via a transatrial approach in order to avoid a ventriculotomy.[6]

Patients and Methods

Between September 1980 and September 1987, 15 patients with double-chambered right ventricle underwent surgical repair. There were 11 girls and 4 boys, and their ages ranged from 9 months to 22 years (mean 9.2 years). Twelve patients were symptomatic (9 in class II, 2 in class III, 1 in class IV). Exercise intolerance was the commonest symptom. Only 3 patients (aged 9

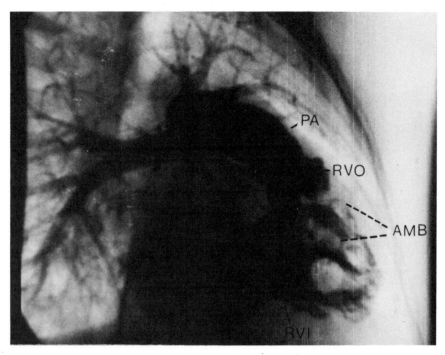

Figure 1. Preoperative right ventricular angiocardiography. (RVI = right ventricular inflow; RVO = right ventricular outflow; PA = pulmonary trunk. AMB = anomalous muscle bands).

months, 1.3 years, and 3 years) had failed to thrive and were in congestive heart failure. In addition, one patient with associated double outlet right ventricle and a right-sided heart was cyanotic.

All patients had right ventricular hypertrophy in the electrocardiogram. Chest X-rays showed mild or moderate cardiomegaly with severe enlargement in the small infant. Increased pulmonary blood flow was evident in 8 patients. Preoperative echocardiography revealed a large oblique muscle bundle crossing the body of the right ventricle in all cases. Cardiac catheterization revealed a midventricular gradient ranging from 25 to 90 mmHg (mean 52.8 mmHg). The obstruction was clearly visualized by right ventricular angiocardiography in the elongated right anterior oblique and lateral views (Fig. 1). A ventricular septal defect, communicating the left ventricle with the proximal chamber of the right ventricle, was present in 14 patients. The shunt fraction

ratio ranged from 1.1 to 3.4 (mean 1.75:1). Other associated intracardiac defects present were: double-outlet right ventricle in 3 patients, atrial septal defect in 1 patient, discrete subaortic stenosis in 1 patient, and prolapse of the aortic valve with insufficiency in 1 patient (Tables 1 and 2).

Surgical Treatment

Repair was performed in all patients using cardiopulmonary bypass and moderate hypothermia. Circulatory arrest with deep hypothermia was used in a 9-month-old infant who weighed 4 kg and had associated double outlet right ventricle. Cold crystalloid cardioplegic solution was used for myocardial protection. Two different approaches were used. Until April 1984, a vertical right ventriculotomy was done routinely (6 patients). Another patient with right-sided heart and double outlet right

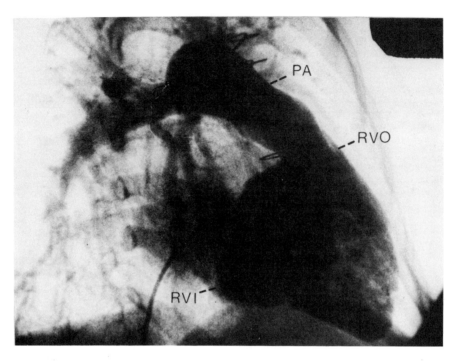

Figure 2. Postoperative right ventricular angiocardiography. (RVI = right ventricular inflor; RVO = right ventricular outflow; PA = pulmonary trunk.

ventricle, operated in 1986, required a right ventriculotomy for accurate assessment and repair of the lesion (Table 1). Since May 1984, a right atrial approach was employed in 8 patients (Table 2). In both groups of patients the operation consisted of resection of the obstructive fibromuscular tissue and the anomalous hypertrophic bands with simultaneous correction of the associated intracardiac defects. The ventricular septal defect, located in the perimembranous area of the septum, was closed with a prosthetic patch in 5 patients, and sutured directly with a reinforced U stitch in 6 cases. In the three

Table 1

Right Ventricular Approach for Resection of Obstructive Bands

| Age | Sex | Assoc. defect | VSD closure | RV Gradients | | Functional class | |
				Preop.	Postop.	Preop.	Postop.
12	M	VSD	No patch	58	10	I	I
11	M	VSD	No patch	50	22	I	I
8	F	VSD	No patch	40	5	II	I
3	F	VSD	Patch	85	13	I	I
15	F	VSD	No patch	80	10	II	I
2	F	VSD	Patch	45	10	II	I
15	F	DORV, right-sided heart	Baffle	90	5	III	I

VSD = ventricular septal defect; DORV = double outlet right ventricle.

Table 2
Right Atrial Approach for Resection of Obstructive Bands

Age	Sex	Assoc. defect	VSD closure	RV Gradients		Functional class	
				Preop.	Postop.	Preop.	Postop.
3	F	VSD	Patch	45	8	II	I
9m	F	DORV	Baffle	30	5	IV	I
20	F	VSD, AI	Patch	30	0	II	I
1	F	VSD, ASD	Patch	25	10	III	I
22	M	VSD	No patch	60	10	II	I
4	F	DORV, DSAS	Baffle	35	0	II	I
8	F	—	—	70	10	II	I
13	M	VSD	No patch	50	20	II	

VSD = ventricular septal defect; DORV = double outlet right ventricle; AI = aortic incompetence; ASD = atrial septal defect; DSAS = discrete subaortic stenosis.

patients with coexisting double outlet right ventricle, a baffle was used to divert the blood flow from the left ventricle to the aorta (Tables 1 and 2). The atrial septal defect was closed by direct suture and the subaortic shelf was excised through a right atrial approach. The prolapsed aortic leaflets were plicated in the patient with aortic insufficiency (Tables 1 and 2). Following repair, peak systolic pressures were measured in the inflow and outflow portions of the right ventricle and in the pulmonary trunk so as to document any residual gradients.

Results

There were no hospital deaths. Normal sinus rhythm with right bundle-branch block was present in every case in both groups. Only one patient with a ventriculotomy had transient ventricular premature beats. Residual gradients measured after repair ranged from 5 to 22 mmHg (mean 10.7 mmHg) in the group with ventriculotomy (Table 1), and from 0 to 20 mmHg (mean 7.8 mmHg) in the group without ventriculotomy (Table 2). The difference is not statistically significant.

Follow-up ranged from 8 to 73 months (mean 38.5 months). All patients are asymptomatic without medications and normally active (Tables 1 and 2). One infant died because of meningitis 1 year after surgery but was asymptomatic and gaining weight adequately until then. Nine patients have a 1 2/6 systolic murmur, which is clinically insignificant. There are no residual ventricular septal defects as judged by noninvasive studies. Postoperative echocardiography shows no evidence of obstruction. Only two patients with transatrial repair were electively recatheterized. The peak systolic gradients between the inflow and outflow portions of the right ventricle were 5 and 15 mmHg respectively, and postoperative angiocardiography (Fig. 2) was normal.

Discussion

Surgical treatment is indicated in all patients with double-chambered right ventricle who are symptomatic, or who have a significant gradient within the right ventricle. The first successful surgical repair was performed in 1960 and reported by Lucas and his associates.[1] Several publications have stressed the difficulty in correctly identifying the ventricular septal defect by a standard right ventriculotomy.[1,3,4,6,9] Rather than closing the septal defect, the stenotic area within the right ventricle may be sutured by mistake.[1,3] The papillary muscles of the tricuspid valve may also be difficult to visualize and can be damaged as a result of poor exposure.[6] For this reason, Penkoske and her colleagues[6] suggested a transatrial approach, which has the additional advantage of preserving right ventricular function by avoiding a ventriculotomy. We have found that the obstructive bands are easier to identify and resect when the transatrial approach is used and, this is now our technique of choice. Other associated defects can also be repaired without a ventriculotomy.

References

1. Lucas RV, Varco RL, Lillehei CW, et al. Anomalous muscle bundle of the right ventricle. Hemodynamic consequences and surgical considerations. Circulation 1962;25:443–5

2. Becker AE, Anderson RH. Miscellaneous right ventricle anomalies. In: Becker AE, Anderson RH, (eds), Cardiac Pathology. New York, NY., Raven Press, 1983, pp 12.8–12.10

3. Hartmann AF, Tsifutis AA, Arvidsson H, Goldring D. The two-chambered right ventricle. Report of nine cases. Circulation 1962;26:279–7.

4. Warden HE, Lucas RV, Varco RL. Right ventricular obstruction resulting from anomalous muscle bundles. J Thorac Cardiovasc Surg 1966;51:53–65.

5. Judson JP, Danielson GK, Ritter DG, Hagler DJ. Successful repair of coexisting double-outlet right ventricle and two-chambered right ventricle. J Thorac Cardiovasc Surg 1982;84:113–21.

6. Penkoske PA, Duncan N, Collins-Nakai RL. Surgical repair of double-chambered right ventricle with or without ventriculotomy. J Thorac Cardiovasc Surg 1987;93:385–93.

7. Simpson WF, Sade RM, Crawford FA, et al. Double-chambered right ventricle. Ann Thorac Surg 1987;44:7–10.

8. Baumstark A, Fellows KE, Rosenthal A. Combined double-chambered right ventricle and discrete subaortic stenosis. Circulation 1978;57:299–303.

9. Rowland TW, Rosenthal A, Castaneda AR. Double-chambered right ventricle: experience with 17 cases. Am Heart J 1975;89:455–62.

10. Hartmann AF, Goldring D, Ferguson TB, et al. The course of children with the two-chambered right ventricle. J Thorac Cardiovasc Surg 1970;60:72–83.

Early and Late Results of Radical Surgery for Annulo-Aortic Ectasia in Three Children

T. Savunen and M. Inberg

Introduction

Annulo-aortic ectasia[1] consists of aneurysmal formation of the ascending aorta and dilatation of the ventriculo-aortic junction, leading to progressive aortic valvar incompetence. Radical surgery (total replacement of the ascending aorta and aortic valve with a composite graft, including reimplantation of the coronary orifices to the tube prosthesis) has become an established mode of treatment for the lesion when seen in adults.[2,3,4] Because of the hereditary native of the malformation in Marfan's syndrome, or even in an idiopathic form,[5] the anomaly may also become manifest in childhood. There are only a few reports concerning corrective surgery in children. Proper timing, as well as the late results of the radical operation, are still in doubt. With this in mind, we describe in this article our experience with three children having this anomaly.

Operative Technique

Cardiopulmonary bypass was instituted utilizing the Rygg-Kyvsgaard bubble oxygen-ator. Myocardial protection was achieved by means of systemic moderate hypothermia (28°C), with cardioplegia and topical cooling with ice-cold saline using a topical cooling device. A single period of aortic crossclamping was used. The myocardial temperature was continuously monitored and kept below 20°C. A composite graft was made by sewing a Bjork-Shiley aortic valve prosthesis into a soft low-porosity Dacron tube. Both coronary orifices were dissected free, the aneurysmal sac was removed, and the coronary arteries were reimplanted into the prosthetic tube using continuous 4–0 Prolene sutures. No wrapping procedure was used (Figs. 1a and 1b). Dicloxacillin was administered prophylactically and permanent anticoagulant therapy was started on the second postoperative day. Each patient underwent follow-up aortography 6 months after surgery and a further aortogram at least 3 years after the operation.

Case Reports

Case 1

This 10-year-old girl exhibited the classic signs of Marfan's syndrome in the mus-

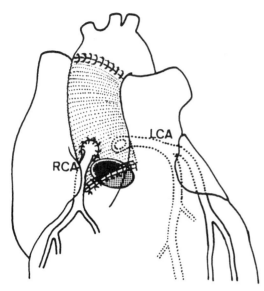

Figure 1a. Technique of total repair. The aneurysm is resected. The origins of the coronary arteries are dissected free and the composite graft is sutured to the ventriculo-aortic junction. (RCA = right coronary artery; LCA = left coronary artery).

culo-skeletal, ocular, and cardiovascular systems. These signs were first noticed at the age of 5 years. Cardiologic evaluation revealed a grade 4/6 diastolic murmur, and chest-roentgenogram demonstrated enlargement of the left ventricle. Aortic valvar regurgitation was suspected and treatment was started with digoxin. The patient was thereafter reevaluated at 6-month intervals.

Left ventricular angiocardiography and aortography at the age of 7 years revealed enlargement and hypertrophy of the left ventricle, a fusiform aneurysm of the ascending aorta, and moderate aortic valvar regurgitation. Left ventricular hypertrophy was also seen in the electrocardiogram. The patient was operated upon in November 1979 because of rapid clinical deterioration. The heart size was twice the normal and the diameter of the aneurysm was 8 cm. The sinuses of Valsalva were greatly dilatated. Reconstruction was performed with a No. 27 Bjork-Shiley tilting disc valve and a No. 30 Cooley low-porosity Dacron graft. The aorta

was crossclamped for 99 minutes. The postoperative period was straightforward and the patient was discharged 15 days after surgery without therapy. Aortography performed 6 months after the operation showed a normal prosthetic function and a marked decrease in the heart size. A second elective aortography, however, performed in June 1987 (7 ½ years after surgery) while the patient was in excellent general condition showed the orifice of the left coronary to be dilated to 75% of its diameter.

Case 2

This patient was a 13-year-old girl with classic Marfan's syndrome without any family history of the condition. The first sign of the disease, severe myopia, had been detected at the age of 5 years. Five years later, a grade 3/6 diastolic murmur was heard at routine examination and she was referred for further investigation. M-mode echocardiography showed dilatation of the aortic root (a diameter of 42 mm compared with the normal 29 mm). The chest roentgenogram revealed an increased heart size, while angiography revealed a fusiform aneurysm

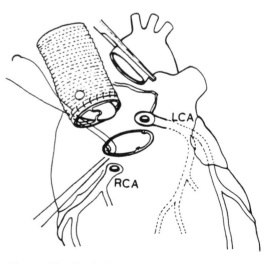

Figure 1b. Technique of total repair. Reconstruction accomplished.

of the left ventricle, and grade III aortic valvar regurgitation.

The patient deteriorated rapidly and operation was carried out in January 1981. The composite graft used for reconstruction was made from a No. 25 Bjork-Shiley tilting disc valve and a No. 26 Cooley low-porosity Dacron tube. The aortic valve was bicuspid and the junction supporting the right leaflet was very poorly developed. The period of aortic crossclamping was 100 minutes. Resternotomy was required because of excessive mediastinal bleeding. Complete atrioventricular block, which occurred immediately after the operation, required insertion of a permanent pacemaker 2 weeks after surgery.

Aortography performed 6 months after surgery showed a well-functioning composite graft and a decrease in heart size. The orifice of the right coronary artery was greatly dilatated in its first centimeter. Repeated aortography done in February 1987, over 7 years after the operation, showed no change in the cardiac status. The patient remains in good general condition.

Case 3

This 12-year-old boy had no classic signs of Marfan's syndrome, but had a strong family history of the condition. His father died at the age of 38 due to a sudden rupture of an aneurysm of the ascending aorta. The boy had, subjectively, always been in excellent health but, after his father's death, he underwent a thorough cardiologic evaluation. The chest roentgenogram demonstrated cardiomegaly and review of previous films showed evidence of a prominent ascending aorta already present at the age of 6 months. Aortography revealed a fusiform aneurysm of the ascending aorta, elongation of the aortic arch, and grade II-III aortic valvar regurgitation. At echocardiography, the left ventricle was found to be dilatated and the diameter of the ascending aorta was 38 mm (upper normal limit:28 mm).

At operation in April 1981 the aneurysm was found to be further enlarged, with a diameter of about 10 cm. The aneurysm and the incompetent three-leaflet aortic valve were excised and replaced with a composite graft comprising a No. 23 Bjork-Shiley tilting disc valve and No. 26 Dacron tube graft. The period of aortic clamping was 87 minutes. The patient was discharged on the 17th postoperative day.

Six months postoperatively there was good performance of the disc valve, as judged by aortography, and the heart size had diminished satisfactorily. At the second follow-up performed in October 1987, 5 ½ years after the operation, the angiogram revealed a slight dilatation (15%) of the orifice of the left coronary artery.

Discussion

The goal of management in annulo-aortic ectasia, in children as well as in adults, is to prevent irreversible left ventricular dysfunction, and rupture or acute dissection of the aortic aneurysm. Repair, when needed in childhood, however, poses some specific problems. Although almost all children affected by Marfan's syndrome have some degree of enlargement of the aortic root, only 10% to 15% show aortic regurgitation or dissection, and rupture of the aneurysm before the age of 21.[6,7] On the other hand, the age of the youngest patients with Marfan's syndrome who die with such complications was only 7 months.[8]

While controversy continues concerning the timing of valvar replacement for chronic aortic regurgitation, the situation is even more complex in the annulo-aortic ectasia. In this disease, the development of aortic regurgitation tends to be more rapid and progressive than in chronic aortic regurgitation and, also, is less predictable. Most patients with annulo-aortic ectasia in combination with Marfan's syndrome also have prolapse of the mitral valve. In many of them, even severe mitral valve regurgitation will develop and, it may be difficult to evaluate aortic regurgitation in the presence of severe mitral regurgitation.[6]

Regarding the timing of surgery, our three patients were old enough to avoid the problem of outgrowing prosthesis, arising later in life. Operation was performed when they had large fusiform aneurysms and grade III-IV aortic regurgitation. In adults, delay of surgery has been recommended until the aortic root has reached a diameter of 6 cm.[9] Others, however, in keeping with our experience,[10] concluded that the relative risk of dissection or rupture cannot be predicted on the basis of the diameter of the aortic root, but is likely to be heterogenous.[6]

Our technique of composite grafting[3] is a modification of the technique devised by Bentall and De Bono.[2] We dissect free the coronary arteries and do not use any wrapping. Our three patients described here are part of a series of 66 adult patients with annulo-aortic ectasia operated on with a comparable technique. Of the overall series, 31 have already undergone repeated follow-up, including aortography at least three years after their operations. Excluding the slight dilatation of the coronary orifices, also seen in our pediatric patients, the late results of the technique are excellent.

References

1. Ellis PR, Cooley DA, DeBakey ME. Clinical considerations and surgical treatment of an-nulo-aortic ectasia. J Thorac Cardiovasc Surg 1961;42:363–70.

2. Bentall HH, DeBono A. A technique for complete replacement of the ascending aorta. Thorax 1968;3:338–9.

3. Inberg MV, Niikoski J, Savunen TJA, Vanttinen E. Total repair of annulo-aortic ectasia with composite graft and reimplantation of coronary ostia: a consecutive series of 41 patients. World J Surg 1985;9:493–9.

4. Kouchoukos NT, Marshall WG, Wedige-Stecher TA. Eleven year experience with composite graft replacement of the ascending aorta and aortic valve. J Thorac Cardiovasc Surg 1986;92:691–705.

5. Savunen T. Annulo-aortic ectasia: a clinical, structural and biochemical study. Scand J Thorac Cardiovasc Surg 1986;37:(Suppl):1–45.

6. Pyeritz RE, Gott VL, Mc Donald GR, et al. Surgical repair of the Marfan aorta: technique, indications and complications. Johns Hopkins Med J 1982;151:71–82.

7. Pyeritz RE, Mc Kusik WA. The Marfan syndrome: diagnosis and management. N Engl J Med 1979;300:772–7.

8. Phornphutkul C, Rosenthal A, Nadas AS. Cardiac manifestations of Marfan syndrome in infancy and childhood. Circulation 1973;47:587–96.

9. Modry DL, Limacher J, Dobell ARC. Surgical treatment for the dilated aortic root in a child with Marfan's syndrome. Can J Surg 1981;24:500–2.

10. Savunen T. Cardiovascular abnormalities on the relatives of patients operated upon for annulo-aortic ectasia. A clinical and echocardiographic study of 40 families. Eur J Cardio-Thorac Surg 1987;1:3–10.

A Surgical Procedure for the Prevention of Atrioventricular Block in Septation for Double Inlet Ventricle

Y. Naito, K. Fujiwara, S. Higashiue, T. Yagihara, and T. Fujita

Introduction

It is well-established that atrioventricular block occurs frequently after septation of double inlet ventricle.[1-4] Since using this approach, we have devised, in 1982, a new technique for positioning the suture line for septation. Since then, we have performed septation with this new technique in four consecutive patients and all maintained normal sinus rhythm postoperatively. In this article, we will describe our surgical technique and discuss our studies on cardiac function after the septation procedure.

Patients

During the period from 1982 to 1985, 4 patients with double inlet ventricle underwent septation using the new procedure at the National Cardiovascular Center (Table 1). All had a dominant left ventricle with two atrioventricular valves, a left-sided anterior rudimentary right ventricle, and a discordant ventriculo-arterial connection. The patients' ages ranged from 4 to 22 years. The 22-year-old patient also had pulmonary stenosis and underwent simultaneous reconstruction of the pulmonary trunk using a porcine valved conduit. A 7-year-old boy had interruption of the aortic arch and straddling of the right-sided atrioventricular valve. Simultaneous reconstruction of the aortic arch was performed at his operation.

Surgical Technique

The location of the conduction axis in double inlet left ventricle with left-sided rudimentary right ventricle was clarified by Anderson and his colleagues,[5,6] and the pathway of conduction is shown in Fig. 1. The atrioventricular node lies anterior, and a long nonbranching bundle penetrates in anterior position, encircles the cephalad quadrants of the pulmonary valve and, when seen from the dominant ventricle, runs cephalad to the ventricular septal defect and branches on its superior border.

To assure the prevention of surgical heart block, it is most important that the line of septation never crosses the nonbranching bundle. To accomplish this, we have kept

Table 1

Clinical Summary of Four Patients who Underwent Septation Using New
Technique for Positioning the Suture Line

Case	Age	Sex	PS	Approach	Postop. AV block	Result	Remarks
1 Y.H.	4	F	−	trans	RA	−	survived
2 S.I.	4	F	−	trans RA	−	survived	
3 J.M.	22	M	+	trans RA	−	survived	PA conduit
4 H.T.	7	M	−	trans RA	−	survived	IAA, (A), straddling

PS, pulmonary stenosis; RA, right atrium; PA conduit, reconstruction of pulmonary trunk using external conduit; IAA (A), interruption of the aortic arch at the isthmus (Type A); Straddling, straddling of atrioventricular valve.

the suture line parallel to this axis, as shown in Fig. 1. In the area of ventricular septal defect, all sutures are placed at the margin of the defect from inside the rudimentary right ventricle and, after reaching the branching bundle, the pathway of the suture line transfers to the free wall of the dominant left ventricle. The landmark of this point of transfer is the area in which the dimensions of the ventricular septum are seen to change. If necessary, the ventricular septal defect is enlarged by resection of its inferior

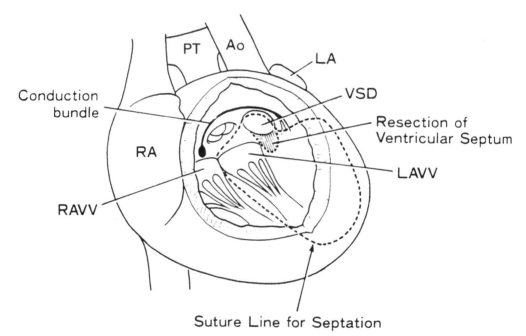

Figure 1. The conduction pathway relative to the proposed suture line for septation of double inlet left ventricle with left-sided and anterior rudimentary right ventricle and discordant ventriculoarterial connection. (PT = pulmonary trunk; Ao = aorta; RA = right atrium; LA = left atrium; VSD = ventricular septal defect; RAVV = right atrioventricular valve; LAVV = left atrioventricular valve.

margin. The patch for septation is sutured using interrupted stitches inserted through the right AV valve.

Results

All 4 patients survived the operation without developing atrioventricular block. Their postoperative electrocardiogram showed normal sinus rhythm, and P-R and QRS intervals were both within normal limits. The postoperative cardiac function was studied in the first three cases. Their new left ventricular end-diastolic volumes were 155 mL/m (235% of normal), 137 mL/m (186% of normal) and 171 mL/m (175% of normal), respectively. The left ventricular ejection fractions were 0.34, 0.50 and 0.40, respectively. The new right ventricular end-diastolic volumes were 83 (129% of normal), 74 (102% of normal), and 76 mL/m (76% of normal), respectively. The right ventricular ejection fraction was measured at 0.26, 0.58, and 0.43 respectively.

Discussion

The recent trend in the intracardiac repair of double inlet ventricle has been toward the modified Fontan procedure, even if the indications for septation have existed. One of the reasons for this approach is that atrioventricular block has been shown to occur frequently after septation. Septation, nonetheless, is a more physiological correction for this entity than is the Fontan procedure. The techniques of septation reported by McGoon, et al.[1] and McKay and his colleagues,[3] who have the most experience with this technique, both use a suture line that crosses the nonbranching bundle. There is, therefore, a strong possibility of injuring the atrioventricular bundle if their procedures are followed. Indeed, we had used their technique in 4 patients before developing the technique described in this ar-

ticle, and all of them developed complete atrioventricular block postoperatively. It was for this reason that, in 1982, we devised the procedure for septation in which the suture line never crosses the nonbranching bundle. A similar procedure was reported by Danielson in 1983.[7] High incidence of postoperative atrioventricular block, however, is still not clear. All of our patients who underwent septation as previously described maintained normal sinus rhythm. This certainly suggests that the technique is a reasonable one for the prevention of atrioventricular block in septation for double inlet left ventricle. We consider that our concept may be applicable to septation of other types of double inlet ventricle for the prevention of surgically induced heart block.

It may be thought that after septation, the left ventricular volume would become smaller. In reality, the postoperative left ventricular end-diastolic volumes were enlarged rather than small, while the new right ventricular end-diastolic volumes were nearly normal. Left ventricular ejection fraction, however, was low compared with normal values, but not disastrously so. These results suggest that cardiac function is also acceptable after septation of double inlet left ventricle.

References

1. McGoon DC, Danielson GK, Ritter DG, et al. Correction of the univentricular heart having two atrioventricular valves. J Thorac Cardiovasc Surg 1977;74:218–26.
2. Feldt R, Mair DD, Danielson GK, et al. Current status of the septation procedure for univentricular heart. J Thorac Cardiovasc Surg 1981;82:93–7.
3. McKay R, Pacifico AD, Blackstone EH, et al. Septation of the univentricular heart with left anterior subaortic outlet chamber. J Thorac Cardiovasc Surg 1982;84:77–87.
4. Pacifico AD, Naftel DD, Kirklin JW, et al. Ventricular septation within the spectrum of surgery for double inlet ventricles. J Jpn Assoc Thorac Surg 1985;33:593–601.
5. Becker AE, Wilkinson JL, Anderson RH. Atrio-

ventricular conduction tissues in univentricular hearts of left ventricular type. Herz 1979;4:166–75.

6. Anderson RH, Becker AE, Ho SY, et al. Disposition of conduction tissues. In: Anderson RH, Crupi G, Parenzan L, (eds) Double inlet ventricle. Tunbridge Wells, Kent, Castle House Publishers, 1987, pp 72–97.

7. Danielson GK. Univentricular heart. In: Stark J, de Leval M, (eds) Surgery for Congenital Heart Defects. London, Grune and Stratton, 1983, pp 427–37.

Index